QUICK FIND GUIDE

COLOR ATLAS of
Common Oral Diseases

ENHANCED

FIFTH EDITION

COLOR ATLAS of
Common
Oral Diseases

ENHANCED
FIFTH EDITION

ROBERT P. LANGLAIS, BA, DDS, MS, PhD, FRCD(c)
Professor Emeritus
Department of Dental Diagnostic Science
University of Texas Health Science Center at San Antonio
School of Dentistry
San Antonio, Texas

CRAIG S. MILLER, DMD, MS, FACD
Professor of Oral Medicine
Department of Oral Health Practice and Department
of Microbiology, Immunology and Molecular Genetics
College of Dentistry, College of Medicine
University of Kentucky
Lexington, Kentucky

JILL S. GEHRIG, RDH, MA
Dean Emeritus, Division of Allied Health
Asheville-Buncombe Technical Community College
Asheville, North Carolina

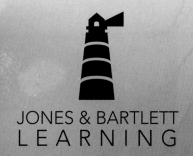

JONES & BARTLETT
LEARNING

World Headquarters
Jones & Bartlett Learning
5 Wall Street
Burlington, MA 01803
978-443-5000
info@jblearning.com
www.jblearning.com

Jones & Bartlett Learning books and products are available through most bookstores and online booksellers. To contact Jones & Bartlett Learning directly, call 800-832-0034, fax 978-443-8000, or visit our website, www.jblearning.com.

24099-3

Production Credits

VP, Product Management: Amanda Martin
Product Manager: Sean Fabery
Content Strategist: Rachael Souza
Content Coordinator: Elena Sorrentino
Digital Project Specialist: Angela Dooley
Director of Marketing: Andrea DeFronzo
Marketing Manager: Dani Burford
Production Services Manager: Colleen Lamy

VP, Manufacturing and Inventory Control: Therese Connell
Composition: S4Carlisle Publishing Services
Project Management: S4Carlisle Publishing Services
Cover Design: Kristin E. Parker
Senior Media Development Editor: Troy Liston
Rights Specialist: Rebecca Damon
Printing and Binding: LSC Communications

Library of Congress Cataloging-in-Publication Data
Library of Congress Cataloging-in-Publication Data unavailable at time of printing.

LCCN: 2020936068

6048

Printed in the United States of America
24 23 22 21 20   10 9 8 7 6 5 4 3 2 1

To our spouses,

Denyse, Sherry, and Dee

Reviewers

F. John Firriolo, DDS, PhD
Professor, Director, Division of Oral Medicine
University of Louisville
Louisville, Kentucky

John Girald, DMD
Supervising Dentist for Allied Dental Education
Dental Hygiene Department
NHTI, Concord's Community College
Concord, New Hampshire

Garland Novosad, DDS
Dental Hygiene Instructor
Wharton County Junior College
Wharton, Texas

Elizabeth Riccio, DDS
Professor, Dental Hygiene Department
Hudson Valley Community College
Troy, New York

Barbara Sullivan, RDH, MEd
Dental Hygiene Instructor
Tarrant County College
Fort Worth, Texas

Tracy Zang, DDS
Assistant Professor
Dental Hygiene Program
West Liberty University
West Liberty, West Virginia

Ximena Zornosa, DMD
Professor of Dental Hygiene
Clayton State University
Morrow, Georgia

Foreword

I take notice of books that are written with the learner in mind. In fact, most of my career as an educator has been spent observing and helping students learn. Since most dental professionals are lifelong learners, the books that get my foremost attention have a distinct methodical format that is user-friendly for students and seasoned practitioners.

In the past 15 years, our annual "Summer Bootcamp for Dental Educators" has brought together faculty members from over 250 dental and allied dental schools to determine how to provide learner-centered experiences for our students. We focus on teaching methodology and frequently discuss books and techniques that help us educators impart superior assessment skills and critical thinking skills to students. Astute assessment skills must be so valued by the learner that he/she employs the skills routinely in an organized and sequential way throughout a lifetime of practice. In doing so, educators often refer to excellent resources such as the *Color Atlas of Common Oral Diseases, Enhanced Fifth Edition (The Color Atlas)*.

The Color Atlas is a prime example of a book written with attention to the needs of the learner, student, and clinician. The whole concept of the book format, which presents similar-appearing diseases grouped together, leads the learner through the process of higher order of thinking that is required for astute differential assessment and diagnosis. Few other oral pathology/oral diagnosis/oral medicine books compare in this respect.

You know a book is written with the learner in mind when the authors of a book are world renown as experts in oral medicine, oral diagnosis, radiology, and dental hygiene. They know how to simplify complex topics and bring the learner along an easy path to understanding of the subject matter. Consistent with this, the authors of *The Color Atlas* have proven track records as expert clinicians and teachers in college and university classrooms as well as in presentations at national and international conferences.

It is interesting to note how these authors who are educators as well as clinicians and researchers came together to coauthor the *Color Atlas of Common Oral Diseases*. The first author, Bob Langlais, is Board Certified in Oral Medicine in the United States and Canada, FRCD(C) and Board Certified in Oral & Maxillofacial Radiology in the United States, and Professor Emeritus at the University of Texas at San Antonio (UTHSCSA). Bob was on the faculty with Jill S. Nield-Gehrig at UTHSCSA for years. Bob taught in the Dental and Dental Hygiene programs and Jill in the Dental Hygiene Education Department. Craig Miller studied under Bob Langlais at UTHSCSA. Craig, being a son of an educator, was soon invited to join Bob in speaking engagements and coauthoring *The Atlas*. Craig is currently a Professor of Oral Medicine, Microbiology, Immunology & Molecular Genetics at the University of Kentucky, College of Dentistry and College of Medicine, and has received several lifetime achievement awards in the fields of Oral Diagnosis and Oral Medicine. He is also a coauthor of several other textbooks.

Jill also has published several textbooks, the most famous of which is her first *Periodontal Instrumentation and Advanced Root Instrumentation*. Her textbook writing style and format was so effective that her first textbook became and still is the biggest selling dental hygiene textbook in the world. Bob and Craig invited Jill to coauthor the *Color Atlas of Common Oral Diseases, Fourth Edition*. Her contributions were of tremendous value, not only because of her unique writing style but also because of her background in dental hygiene, patient assessment, periodontics, and communication. The outstanding work of Bob Langlais and Craig Miller in this *Color Atlas* has been magnified with Jill's contributions in the form of formatting, editing, and case presentations.

What these authors have in common is their understanding of how students and clinicians learn. They know that most students are visual learners and best practices in teaching allow students to assimilate what they learn in the classroom into their clinical learning experiences. Color coding is what makes the fifth edition so organized for the learner. And, the cases and disease groupings take the reader on a journey through clinical associations that make learning fun. These are but a few of the excellent strategies utilized throughout *The Color Atlas* that make this resource extremely user-friendly. The authors are to be commended for adding current evidenced-based information and incorporating the recommendations from many readers and teachers making the fifth edition a gold mine for learning and investigating key clinical features of oral diseases.

CYNTHIA BIRON LEISECA, RDH, EMT, MA

PRESIDENT OF DH METHODS OF EDUCATION, INC.

AMELIA ISLAND, FLORIDA

Preface

The enhanced fifth edition of *Color Atlas of Common Oral Diseases* benefits from keeping some of the old, yet bringing in the new. One prominent thing that remains is the *format*. Our Oral Disease Atlas is one of the few whose format is arranged by disease appearance, such that similar-appearing diseases are grouped together. Why do we do this? Because the patient benefits from this assessment approach. It also makes learning easier. Consistent with this, efforts have been made to keep the book user-friendly by exploiting the use of color-coded tabs at the outer edge of the page margins for easy location of similar-appearing diseases and disorders. The color of the tab was selected to be similar in appearance to the types of diseases found within that section (e.g., caries: tan-brown; periodontium: pink; radiographs: black). The color of the tab also is matched with the page headers on the left-hand page within each section so readers will easily identify the section they are reading. Further, the table of contents has been moved to inside the jacket cover, for easier reference and quick locating of any section of the book. As in the past, high-quality color images are presented eight to a page and always on the right side. Found on the matching left-hand side are the concise, focused, and detailed descriptions that enhance student learning. Images continue to be selected with the intent to be highly representative of the most common appearance of that disease entity, so students of dentistry, dental hygiene, and dental assisting can recognize the most common appearance of that particular disease.

While unyielding on the format, images, and descriptions, this edition represents several significant evolutionary improvements and expanded coverage as compared with our previous editions. Careful consideration was given to expand areas previously underrepresented, select highly representative cases, use new illustrations, exploit the electronic format for visualization and learning, and utilize web-based resources.

The most significant changes to be discovered in the fifth edition are the inclusion of tooth development and eruption, expansion of the radiographic diseases, expansion of the case studies, rearrangement of periodontal conditions, and the inclusion of dental implants. Key words remain highlighted in color throughout the text of the book. The key words help the student focus on important concepts and critical information and are directly linked to the Glossary at the end of the book, where simplified definitions appear. The text, in addition to being updated with the latest scientific information, has been reviewed extensively to make it an easy to read and understand book for all levels of students in dental school, dental hygiene, and dental assisting programs.

In terms of content, this is one of our most extensive revisions. We have included *22* new full pages of text and illustrations and *33* new thought-provoking cases. Thus, the entire book now contains more than 800 color and radiographic images. The new pages provide text and clinical examples of the following topics: tooth development and eruption, hypodontia, oligodontia, and syndromic hypodontia, alterations in pulp and root structure, dental caries by type and stage of invasion, conditions that appear as radiopacities, unilocular radiolucencies, periapical unilocular radiolucencies, interradicular unilocular radiolucencies, multilocular radiolucencies, mixed radiolucent-radiopaque lesions, generalized rarefactions, floating teeth, radiographic diseases that alter the periodontal ligament and/or cause loss of lamina dura, and dental implants. Throughout the book, the authors and editors scrutinized the reproduction quality of the existing images and have provided numerous color corrections. In several cases, images were improved or replaced to achieve a higher standard. In terms of achieving the highest quality, several artist renditions were added to better illustrate the subject matter for the ultimate edification of the student. Several other existing diagrams have also been revised for format improvement and for content corrections.

A major content addition for this edition is the expansion of the case-based application questions that will help students prepare for National Board examinations. To maximize the utility of this new content, we consulted with educators and studied the curricular guidelines and released National Board Examinations. This new material now involves more than 55 high-quality clinical photos or radiographs or both. These have been placed at the end of each section so that the cases can be reviewed as the material is completed. The clinical cases are provided so students can review the information such that they can (1) describe the lesion; (2) determine if it is normal, variant of normal, or disease; (3) provide a list of other diseases that look similar (i.e., differential diagnosis); (4) provide an assessment work-up plan; (5) provide a management plan for each case, and (6) communicate with the dentist and patient regarding the findings. The latter being a new accreditation requirement for dental and dental hygiene education.

In order to accommodate the many revisions and yet limit the size of the text, the "Clinical Applications and Resources," with the drug prescription information, appears in a compressed, but detailed, format. The Guide to Diagnosis and Management of Common Oral Lesions section remains a study guide favorite for students and has been updated.

Support for course directors remains an important focus for the authors and publisher. We understand from listening to the many participants of our Summer Workshops and continuing education courses (e.g., Summer Camp Amelia Island) that many institutions and faculty do not have sufficient high-quality oral pathology material, cases, or information on hand to support faculty needs. To meet this formidable need in a truly unprecedented and "expansive" way, we continue to enlist a "team of educational and publication experts." The team includes the three authors, an independent dental hygienist, our editor, and the publisher. Together our team has created and made available electronic PowerPoint lectures for each chapter. Jane N. Gray, who is highly experienced in this specialized field, has incorporated the appropriate text information into PowerPoint lectures. Individual course directors and instructors who adopt this text can access the complete PowerPoint package free of charge through our publisher's Navigate 2 Advantage Access site. Further, course directors and instructors can add or delete information and illustrations to suit their needs by accessing the Atlas image bank through the same Navigate 2 Advantage Access site.

The answers to the Case Studies will only be available Online to instructors so they can better challenge their students' by not including the answers in the book. In addition, multiple reference materials will be listed for quick access by students and faculty alike. As time progresses, the authors and publisher will expand the variety of online Internet support. We remain committed to providing continuing education opportunities to our readers and teachers through summer workshops, seminars, and presentations at national meetings and locally.

It is with reference to these concepts that we thank all those who have contributed ideas, suggestions, reviews, editorial comments, and images for this edition. Many of these concepts have improved the Atlas and in turn contributed to the growing number of people who use this book on a daily basis. Thank you for using this resource. Remember, we encourage you to contact us regarding ways that we can help you or improve this text.

ROBERT P. LANGLAIS, BA, DDS, MS, PHD, FRCD(C)

CRAIG S. MILLER, DMD, MS

JILL S. GEHRIG, RDH, MA

Acknowledgments

We are extremely grateful to our many colleagues who have graciously provided material for publication in this atlas. Without their contributions, this fine quality text would not have been possible. We are also grateful to all practicing dentists and physicians who have referred patients throughout the years to the University of Texas Health Science Center at San Antonio, Department of Dental Diagnostic Science Referral Clinic, and the University of Kentucky College of Dentistry.

To Jill Nield-Gehrig, who completely reviewed this text, we extend our thanks for her valuable comments and contributions. In addition, we are grateful for the objectives and suggestions she provided for each section.

Marnie Palacios, Christopher McKee, Sam Newman, and David Baker of the Photographic Services Section of Education Resources of The University of Texas Health Science Center receive a special thank you for their masterful job of cropping, background adjustments, and recreating the proper color balance on our illustrations. Also, thanks are offered to Matt Hazzard of the University of Kentucky for creating five new illustrations found in this edition.

We wish to express our appreciation to the following persons for contribution of their clinical photographs and radiographs used in this text:

Dr. Kenneth Abramovitch
Dr. A.M. Abrams
Dr. Marden Alder
Dr. Robert Arm
Dr. Ralph Arnold
Dr. Tom Aufdemorte
Dr. Bill Baker
Dr. Douglas Barnett
Dr. Pete Benson
Dr. Ashley Betz
Dr. Howard Birkholz
Dr. Steve Bricker
Dr. Dale Buller
Dr. James Cecil
Dr. Israel Chilvarquer
Dr. Jerry Cioffi
Dr. Laurie Cohen
Dr. John Coke
Dr. Walter Colon
Dr. Herman Corrales
Dr. James Cottone
Dr. Robert Craig Jr
Dr. Stephen Dachi
Dr. Douglas Damm
Dr. Maria de Zeuss
Dr. Anna Dongari
Dr. S. Brent Dove
Dr. Pinar Emecen-Huja
Dr. John Francis
Dr. David Freed
Dr. Franklin Garcia-Godoy
Dr. Birgit Glass
Dr. Tom Glass
Dr. Michael Glick
Dr. Kirsten Gosney
Dr. Ed Heslop
Dr. Michaell Huber
Dr. Sheryl Hunter
Dr. Ce.E. Hutter
Dr. J.L. Jensen
Dr. Nate Johnson
Dr. Ron Jorgenson
Dr. Jerald Katz
Dr. George Kaugers
Dr. Gary Klasser
Dr. Tom Kluemper
Dr. Eric Kraus
Dr. Ahmad Kutkut
Dr. Olaf Langland
Dr. Al Lugo
Dr. Curt Lundeen
Dr. Carson Mader
Dr. Nancy Mantich
Dr. Tom McDavid
Dr. John McDowell
Dr. Monique Michaud
Dr. Dale Miles
Dr. John Mink
Dr. David F. Mitchell
Dr. David Molina
Dr. Charles Morris
Dr. Rick Myers
Dr. Stanley Nelson
Dr. Christoffel Nortjé
Dr. Pirkka Nummikoski
Dr. D. Nugyyen
Dr. Linda Otis
Dr. Garnet Pakota
Dr. Joe Petrey
Dr. Michael Piepgrass
Dr. Roger Rao
Dr. Tom Razmus
Dr. Spencer Redding
Dr. Terry Rees
Dr. Michael Rollert
Dr. Elias Romero
Dr. Michele Saunders
Dr. Stanley Saxe
Dr. Tom Schiff
Dr. James Scuibba
Dr. Jack Sherman
Dr. Sol Silverman
Dr. Larry Skoczylas
Dr. D.B. Smith
Dr. John Tall
Dr. George Taybos

Dr. Geza Terezhalmy
Dr. Mark Thomas
Dr. Nathaniel Triester
Dr. Martin Tyler
Dr. Margot Van Dis
Dr. Michael Vitt
Dr. Elaine Winegard
Dr. Donna Wood
Dr. John Wright
Dr. Terry Wright
Dr. Juan F. Yepes
Dr. Jim Zettler

We also wish to express our appreciation to the following educators for attending our Summer Workshops and providing helpful suggestions regarding the format and content of this text over the many editions:

Dr. William Batson
Dr. Suzanne M. Beatty
Dr. G. David Byers
Michael Campo
Janita D. Cope
Nancy Cuttic
Leslie A. DeLong
Dr. Robert C. Dennison
Dr. Art DiMarco
Kathy Duff
Dr. Robert S. Eldridge
Dr. Marie English
Diana Cooke Gehrke

Deborah Goldstein
Dr. Joel Grand
Jane Gray
Donna Hamil
Rosemary Herman
Dr. Stanley L. Hill
Debbie Hughes
Brenda Knutson
Susan Luethge
Debbie Lyon
Mattie Marcum
Joan McClintock
Patty McGinley
Julie Mettlen
Dr. John A. Olsen
Polly Pope
Carol Roberton
Donna Rollo
Donna Thibodeau
Dana Wood
Mary Ellen Young
Anita Weaver
Karen Sue Williams

Finally, we would like to thank our wives, Denyse and Sherry, for their continuing support throughout this project. Authorship of a high-quality text requires numerous off-duty hours; without the understanding of these two most important people in our lives, this work might never have been completed.

Figure Credits

Fig. 1.5	Dr. Kirsten Gosney
Fig. 2.2	Dr. James Cottone
Fig. 2.8	Dr. Linda Otis
Fig. 3.3	Dr. Kirsten Gosney
Fig. 3.4	Dr. Kirsten Gosney
Fig. 3.7	Dr. Ralph Arnold
Fig. 4.1	Dr. Jim Zettler
Fig. 4.2	Dr. Jim Zettler
Fig. 4.3	Dr. Jim Zettler
Fig. 4.4	Dr. Tom Kluemper
Fig. 4.5	Dr. Tom Kluemper
Fig. 4.6	Dr. Tom Kluemper
Fig. 4.7	Dr. Joe Petrey
Fig. 4.8	Dr. Joe Petrey
Fig. 4.9	Dr. Joe Petrey
Fig. 4.10	Dr. Tom Kluemper
Fig. 4.11	Dr. Tom Kluemper
Fig. 4.12	Dr. Tom Kluemper
Fig. 7.3	Dr. Stanley Nelson
Fig. 7.4	Dr. Stanley Nelson
Fig. 7.5	Dr. Stanley Nelson
Fig. 13.4	Dr. Michael Huber
Fig. 13.8	Dr. John Wright
Fig. 13.9	Dr. Nancy Mantich
Fig. 15.1	Dr. Sheryl Hunter
Fig. 15.2	Dr. Christoffel Nortjé
Fig. 15.4	Dr. Ron Jorgenson
Fig. 15.5	Dr. Franklin Garcia-Godoy
Fig. 15.6	Dr. Ron Jorgenson
Fig. 15.7	Dr. Ron Jorgenson
Fig. 15.8	Dr. Al Lugo
Fig. 15.10	Dr. Barney Olsen
Fig. 15.13	Dr. Juan F. Yepes
Fig. 17.3	Dr. Birgit Glass
Fig. 17.7	Dr. Terry Rees
Fig. 18.7	Dr. Juan F. Yepes
Fig. 18.8	Dr. Juan F. Yepes
Fig. 19.3	Dr. John Mink
Fig. 19.4	Dr. John Mink
Fig. 19.7	Dr. John Francis and Dr. Ashley Betz
Fig. 20.3	Dr. Ralph Arnold
Fig. 20.7	Dr. Geza Terezhalmy
Fig. 21.6	Dr. Kenneth Abramovitch
Fig. 22.3	Dr. Rick Myers
Fig. 22.6	Dr. Ralph Arnold
Fig. 22.8	Dr. Israel Chilvarquer
Fig. 24.3	Dr. Jerry Katz
Fig. 24.7	Dr. Pirkka Nummikoski
Fig. 24.8	Dr. Pirkka Nummikoski
Fig. 25.2	Dr. Charles Morris
Fig. 26.6	Dr. Ralph Arnold
Fig. 26.8	Dr. David Molina
Fig. 29.7	Dr. David F. Mitchell
Fig. 29.9	Dr. C.E. Hutton
Fig. 29.12	Dr. Juan F. Yepes
Fig. 31.7	Dr. Birgit Glass
Fig. 32.3	Dr. Ralph Arnold
Fig. 36.8	Dr. Garnet Pakota
Fig. 38.5	Dr. Kenneth Abramovitch
Fig. 39.2	Dr. Pirkka Nummikoski
Fig. 40.2	Dr. Christoffel Nortjé
Fig. 41.1	Dr. Israel Chilvarquer
Fig. 41.2	Dr. Elias Romero
Fig. 41.8	Dr. Robert Arm
Fig. 43.10	Dr. D. Nugyyen
Fig. 44.4	Dr. Charles Morris (Deceased)
Fig. 45.3	Dr. Tom McDavid
Fig. 45.6	Dr. Ralph Arnold

Contents

Anatomic Landmarks

Objectives:

- Recognize, define, and describe the soft tissue structures and landmarks of the anterior and posterior oral cavity.
- Recognize, define, and describe the soft tissue structures and landmarks of the floor of the mouth, tongue, and palate.
- Recognize, define, and describe the soft tissue structures and landmarks of the periodontium.
- Recognize, define, and describe the bony structures and landmarks of the maxilla and mandible and adjacent regions.
- Recognize, define, and describe common variants of normal.
- In the clinical setting, identify intraoral soft tissue structures and anatomic landmarks in a patient's mouth.

LANDMARKS OF THE ORAL CAVITY

Lips (Fig. 1.1) The lips form the outer border of the oral cavity. They are covered by mucosa and a surface layer of parakeratin. Beneath this is connective tissue and rich blood supply. Deeper are muscles that control lip movement (orbicularis oris, levator, and depressor oris). Lips appear pink-red but can vary in color depending on the age and pigmentation of the patient, sun exposure, and history of trauma. The junction of the lips with the labial mucosa is the **wet line**, the point of contact of the upper and lower lips. The **vermilion** is the portion external to the wet line. The **vermilion border** is the junction of the lip with the skin. The lips should be visually inspected and palpated by everting during the oral examination. The surface should be smooth and uniform in color; the border should be smooth and well delineated.

Labial Mucosa (Fig. 1.2) is the thin, pink parakeratotic epithelium lining the lips. The **labial mucosa** is usually pink or brownish-pink with small red capillaries nourishing the region. Minor **salivary gland ducts** empty onto the surface of the mucosa. These ducts appear as small orifices that emit mucinous saliva.

Buccal Mucosa (Fig. 1.3) is the inner epithelial lining of the cheeks. The **buccal mucosa** broadens bilaterally from the labial mucosa to the retromolar pad and extends to the pterygomandibular raphe. Deposits of fat within the buccal connective tissue can make it appear yellow or tan. Accessory salivary glands are present in this region and moisten the oral mucosa. The **caliculus angularis** is a normal pinkish papule located in the buccal mucosa at the commissure.

Parotid Papilla (Fig. 1.4) is a triangular, raised, pink papule on the buccal mucosa adjacent to the maxillary first molars bilaterally. The **parotid papilla** forms the end of **Stensen duct**, the excretory duct of the parotid gland. The gland is milked by drying the papilla with gauze, pressing the fingers below the mandible, and extending pressure upward and over the gland. In health, clear saliva should flow from the duct.

Floor of the Mouth (Fig. 1.5) is the region below the front, anterior half of the tongue. It is composed of thin, pink parakeratinized epithelium, connective tissue, salivary glands, and associated nerves and blood vessels. The **floor of the mouth** has U-shaped boundaries bordered anterolaterally by the dental arch and posteriorly by the ventral tongue surface. The anterior portion is smooth, uniform, and covered by mucosa. The **lingual frenum** is located along the midline of the posterior portion. Between the two halves is an elevated area under which **Wharton duct** of the submandibular gland lies. Saliva from the submandibular gland exits through an elevated papilla called the **sublingual caruncle** to moisten the floor of the mouth. Along the posterior portion of the caruncle are multiple small openings, the "**ducts of Rivinus**," that carry saliva from the sublingual salivary gland. Beneath these structures lies a pair of **mylohyoid muscles** that function in lifting the tongue and hyoid bone.

Hard Palate (Fig. 1.6) forms the roof of the oral cavity. The **hard palate** is composed of squamous epithelium, connective tissue, minor salivary glands and ducts (in the posterior two thirds only), **periosteum**, and the palatine processes of the maxilla. Anatomically, it consists of several structures. The **incisive papilla** is directly behind and between the maxillary incisors. It is a raised, pink ovoid structure that overlies the nasopalatine foramen. The **rugae** are fibrous ridges that are located slightly posterior to the incisive papilla, in the anterior third of the palate. They run laterally from the midline to within several millimeters of the attached gingiva of the anterior teeth. A little further back are the **lateral vaults**, alveolar bones that support the palatal aspects of the posterior teeth. In the center of the hard palate is the **median palatal raphe**, a yellow-white fibrous band that appears at the junction of the right and left palatine processes.

Soft Palate (Fig. 1.7) is located posterior to the hard palate. It is unique from the hard palate in that the soft palate lacks bony support and has more minor salivary glands and lymphoid and fatty tissue than the hard palate. The **soft palate** functions during mastication and swallowing. It is elevated during swallowing by the levator palati and tensor palati muscles and motor innervated by cranial nerves IX and X. The **median palatal raphe** is more prominent and thicker in the soft palate. Just lateral to the raphe are the **fovea palatinae**. The foveae are 2-mm excretory ducts of minor salivary glands. They are landmarks of the junction between the hard and soft palates. At the midline distal aspect of the soft palate is the **uvula**, which hangs down.

Oropharynx and Tonsils (Fig. 1.8) The **oropharynx** is the junction between the mouth and the esophagus. The borders of the oropharynx are the uvula along the anterior aspect, the two tonsillar pillars (fauces) along the anterolateral aspect, and the pharyngeal wall at the posterior aspect. The tonsils are lymphoid tissue located within two pillars. The anterior tonsillar pillar is formed by the palatoglossus muscle that runs downward, outward, and forward to the base of the tongue. The posterior pillar is larger and runs posteriorly. It is formed by the palatopharyngeus muscle. The **tonsils** are dome-shaped soft tissue structures that have surface crypts and invaginations (folds), which serve to capture invading microbes. Tonsils enlarge during adolescence (a lymphoid growth period) and during infectious, inflammatory, and neoplastic processes. Islands of tonsillar tissue are seen on the surface of the posterior pharyngeal wall. **Waldeyer ring** is the ring of adenoid tissue formed by the tonsillar tissue found on the posterior tongue (lingual tonsils), pharynx (pharyngeal tonsils), and fauces (tonsillar pillars).

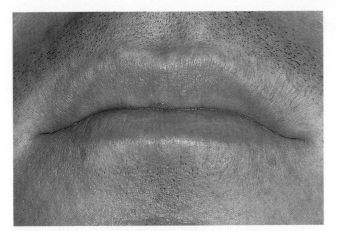

Fig. 1.1. Lips: normal, healthy appearance.

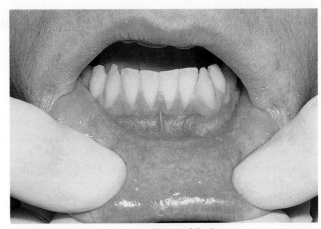

Fig. 1.2. Labial mucosa: inner lining of the lips.

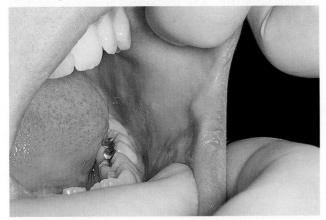

Fig. 1.3. Buccal mucosa: and caliculus angularis.

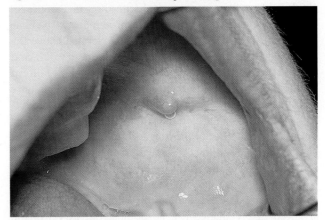

Fig. 1.4. Parotid papilla: adjacent to maxillary first molar.

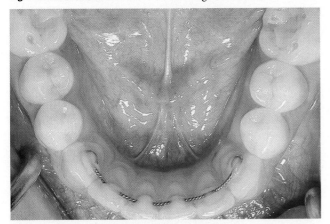

Fig. 1.5. Floor of the mouth: with central lingual frenum.

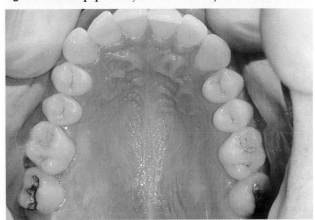

Fig. 1.6. Hard palate: incisive papilla and rugae in anterior third.

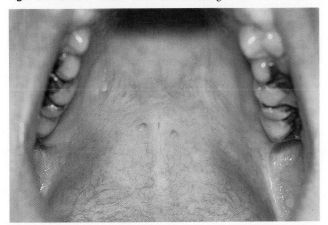

Fig. 1.7. Soft palate: fovea palatinae and median palatal raphe.

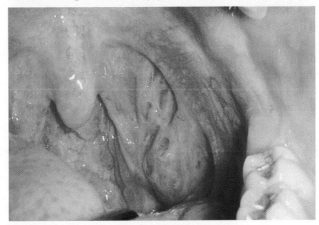

Fig. 1.8. Oropharynx and tonsillar pillars.

Normal Tongue Anatomy (Figs. 2.1–2.5) The tongue is a compact organ composed of skeletal muscles that has important functions in taste, chewing, swallowing (deglutition), and speech. The **dorsum** (upper surface) of the tongue is covered by a protective layer of stratified squamous epithelium and numerous mucosal projections that form papillae. Four types of papillae cover the dorsum of the tongue: filiform, fungiform, circumvallate, and foliate papillae. **Filiform papillae** are the smallest but the most numerous. They are slender, hairlike, cornified stalks that serve to protect the tongue. They appear pink in patients with good oral hygiene but may be red or white if irritated or inflamed. Elongated papillae or atrophy/loss of papillae are associated with disease. **Fungiform papillae** are noncornified, round, mushroom-shaped papillae found interspersed between and slightly elevated above the filiform papillae. They are brighter red, broader in width, and fewer in number (approximately 300 to 500) than the filiform papillae. Each fungiform papilla contains two to four taste buds that confer the ability to taste (salty, sweet, sour, and bitter). Fungiform papillae are most numerous on the anterior tip and lateral border of the tongue and can be stained with blue food color and viewed. Fungiform papillae sometimes contain brown pigmentation, especially in melanoderms.

The largest papillae, the **circumvallate papillae**, also contain taste buds. There are 8 to 12 circumvallate papillae arranged in a V-shaped row at the posterior aspect of the dorsum of the tongue. They appear as 2- to 4-mm pink elevations surrounded by a narrow trench, the **sulcus terminalis**.

Careful examination of the lateral border of the posterior region of the tongue reveals the **foliate papillae**. These papillae are leaflike projections oriented as vertical folds. Foliate papillae are more prominent in children and young adults than in older adults. Corrugated hypertrophic lymphoid tissue (**lingual tonsil**) extending into this area from the posterior dorsal root of the tongue may sometimes be mistakenly called foliate papillae.

On the ventral surface (underside) of the tongue are linear projections known as the **plica fimbriata**. The plica fimbriata has little known function in humans but contains taste buds in newborns and other primates. Occasionally, the fimbriata is brown in dark-skinned individuals.

Fissured Tongue (Plicated Tongue, Scrotal Tongue) (Fig. 2.6) is a variation of normal tongue anatomy that consists of a single midline fissure, double fissures, or multiple fissures of the anterior two thirds of the dorsal surface of the tongue. Various patterns, lengths, and depths of fissures have been observed. The cause of **fissured tongue** is often unknown, but it often develops with increasing age and in patients who have hyposalivation. About 1% to 5% of the population is affected. The frequency of the condition is equal in men and women. It occurs commonly in patients with Down syndrome and in combination with geographic tongue. Fissured tongue is a component of the **Melkersson-Rosenthal syndrome** (fissured tongue, cheilitis granulomatosa, and unilateral facial nerve paralysis).

Tongue fissures may become secondarily inflamed and cause halitosis as a result of food impaction; thus, brushing the tongue to keep the fissures clean is recommended. The condition is benign and does not cause pain.

Ankyloglossia (Fig. 2.7) The **lingual frenum** is normally attached to the ventral tongue and genial tubercles of the mandible. If the frenum fails to attach properly to the tongue and genial tubercles, but instead fuses to the floor of the mouth or lingual gingiva and the ventral tip of the tongue, the condition is called **ankyloglossia** or "tongue-tie." This congenital condition is characterized by (i) an abnormally short, malpositioned, and thickened lingual frenum and (ii) a tongue that cannot be extended or retracted. The fusion may be partial or complete. Partial fusion is more common. If the condition is severe, speech may be affected. Surgical correction and speech therapy are necessary if speech is defective or if a mandibular denture or removable partial denture is planned. The estimated frequency of ankyloglossia is one case per 1,000 births.

Lingual Varicosities (Phlebectasia) (Fig. 2.8), enlarged dilated veins on the ventral surface of the tongue, are a common finding in elderly adults. The cause of these vascular dilatations is either a blockage of the vein by an internal foreign body, such as an atherosclerotic plaque, or the loss of elasticity of the vascular wall as a result of aging. Intraoral **varicosities** most commonly appear superficially on the ventral surface of the anterior two thirds of the tongue and may extend onto the lateral border and floor of the mouth. Men and women are affected equally.

Varicosities appear as red-blue to purple fluctuant papules or nodules. Individual varices may be prominent and tortuous or small and punctate. Palpation does not elicit pain but can move the blood temporarily out of the vessel, thereby flattening the surface appearance. **Diascopy** (pressing against the lesion with a clear plastic tube or glass slide) causes varices to blanch. When many lingual veins are prominent, the condition is called "**phlebectasia linguae**" or "**caviar tongue**." The lip and labial commissure are other frequent sites of phlebectasia. Treatment of this condition is not required, unless for cosmetic reasons.

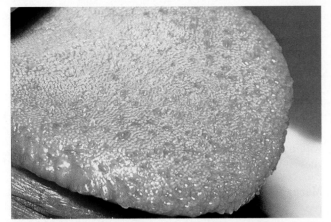

Fig. 2.1. Filiform and fungiform papillae of the tongue.

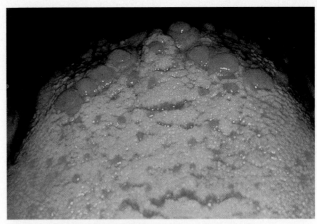

Fig. 2.2. Circumvallate papillae forming a V-shaped row.

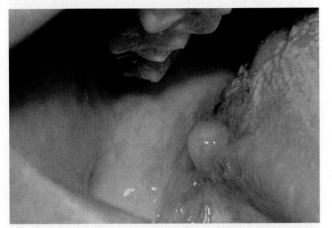

Fig. 2.3. Foliate papilla: posterolateral aspect of the tongue.

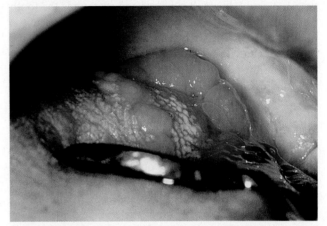

Fig. 2.4. Lingual tonsil at dorsolateral aspect of the tongue.

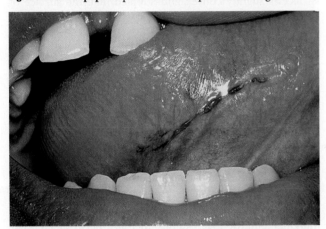

Fig. 2.5. Plica fimbriata in person who is pigmented.

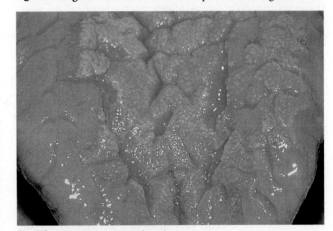

Fig. 2.6. Fissured tongue: dorsal aspect.

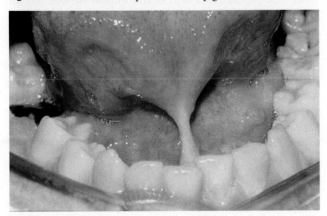

Fig. 2.7. Ankyloglossia: not causing a speech impediment.

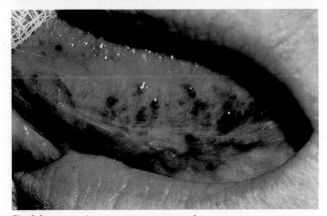

Fig. 2.8. Lingual varicosities: on ventral tongue.

LANDMARKS OF THE PERIODONTIUM

Periodontium (Figs. 3.1 and 3.2) is the tissue that immediately surrounds and supports the teeth. It consists of alveolar bone, periosteum, periodontal ligament, gingival sulcus, and gingiva; each of these components contributes to stabilizing the tooth within the jaws. The **alveolar bone** is composed of cancellous or spongy bone. It is located between the cortical plates and is penetrated by blood vessels and marrow spaces. The **periosteum** is the dense connective tissue attached to and covering the outer surface of the alveolar bone. Teeth are anchored to alveolar bone by the periodontal ligament that attaches to the cementum that covers the roots of teeth. The **periodontal ligament** is composed of cells and collagen type 1, 3, and 5 fibers. It supports and surrounds the tooth root and extends from the apex of the root to the base of the **gingival sulcus**. The gingival sulcus, the space between the free gingiva and the tooth surface, is lined internally by a thin layer of epithelial cells. The base of the sulcus is formed by the **junctional epithelium**, a specialized type of epithelium that attaches the gingiva to the root. This epithelium provides the barrier to the ingress of bacteria. In health, the gingival sulcus is less than 3 mm deep as measured by a periodontal probe from the **cementoenamel junction (CEJ)** to the base of the sulcus. Colonization of bacteria within the sulcus promotes inflammation that eventually leads to breakdown of the **epithelial attachment**. Evidence of chronic inflammation is the apical extension of the epithelial attachment beyond 3 mm. Although accumulation of **bacterial plaque** is the most important factor influencing the health of the **periodontium**, position of the tooth within the arch, occlusal loading, parafunctional habits, appliances, drugs, and frenal attachments also affect periodontal health and the development of periodontal pockets.

Alveolar Mucosa and Frenal Attachments (Figs. 3.3 and 3.4)

The **mucosa** is the epithelium and loose connective tissue covering the oral cavity. The **alveolar mucosa** is a movable mucosa that overlies alveolar bone and borders the apical extent of the periodontium. It is movable because it is not bound down to the underlying periosteum and bone. The alveolar mucosa is thin and highly vascular. Accordingly, it appears pinkish-red, red, or bright red. On close inspection, small arteries and capillaries can be seen within the alveolar mucosa. These vessels provide nutrients, oxygen, and blood cells to the region. The mucosa is generally identified as either **buccal mucosa** (if it is located laterally or posteriorly) or **labial mucosa** (if it is located anteriorly).

Frena are lip and cheek muscle attachments at specific locations within the alveolar mucosa. They appear as arclike rims of flexible fibrous tissue when the lips or cheeks are distended. Six oral frena have been identified. The **maxillary labial frenum** is located at the midline between the maxillary central incisors, about 4 to 7 mm apical to the interdental region.

The **mandibular labial frenum** appears similarly below and between mandibular central incisors within the alveolar mucosa. The two **maxillary** and two **mandibular buccal frena** are located within the alveolar mucosa near the first premolar on the right and left sides. Although frena do not directly contribute to periodontal support, those that attach within 3 mm of the CEJ of a tooth can pull on periodontal tissues and contribute to the development of gingival recession.

Mucogingival Junction (Fig. 3.5)

is an anatomic landmark representing the border between the unattached alveolar mucosa and the attached gingiva. The **mucogingival junction** is about 3 to 6 mm below the CEJ and extends around the buccal and lingual aspects of the arches. Visibility of the junction depends on the difference in vascularity and color of the two tissues. It is easily distinguished when the alveolar mucosa is red and the attached gingiva is pink and because it is the junction between the moveable alveolar mucosa and the nonmoveable attached gingiva.

Attached Gingiva and Free Marginal Gingiva (Figs. 3.6–3.8)

The attached gingiva and free marginal gingiva cover the outer aspect of the gingival sulcus. The **attached gingiva** extends coronally from the alveolar mucosa to the free marginal gingiva. It is covered by keratinized epithelium, is bound down to periosteum, and cannot be moved. In health, the attached gingiva is pink, firm, and 2 to 7 mm wide. Its surface is slightly convex and stippled, like the surface of an orange. **Interdental grooves** can be seen in the attached gingiva as vertical grooves or narrow depressions located between the roots of the teeth.

The **marginal gingiva** provides the gingival collar around the cervix of the tooth. It is pink and keratinized like the attached gingiva, with a smooth rounded edge. Unlike the attached gingiva, the marginal gingiva is not attached to periosteum, nor is it stippled. Its freely movable nature allows a periodontal probe to be passed under it during pocket depth assessment. Accordingly, it is also termed the **free marginal gingiva**. The junction between the marginal gingiva and the attached gingiva is called the **free gingival groove**.

The **interdental papilla** is the triangular projection of marginal gingiva that extends incisally between adjacent teeth. The papilla has a buccal and lingual surface and an interdental region (the **col**) that is concave, depressed, and covered by free marginal gingiva. In health, papillae are pink and knife-edged, can barely be moved by the periodontal probe, and extend near to the interdental contact region. The presence of inflammation and disease (i.e., gingivitis) alters the color, contour, and consistency of the free marginal gingiva and interdental papillae, causing the marginal gingiva to appear red-purple, soft, swollen, and tender, and the papillae to relax away from the tooth.

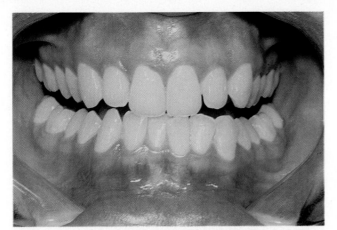

Fig. 3.1. **Healthy periodontium:** anterior view.

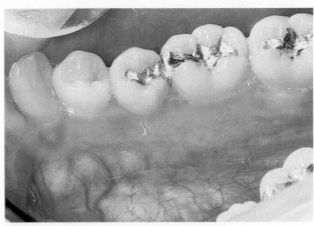

Fig. 3.2. **Healthy periodontium:** lingual aspect.

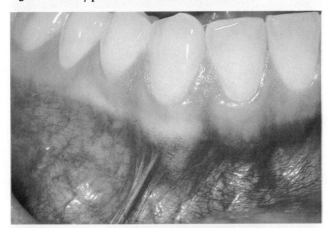

Fig. 3.3. **Healthy periodontium and buccal frenum.**

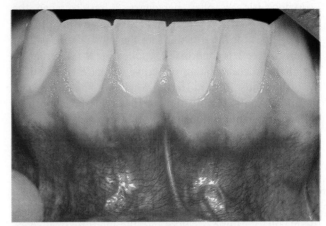

Fig. 3.4. **Red alveolar mucosa and labial frenum.**

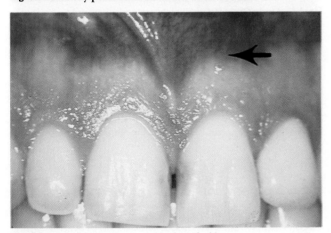

Fig. 3.5. **Mucogingival junction:** identified by *arrow*.

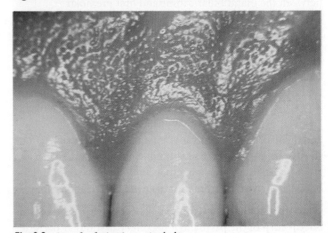

Fig. 3.6. **Attached gingiva:** stippled texture.

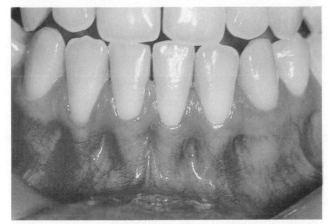

Fig. 3.7. **Interdental grooves.**

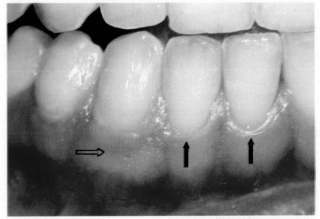

Fig. 3.8. **Marginal gingiva** (*closed arrows*) **and gingival groove** (*open arrow*).

OCCLUSION AND MALOCCLUSION

Occlusion is the relation of the maxillary and mandibular teeth during functional contact. The term is used to describe the way teeth are aligned and fit together. In an ideal occlusion, all the maxillary teeth fit slightly over the mandibular teeth, the cusps of the upper molars fit into the buccal grooves of the lower molars, and the midline is aligned. Few people have perfect occlusion, and **malocclusion** (abnormal positional relationship of the maxillary teeth with the mandibular teeth) is a common reason for patients to seek orthodontic care. Although most malocclusions do not require treatment, correcting a malocclusion can enhance the patient's appearance and ability to clean their teeth and reduce the risk of developing oral disease.

Malocclusion is often hereditary. It results when the upper and lower jaws are disproportionate in size, the size of the teeth is too large or small for the jaws, or the spacing/eruption of teeth is abnormal. The following is a summary of the modified classification of occlusion first established by the orthodontist Edward Hartley Angle, who based his classification (**Angle classification**) on the occlusal relationships of the permanent first molars.

Class I Occlusion (Figs. 4.1–4.3) is considered to be the ideal (normal) occlusion and normal anteroposterior relationship of the jaws. In **Class I occlusion**, the mesiobuccal cusp of the permanent maxillary first molar occludes (fits) into the buccal groove of the permanent mandibular first molar. Also, the maxillary canine occludes into the interproximal space between the mandibular canine and first premolar.

Class II Occlusion (Figs. 4.4–4.9) occurs when the maxillary teeth appear anterior to the normal relationship with the mandibular teeth. In **Class II occlusion**, the mesiobuccal cusp of the permanent maxillary first molar occludes mesial (anterior) to the buccal groove of the permanent mandibular first molar. There are two divisions. **Class II Division 1** is when the maxillary teeth are protruded (labioversion, producing a large overjet) and the maxillary first molar is anterior to the normal relationship. **Class II Division 2** is where the maxillary central incisors are intruded (linguoversion, producing a deep overbite) and the maxillary first molar is anterior to the normal relationship.

Class III Occlusion (Figs. 4.10–4.12) is where the mesiobuccal cusp of the permanent maxillary first molar occludes distal (posterior) to the buccal groove of the permanent mandibular first molar. This condition produces a prognathic profile (the lower jaw projects forward) and occurs in about 3% of the U.S. population.

Overbite: The vertical overlap of the maxillary teeth over the mandibular teeth when the posterior teeth are in contact in centric occlusion.

Overjet: The horizontal overlap (protrusion) of the maxillary anterior/posterior teeth beyond the mandibular teeth when the mandible is in centric occlusion.

Subdivision: A unilateral condition on the left or right side only.

Note: Patients can have different classes of malocclusion on the left and right sides.

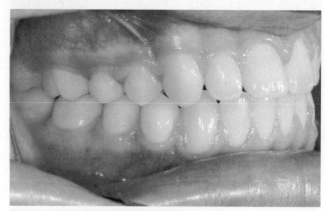

Fig. 4.1. **Angle Class I:** normal occlusion, right.

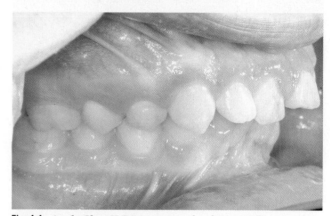

Fig. 4.4. **Angle Class II Division 1:** malocclusion, right.

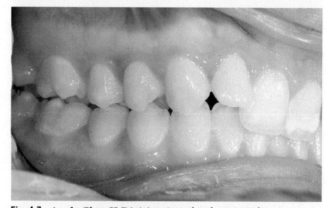

Fig. 4.7. **Angle Class II Division 2:** malocclusion, right.

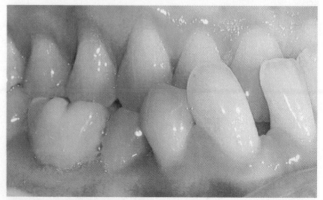

Fig. 4.10. **Angle Class III:** malocclusion, right.

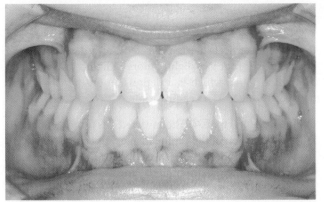

Fig. 4.2. Angle Class I: normal occlusion, center.

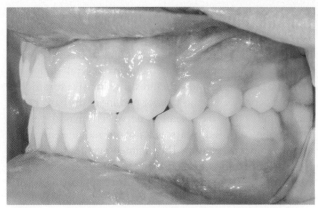

Fig. 4.3. Angle Class I: normal occlusion, left.

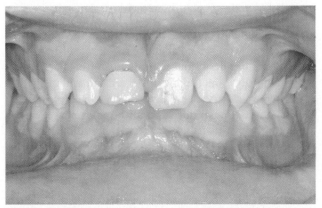

Fig. 4.5. Angle Class II Division 1: malocclusion, center.

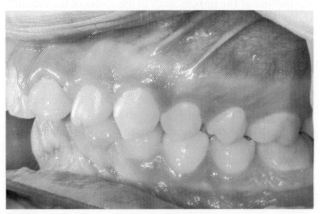

Fig. 4.6. Angle Class II Division 1: malocclusion, left.

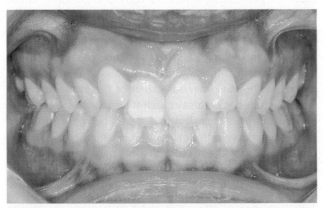

Fig. 4.8. Angle Class II Division 2: malocclusion, center.

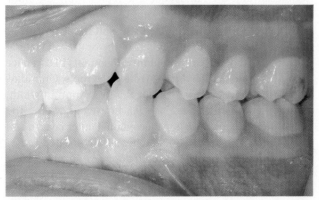

Fig. 4.9. Angle Class II Division 2: malocclusion, left.

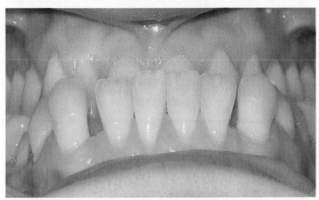

Fig. 4.11. Angle Class III: malocclusion, center.

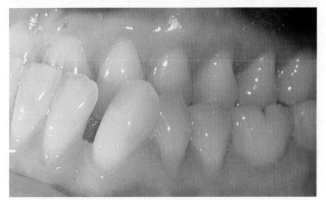

Fig. 4.12. Angle Class III: malocclusion, left.

Anterior Midline Region (Figs. 5.1 and 5.2) The anterior maxillary radiographic image contains several important anatomic landmarks and structures. The **incisive foramen** is an ovoid depression in the anterior midline of the **hard palate** that contains the nasopalatine nerve and blood vessels. Radiographically, it appears as an ovoid radiolucency with a fine radiopaque margin. The foramen overlies the median palatal suture and is located between the roots of the central incisors. The **median palatal suture** appears as a midline radiolucent line bordered by a radiopaque margin. It runs vertically and apically between the roots of the central incisors to the V-shaped **anterior nasal spine**. The **soft tissue outline of the nose** extends to the apices of the incisors, and the **soft tissue outline of the upper lip** is often seen as a light radiopacity bisecting the crowns of the central incisors. Alveolar bone in this region appears as fine, interspersed radiopaque **trabeculae** that surround radiolucent **marrow spaces**. The **cementoenamel junction (CEJ)**, or cervical line, of the incisors is seen as a smooth, curved line delineating the crown and root portions of the tooth. Apically, the CEJ is a more subtle round line above the **crest of the alveolar bone**. In Figure 5.2, the root structure between the CEJ and alveolar crest is not covered by bone owing to destruction by periodontal disease.

Anterior Lateral Region (Fig. 5.3) The **superior foramen of the incisive canal** is seen as a round radiolucent landmark within the **nasal fossa** and above the root apex of the central incisor and the radiopaque line representing the **floor of the nasal fossa**. The radiolucent **incisive canal** runs vertically below the incisive foramen. The **soft tissue outline of the nose** is seen bisecting the roots of the central and lateral incisors. The radiolucent **periodontal ligament (PDL) space** and radiopaque **lamina dura** surround the roots. On radiographs, the PDL space is typically 0.5 to 1.5 mm in width, and the lamina dura is 0.2 and 0.5 in average width. The crowns demonstrate a radiopaque **enamel** outer layer, a less dense inner layer of **dentin**, and a centrally located radiolucent **pulp chamber**. Each tooth root has an outer layer of **cementum** that is not normally visible on radiographs, unless excessive amounts, called **hypercementosis**, are present. Beneath the cementum is the dentin of the root that appears immediately adjacent to the radiolucent periodontal membrane space. Centrally within the root is the **root canal space**, which contains the pulp. In the central and lateral incisors shown in Figure 5.3, note the **cervical line** crossing the junction between the crown and roots of the teeth. Because of the excess vertical angulation of the beam in this example, the buccal cervical line is projected downward and the lingual cervical line is projected upward. Distal to the lateral incisor root is a slightly more radiolucent area called the **lateral fossa**, which is a depression on the labial bone between the lateral and canine roots.

Canine Region (Fig. 5.4) The **inverted Y** is prominently seen in the top portion of the canine image. It is composed of two structures: the floor of the nasal cavity (fossa) and the anterolateral wall of the maxillary sinus. The more anterior arm of the inverted Y consists of the floor of the nasal cavity (fossa); the more posterior curved arm is the anterolateral wall of the maxillary sinus. The **soft tissue outline of the nasal mucosa** is delineated by a thin radiolucent line representing an airspace between the nasal turbinate and nasal mucosa.

Premolar Region (Fig. 5.5) The **floor of the maxillary sinus** is located above the premolar and in molar roots. The normal floor of the maxillary sinus appears as an irregular, slightly wavy radiopaque line. Above the floor and within the lateral sinus wall is the curved radiolucent line representing the **canal of the posterior superior alveolar nerve, artery, and vein**. Notice that this canal has thin radiopaque margins. Above the second molar root is the radiopaque **zygomatic process of the maxilla**, sometimes referred to as the **malar process**. It is the anterior root of the zygomatic arch. Sometimes on a premolar image, the nasolabial fold bisects the root of the first premolar. Note the elongated palatal root of the first molar and the shortened buccal roots owing to incorrect positioning (excessive vertical angulation) of the **beam-indicating device (BID)** during image exposure.

Molar Region (Fig. 5.6) A prominent landmark in the maxillary molar image is the radiopaque U-shaped "malar shadow," which is the **zygomatic process of the maxilla**. It delineates the most anterior extent of the **zygomatic arch** (cheek bone). The zygomatic arch is buccal and lateral to the maxilla and extends horizontally across the upper portion of the molar image. In this example, it extends across the posterior portion of the **maxillary sinus**. Distal to the second molar is the **maxillary tuberosity**—a bony structure covered by connective tissue and mucosa.

Tuberosity Region (Figs. 5.7 and 5.8) Distal to the second molar is the **maxillary tuberosity**, the **lateral pterygoid plate**, and small **hamular process** of the medial pterygoid plate. Superior and lateral to this region is the **zygomatic arch**. The anterior half of the zygomatic arch is delineated from the posterior portion by the **zygomaticotemporal suture** (Fig. 5.7). The **coronoid process** of the mandible can be seen overlying the inferior portion of this region (Figs. 5.6–5.8).

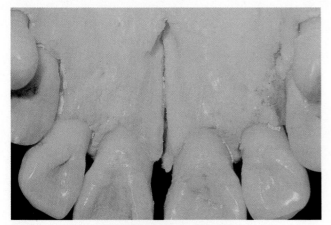

Fig. 5.1. **Maxilla:** lingual aspect of central incisor region.

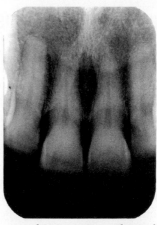

Fig. 5.2. **Maxilla:** central incisor region radiograph.

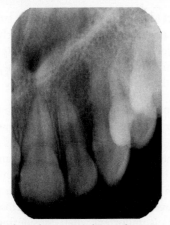

Fig. 5.3. **Maxilla:** lateral incisor radiograph.

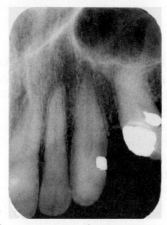

Fig. 5.4. **Maxilla:** canine periapical image.

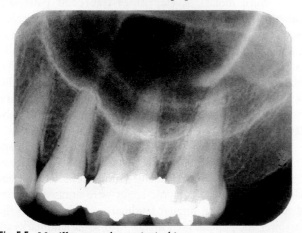

Fig. 5.5. **Maxilla:** premolar periapical image.

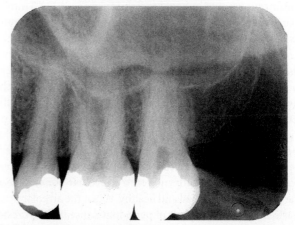

Fig. 5.6. **Maxilla:** molar periapical image.

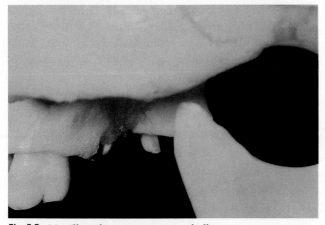

Fig. 5.7. **Maxilla:** tuberosity region on skull.

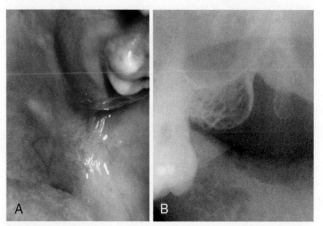

Fig. 5.8. **Maxilla:** clinical photograph (**A**) and radiograph (**B**) of tuberosity region.

Incisor-Canine Region (Figs. 6.1 and 6.2) On the lingual aspect of the mandible, the incisor image reveals the **lingual foramen** located several millimeters below the root apices. This radiolucent landmark is surrounded by the four **genial tubercles**. The superior tubercles serve as the attachment site of the **genioglossus muscle**, and the inferior pair anchors the **geniohyoid muscle**. The **inferior border** of the mandible below this area is delineated by a thick cortex (outer covering). Radiographically, the **genial tubercles** appear as round doughnut-shaped radiopacities. In this case, the **lingual canal** extends inferiorly from this region. Below this is the **inferior cortex** of the mandible. In Figure 6.2, the inverted V-shaped thick radiopaque line that extends posteriorly along the incisor root apices is the **mental ridge**; it is located on the buccal aspect of the mandible.

Premolar and Molar Regions (Figs. 6.3 and 6.4) In the photographs of the skull, the **mental foramen** is located near the root apex of the second premolar, and the **external oblique ridge** is highlighted (i.e., reflecting light from the flash) distal to the second molar. Both are landmarks of the **buccal aspect** of the mandible. On the lingual side of the mandible is the **internal oblique** or **mylohyoid ridge**. It is anterior, more horizontal, and longer than the external oblique ridge. Beneath the mylohyoid ridge is a **fossa** or **depression** within which lies the submandibular salivary gland.

Premolar Region (Fig. 6.5) Radiographically, the **mental foramen** is a round or ovoid radiolucency about 2 to 3 mm in diameter that lacks a distinct radiopaque corticated margin. Its location varies from the distal aspect of the canine to the distal aspect of the second premolar near and below the root apex region. In this radiograph, a mixed **trabecular pattern** is seen with a denser (more radiopaque) pattern toward the alveolar crest and a looser (more radiolucent) pattern in the apical area. Loose and dense trabecular patterns depend on the number of bone trabeculae present in the region. In this radiograph, the radiopaque **lamina dura** and radiolucent **periodontal membrane space** are well illustrated in the second premolar. The radiopaque **crestal alveolar bone** between the premolars is pointed and healthy. When the alveolar bone starts to resorb as a result of periodontal disease, the crestal bone (radiopaque line) is lost. The densely radiopaque material in the crowns of the second premolar and molar is **amalgam**. Notice that the gingival margins of the restorations are smooth and continuous with the remaining tooth structure in the interproximal areas, which helps to maintain proper periodontal health. In this view, the buccal cusps are slightly higher than the lingual cusps owing to excess negative vertical angulation of the BID during the exposure.

Buccal Aspect Molar Region (Fig. 6.6) The **external and internal oblique ridges** are densely radiopaque structures, approximately 2 to 6 mm in width, that sometimes parallel each other. The external oblique ridge is above and posterior to the internal oblique ridge. The smooth, round radiopaque area at the bifurcation of the first molar is frequently mistaken for an enamel pearl or pulp stone. Actually, it is an anatomic artifact (due to superimposition of buccal and lingual root structure at the bifurcation) produced by incorrect horizontal angulation of the BID. The artifact disappears when the correct horizontal angulation of the BID is used—in cases in which it does not disappear, an enamel pearl or pulp stone should be suspected.

Lingual Aspect Molar Region (Fig. 6.7) The **submandibular fossa** is a broad radiolucent area immediately beneath the mylohyoid ridge and above the **inferior cortex** of the mandible. It is seen more often when excessive negative vertical angulation of the BID is used.

Internal Aspect Molar Region (Fig. 6.8) The **inferior alveolar canal** (or mandibular canal)—containing the inferior alveolar nerve and blood vessels—appears as a 6-mm wide radiolucent canal in the molar image. The canal is outlined by parallel radiopaque cortical lines representing the canal walls and often runs below or in close proximity to the molar apices or to developing third molars. This close relationship to third molars is important when considering the removal of the third molars. A **stepladder trabecular pattern** is sometimes seen between the roots of mandibular first molars (and central incisors). This usually represents a variation of normal. However, if generalized in appearance, it may indicate a severe form of anemia. In this instance, the trabeculae are horizontal, in a limited region, and more or less parallel to each other. Note the fractured distal surface of the first molar, the subtle occlusal caries in the second molar, and the developing third molar.

Author comment: We purposely used no. 2 size image in these examples to provide as many landmarks as possible in the limited space available. Some views in the standard full-mouth radiographic series were omitted because of space limitations. Similar landmarks can be seen in the narrower and popular no. 1 image. Also, some landmarks are seen variably, depending on individual patient differences and whether the bisecting angle or paralleling techniques are used or whether excessive vertical or horizontal angulation of the BID is used. Landmarks and structures are not indicated by arrows as they can obscure adjacent anatomic structures.

Remember, the recognition of normal is an absolute prerequisite to recognizing and identifying disorders and diseases. As we have often said, learning should be fun, and we hope this descriptive and illustrative approach helps.

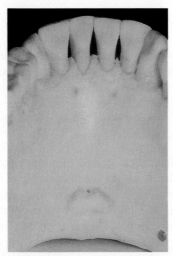

Fig. 6.1. Mandible: lingual aspect incisor-canine region.

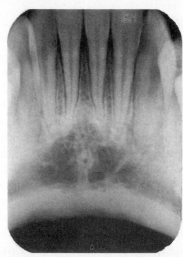

Fig. 6.2. Mandible: incisor-canine periapical image.

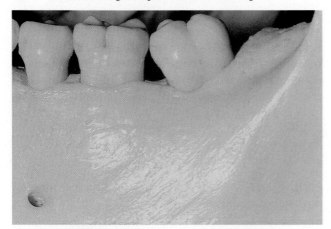

Fig. 6.3. Mandible: external oblique ridge; see Figure 6.6.

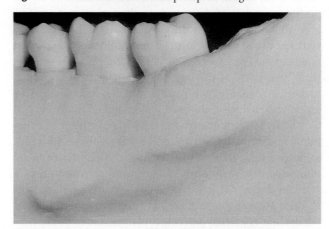

Fig. 6.4. Mandible: internal oblique ridge; see Figure 6.6.

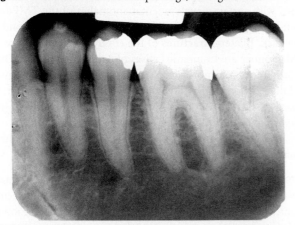

Fig. 6.5. Mandible: premolar periapical image.

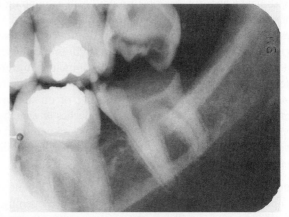

Fig. 6.6. Mandible: molar periapical image.

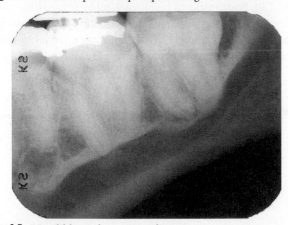

Fig. 6.7. Mandible: molar periapical image.

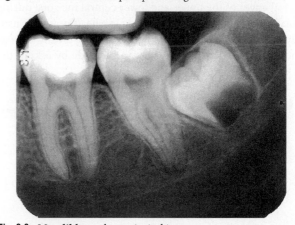

Fig. 6.8. Mandible: molar periapical image.

Normal Anatomy (Figs. 7.1 and 7.2) The **temporomandibular joint (TMJ)** is composed of several major hard and soft tissue structures. The bony structures (visible in radiographic images) include the head of the **condyle** and condylar **neck**. The soft tissue components, shown in the diagram (Fig. 7.1) and anatomic specimen (Fig. 7.2), include the **disk** and **joint capsule**. The disk is made of fibrous cartilage disk, is hourglass shaped, and lies above the condyle and below the glenoid fossa. The disk is located within the joint capsule that contains the synovial fluid. The disk and synovial fluid cushion the head of the condyle from the bones of the glenoid fossa. The disk divides the joint capsule into the upper and lower joint spaces. It is attached posteriorly to the joint capsule, superiorly to the temporal bone, inferiorly to the posterior condyle, and anteriorly to the capsule and external pterygoid muscle. When the jaws are closed, the condyle is centered in the glenoid fossa of the temporal bone. During opening, the condyle first "rotates" in the glenoid fossa and then "translates" as the mouth opens wider. Upon normal maximum opening, the condylar head approximates the articular eminence of the base of the skull.

All of the components of the TMJ are subject to functional and/or pathologic change. Some of the major clinically observable features of TMJ function or dysfunction are illustrated. The major observable **signs** of TMJ disorders are swelling in the TMJ area; redness of the overlying skin; pain/tenderness to palpation of the TMJ; atrophy, hypertrophy, or paralysis or restricted movement of the muscles of mastication; pain on palpation of the muscles of mastication or their attachments; abnormal audible sounds, such as popping or crepitus (grinding); facial asymmetry; occlusal abnormalities, such as unilateral posterior open bite (apertognathia); crossbite; acquired anterior open bite; a shift in the anterior midline; and radiographic changes. Common **symptoms** elicited with TMJ disorders include reports of popping (or crepitus) sounds; pain at rest, on opening, or on chewing; limited opening; ringing in the ear; headaches or earaches; changes in the face, such as "my face or jaw looks crooked or swollen"; inability to chew or eat properly; and the inability to fully open or close the jaw.

Normal Opening (Fig. 7.3) is assessed in terms of the amount of opening and amount of deviation. How much opening is usually expressed in millimeters (mm) measured between the incisal edges of the upper and lower central incisors, during **maximal opening**. Normal opening in a healthy adult is usually at least 40 mm. However, patients vary greatly in size, and a simple quick assessment can be made by asking the patient if he or she can open fully to accommodate three fingers (the index, middle, and ring fingers) between the incisal edges of the maxillary and mandibular teeth. Limited opening consists of a width less than three fingers, but seldom are functional reports made unless the opening is severely restricted (less than two fingers).

Deviation on Opening (Fig. 7.4) The assessment of **deviation** is performed by observing the relationship of the mandibular midline (between the central incisors) with the maxillary midline during opening. When the midlines do not line up during opening, this is called deviation. Deviation on opening can occur to one side only, or first to one side and then the other.

Posterior Open Bite (Fig. 7.5) is also referred to as apertognathia. The term ipsilateral apertognathia is used when the **posterior open bite** is on the same side as the TMJ disorder (usually a tumor). The term contralateral apertognathia is used when the open bite is on the opposite side as the TMJ problem. This may happen after condylectomy or TMJ fractures. In Figure 7.5, the patient is in centric occlusion; he had an ipsilateral apertognathia, deviation of the midline at rest, and a **crossbite** (see Fig. 7.7) that is due to an osteochondroma on his right condyle.

Anterior Open Bite (Fig. 7.6) Patients can have an **anterior open bite** from childhood habits such as tongue thrusting or thumb sucking. In these instances, the mamelons of the incisors may persist well into adult life. Anterior open bite is also seen with certain developmental anomalies of the TMJ and conditions that alter the height of the TMJ condyle or condylar neck. Bilateral fractures of the condyles or bilateral condylectomies are traumatic causes of anterior open bite. One of the most common causes of anterior open bite in aging adults is resorption of the condyles because of degenerative diseases such as rheumatoid arthritis. With this disease, the superior condylar surface is slowly destroyed, producing wear facets and a loss of vertical height of the head of the condyles.

Crossbite (Figs. 7.7 and 7.8) can be a sign of a TMJ abnormality or neoplasm. In this example, a growth deficit resulted in a contralateral crossbite (Fig. 7.7), especially evident in the lower third molar region, which contributed to facial asymmetry (Fig. 7.8). Some patient's hemihypertrophy involves the condylar neck, making this structure longer on one side than the other. In another example (Fig. 56.3), there is a **crossbite** due to unilateral enlargement of the tongue (hemihypertrophy).

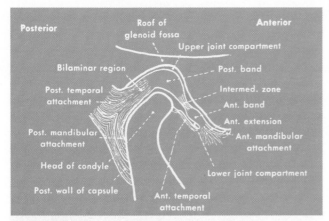

Fig. 7.1. TMJ: anatomy diagram of hard and soft tissues.

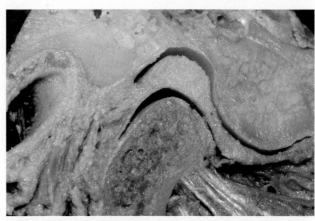

Fig. 7.2. TMJ: anatomic section; correlate with Figure 7.1.

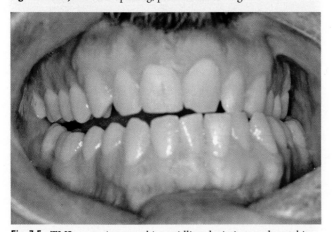

Fig. 7.3. TMJ: normal opening; patient's three fingers.

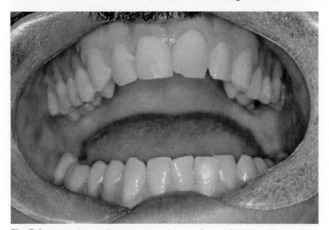

Fig. 7.4. TMJ: limited opening with significant deviation.

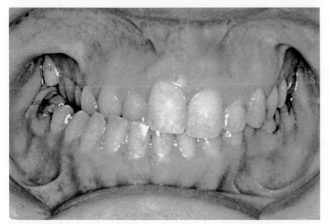

Fig. 7.5. TMJ: posterior open bite, midline deviation, and crossbite.

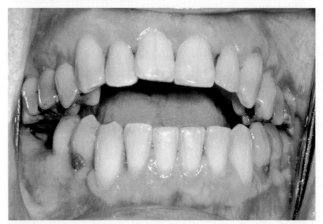

Fig. 7.6. TMJ: anterior open bite in rheumatoid arthritis.

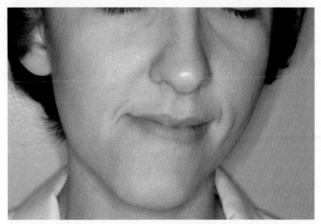

Fig. 7.7. TMJ: developmental crossbite; long condylar neck.

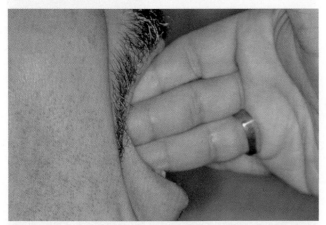

Fig. 7.8. TMJ: facial asymmetry in same patient as Figure 7.7.

CASE STUDIES

CASE 1. (FIG. 7.9)

1. Identify what region is shown in this periapical radiographic image.

2. Identify the structure labeled A.

3. Is this a normal finding of the maxilla?

4. Identify the structures labeled B and E.

5. Identify the structure labeled C.

6. Identify the structure labeled D.

7. Identify the structure labeled by the black arrows.

8. Identify the structure labeled by the yellow arrow.

9. Identify the structures labeled by the green and red arrows.

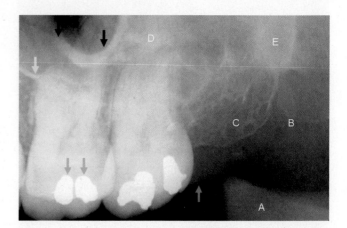

10. Based on this radiographic image, would a dental hygienist need to communicate to the dentist any concerns about anatomic structures or dental caries?

CASE 2. (FIG. 7.10)

This 22-year-old young lady presents to your dental office for routine dental care.

1. Identify the structure labeled A.

2. Identify the structure labeled by the yellow arrows.

3. Identify the structure labeled by the green arrow. Is this structure normal or abnormal, and how is it contributing to the dentition?

4. Identify the gingival tissue that is light brown in color. Why is it brown? Is this a normal finding, a variant of normal, or disease?

5. True or false: The marginal gingiva in this patient is pigmented.

6. Identify the structure labeled by the black arrow.

7. Identify the structure labeled by the red arrow. Is this structure healthy or diseased?

8. What questions might you ask the patient relative to the structure identified by the green arrow?

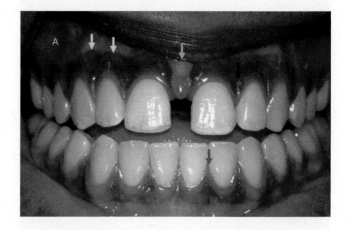

Additional cases to enhance your learning and understanding of this section are available Online through the book's Navigate 2 Advantage Access site.

Diagnostic and Descriptive Terminology

Objectives:

- Recognize, define, and use terms that describe oral lesions and help in the diagnostic process:
  a. Colored or textured lesions that can occur in the skin and oral mucosa
  b. Lesions that denude epithelium
  c. Lesions associated with inflammatory reactions
  d. Clefts and cavities within skin and oral mucosa
  e. Solid raised lesions in the skin and oral mucosa
  f. Fluid-filled lesions in the skin and oral mucosa
- Recognize clinical features of the skin and mucosa associated with infection and inflammatory disease.
- Recognize clinical features of benign and malignant disease.
- Use the descriptive terminology from this section to accurately document extraoral and intraoral findings in a clinical setting.

Macule (Figs. 8.1 and 8.2) is a small confined area of epidermis or mucosa distinguished by color from its surroundings. By definition, it is less than 1 cm in diameter. The **macule** may appear alone or in groups as a red, blue, brown, or black stain or spot. It is neither elevated nor depressed. A macule may represent a normal condition, a variant of normal, or local or systemic disease. The term *macule* would be used to clinically describe the following conditions: oral melanotic macule, ephelis, amalgam, India ink or pencil tattoos, and focal argyrosis. The color and shape of the macule aid in the diagnosis. Conditions that appear as macules are discussed in detail under "Pigmented Lesions" (Figs. 77.1–79.8).

Patch (Figs. 8.3 and 8.4) is a circumscribed area that is larger than the macule and differentiated from the surrounding epidermis by color, texture, or both. Like the macule, the **patch** is neither elevated nor depressed. Focal argyrosis, lichen planus, mucous patch of secondary syphilis, and snuff dipper's patch represent patchlike lesions that may be seen intraorally. Conditions that appear as patches are discussed in detail under "White Lesions" (Figs. 68.1–70.8), "Pigmented Lesions" (Figs. 77.1–79.8), and "Sexually Transmissible Conditions" (Figs. 91.1–93.8).

Erosion (Figs. 8.5 and 8.6) is a clinical term that describes a soft tissue lesion in which the skin or mucosa is denuded (i.e., the epithelium is worn away or destroyed). An **erosion** is moist and slightly depressed and often results from a broken vesicle, epithelial breakdown, or trauma. In the eroded area, the epithelium is lost; however, the basal cell layer (layer above the connective tissue or dermis) is preserved. Thus, it represents a shallow area where only a few layers of the epithelium are lost. Healing rarely results in scarring because the basal layer of the epithelium remains intact. Pemphigus, erosive lichen planus (desquamative gingivitis), and erythema multiforme are diseases that produce mucocutaneous erosions. Conditions that appear as erosions are discussed in detail under "Vesiculobullous Lesions" (Figs. 83.1–87.8).

Ulcer (Figs. 8.7 and 8.8) is a craterlike lesion of the skin or oral mucosa. It is the term used to describe an uncovered wound of cutaneous or mucosal tissue that exhibits gradual tissue disintegration and necrosis. The border of a mucosal **ulcer** is often round but can be irregular. Ulcers are deeper than erosions, extending below the basal layer of the epithelium into the dermis (connective tissue). Scarring may follow healing of an ulcer. Ulcers may result from trauma; aphthous stomatitis; infection by viruses, such as herpes simplex, variola (smallpox), and varicella-zoster (chickenpox and shingles); cancer; or granulomatous disease. Ulcers are usually painful and often require topical or systemic drug therapy for effective management. Conditions that appear as ulcers are discussed in detail under "Vesiculobullous Lesions" (Figs. 83.1–87.8) and "Ulcerative Lesions" (Figs. 88.1–90.8).

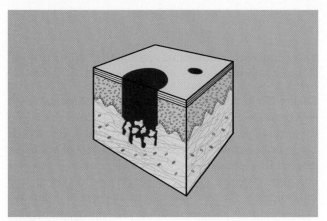

Fig. 8.1. Macule: nonraised area altered in color.

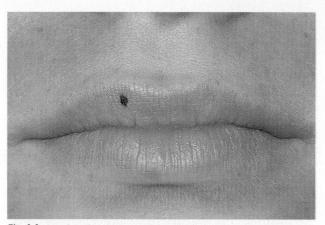

Fig. 8.2. Oral melanotic macule on the lip.

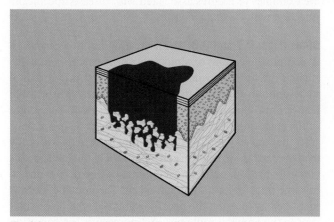

Fig. 8.3. Patch: pigmented area larger than a macule.

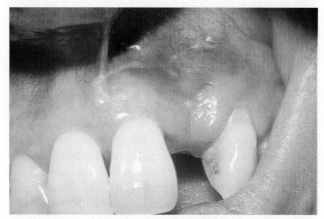

Fig. 8.4. Patch: amalgam tattoo after retrograde amalgam.

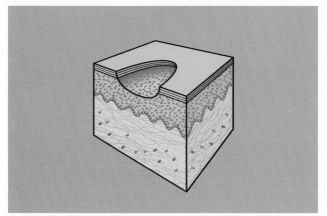

Fig. 8.5. Erosion: denudation above basal layer of epithelium.

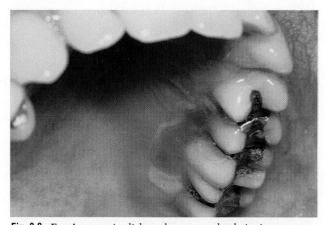

Fig. 8.6. Erosion: erosive lichen planus on palatal gingiva.

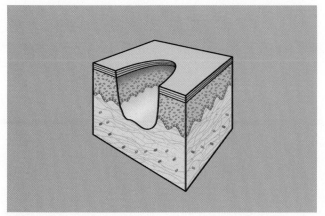

Fig. 8.7. Ulcer: denudation below basal layer of epithelium.

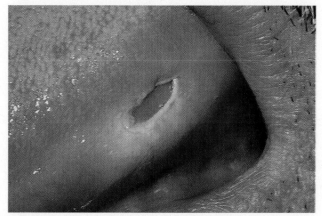

Fig. 8.8. Traumatic ulcer on lateral tongue border.

Wheal (Figs. 9.1 and 9.2) is a raised area of localized tissue swelling (edema). This smooth-surfaced papule or plaque results from acute extravasation of serum into the superficial dermis. A **wheal** is generally pale red, pruritic, and of short duration. By definition, they are only slightly raised and vary in size. While they can appear as a single entity, they more often appear in numbers (wheals) and most commonly in persons with allergies. The wheal develops as a result of histamine release from mast cells or activation of the complement cascade. Wheals are a sign of an allergic reaction that develops shortly after insect bites, consuming a particular food, or mechanical irritation (such as that occurring in patients with dermatographia). They are often very itchy. Conditions that appear as wheals are discussed in detail under "Allergic Reactions" and "Vesiculobullous Lesions" (Figs. 83.1–87.8).

Scar (Figs. 9.3 and 9.4) is a permanent mark or cicatrix remaining after a wound heals. A **scar** is a visible sign of wound repair and indicates a previous disruption in the integrity of the epidermis and dermis and healing of epithelium with fibrous (collagen connective) tissue. Scars are infrequently found in the oral cavity because oral tissue is elastic and less prone to scar formation than skin. When they do occur, they may be of any shape or size. They are distinct from the adjacent tissue. The color of an intraoral scar is usually lighter than that of the adjacent mucosa. Histologically, they are more dense than the adjacent epithelium, lack sweat (or salivary) glands, and have fewer blood vessels. Oral (i.e., periapical) surgery, burns, or intraoral trauma may result in a scar. Scars are discussed in detail under "White Lesions" (Figs. 69.3–69.6).

Fissure (Figs. 9.5 and 9.6) is a normal or abnormal linear cleft or furrow in the epidermis (skin or mucosa) that affects the tongue, lips, and perioral tissues. The presence of a **fissure** can indicate a condition representing a variant of normal or disease. Disease-associated fissures result when pathogenic organisms infect a fissure, causing pain, ulceration, and inflammation. Fissured tongue is an example of a variation of normal that is associated with dry mouth, hyposalivation, and dehydration. Angular cheilitis and exfoliative cheilitis are examples of fissures associated with disease, specifically infection with *Candida albicans*.

Sinus (Figs. 9.7 and 9.8) The term **sinus** has two meanings. A common meaning of sinus is a normal recess or cavity, such as the frontal or maxillary sinus. The term is also used to describe an abnormal dilated tract, channel, or fistula that leads from a suppurative cavity, cyst, or abscess to the surface of the epidermis. An abscessed tooth often produces a sinus tract that travels from the infected root apex to the clinically evident parulis, which is the terminal end of the tract. In this clinical situation, gutta-percha points can be deeply placed into the tract and a radiograph taken. The nonvital tooth is identified by locating the tip of the gutta-percha point adjacent to the nonvital root apex. Actinomycosis is a condition characterized clinically by several yellow sinus tracts exiting onto the mucosa or skin surface.

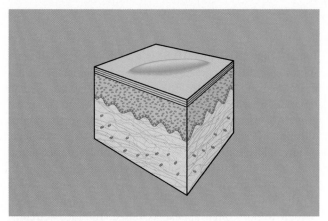

Fig. 9.1. Wheal: serum-filled papule or plaque.

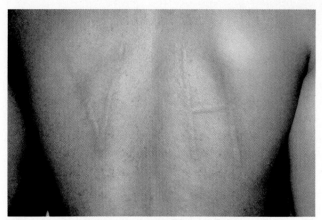

Fig. 9.2. Wheal: dermatographism after rubbing the skin.

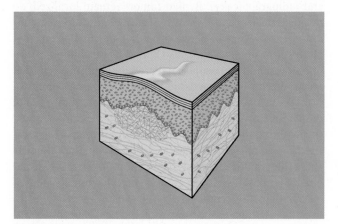

Fig. 9.3. Scar: permanent mark from wound.

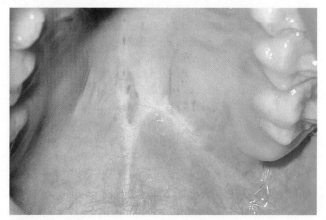

Fig. 9.4. Scar: fibrotic tissue as a result of trauma.

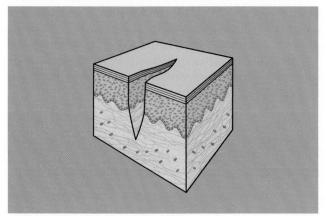

Fig. 9.5. Fissure: a linear crack in the epidermis.

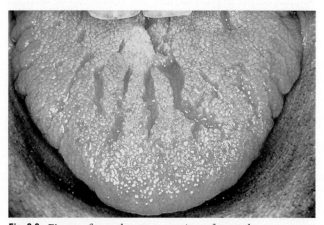

Fig. 9.6. Fissure: fissured tongue, a variant of normal.

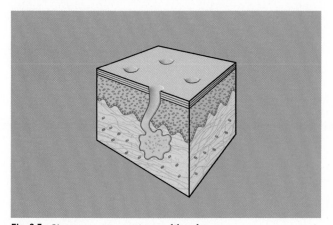

Fig. 9.7. Sinus: a recess, cavity, or dilated tract.

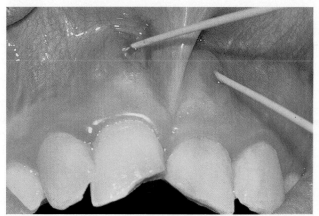

Fig. 9.8. Sinus tracts exiting from nonvital incisors.

Papule (Figs. 10.1 and 10.2) is a small, superficial, elevated, solid lesion or structure that is less than 1 cm in diameter. A **papule** may be of any color and may be attached by a stalk or firm base. Papules often represent a benign or slow-growing lesion that is caused by infection, inflammation, hyperplasia, or neoplasia. Common examples of benign lesions appearing as papules include condyloma acuminatum, parulis, and squamous papilloma. Basal cell carcinoma, a slow-growing skin cancer, can also appear as a papule. Conditions that appear as papules are discussed in the section on "Papulonodules" (Figs. 82.1–82.8).

Plaque (Figs. 10.3 and 10.4) is a flat, solid, raised area of the skin or mucosa that is greater than 1 cm in diameter. Although essentially superficial, a **plaque** may extend deeper into the dermis than a papule. The edges may be sloped, and sometimes, keratin proliferates along the surface (a condition known as lichenification). Lichen planus, leukoplakia, or melanoma may initially appear as a plaque. Lichen planus, a plaque-producing disease, is discussed under "Red and Red-White Lesions" (Figs. 74.1–74.8). As with many medical-dental words, *plaque* has more than one definition. In dentistry, dental plaque is the biofilm of bacteria that builds up on teeth. Dental plaque can be located supra- or subgingivally, and the type of bacteria in plaque varies by location.

Nodule (Figs. 10.5 and 10.6) is a solid and raised lump or mass of tissue that has the dimension of depth. Like a papule, a **nodule** is less than 1 cm in diameter; however, a nodule extends deeper into the dermis. The nodule can be detected by palpation. The overlying epidermis is usually nonfixed and can be easily moved over the lesion. Nodules can be asymptomatic or painful and usually are slow growing. Benign mesenchymal tumors, such as fibroma, lipoma, lipofibroma, and neuroma, often appear as oral nodules. Other examples of nodules are discussed under "Nodules" (Figs. 80.1–81.8).

Tumor (Figs. 10.7 and 10.8) is a term used to indicate a solid mass of tissue greater than 1 cm in diameter that has the dimension of depth. The term **tumor** is also used to represent a **neoplasm**—a new, independent, and abnormal growth of tissue with uncontrolled and progressive multiplication of cells that have no physiologic use. Tumors may be any color and may be located in any intraoral or extraoral soft or hard tissue. Tumors are classified as **benign, in situ**, or **malignant neoplasms**. Benign tumors grow more slowly and are less aggressive than malignant tumors. Benign tumors often appear as raised, rounded (circumscribed) lesions that have well-defined margins (clinically and radiographically). Benign tumors remain localized, do not metastasize, and do not transform into cancer. A condition that occurs in between benign and malignant neoplasms is *in situ neoplasia*, also known as **carcinoma in situ** or precancer. In situ neoplasm represents abnormal cells that are localized within one tissue and have a high probability of progressing onto cancer. Malignant tumors are comprised of numerous neoplastic cells that have enlarged dark-staining (hyperchromatic) nuclei. Malignant tumor cells are aggressive, invade adjacent tissues, and spread rapidly. Clinically and radiographically, malignant tumors often have ill-defined margins. Persistent tumors may be umbilicated or ulcerated in the center. The term *tumor* is often used to describe a benign tissue mass such as a neurofibroma, granular cell tumor, or pregnancy tumor. The term **carcinoma** is reserved for malignant cancers/neoplasia of epithelial tissue (Figs. 90.3 and 90.4). The term **sarcoma** is reserved for a malignant neoplasm/neoplasia of embryonic connective tissue origin, such as osteosarcoma, a malignant neoplasm of bone. Malignancies destroy tissue by direct invasion and extension and by spread to distant sites by metastasis through blood, lymph, or serosal surfaces.

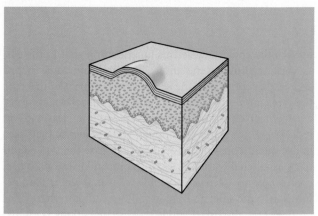

Fig. 10.1. Papule: elevated, solid lesion less than 1 cm wide.

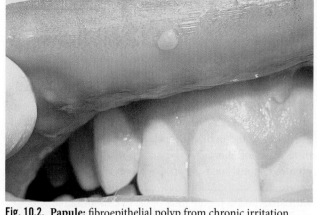

Fig. 10.2. Papule: fibroepithelial polyp from chronic irritation.

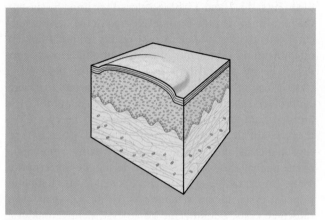

Fig. 10.3. Plaque: flat, raised area greater than 1 cm in diameter.

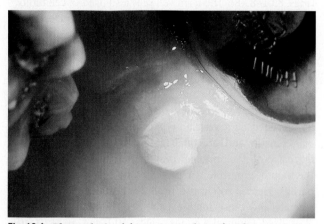

Fig. 10.4. Plaque: leukoplakia owing to clasp of appliance.

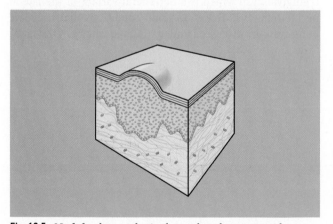

Fig. 10.5. Nodule: deep and raised mass less than 1 cm wide.

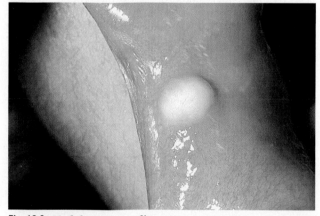

Fig. 10.6. Nodule: irritation fibroma at commissure.

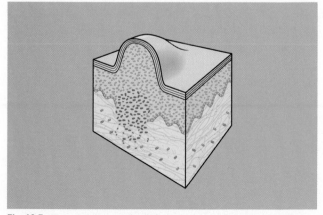

Fig. 10.7. Tumor: deep and solid mass greater than 1 cm wide.

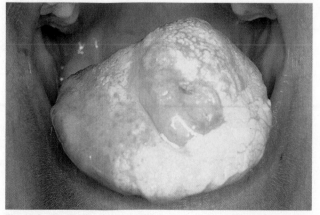

Fig. 10.8. Tumor: squamous cell carcinoma of the tongue.

Vesicle (Figs. 11.1 and 11.2) is a small, fluid-filled elevation (blister) in the epidermis (skin or mucosa). They are often the size of a pin but, by definition, extend up to 1 cm in diameter. The fluid of a vesicle generally consists of lymph or serum but may contain blood and infectious agents. The epithelial lining of a vesicle is thin and will eventually break down, thus causing an ulcer and eschar (surface slough). Vesicles are a common result of allergic reactions or inflammation caused by viral infections, such as herpes simplex, herpes zoster, chickenpox, and smallpox. In viral infections, the vesicle is laden with virus and is highly infectious. Conditions characterized by vesicles are discussed under "Vesiculobullous Lesions" (Figs. 83.1–83.8). The term *vesicle* is also used in cell biology to mean an organelle within a living cell that is enclosed by a lipid bilayer member and used to transport materials.

Pustule (Figs. 11.3 and 11.4) is a circumscribed elevation filled with pus—a purulent exudate consisting of a mixture of inflammatory cells and liquid—resulting from an infection. Pustules are small, less than 1 cm in diameter, and may be preceded by a vesicle or papule. They are creamy white or yellowish and are often associated with acne—an epidermal pore (i.e., pimple) or inflamed sweat gland. Within the mouth, a pustule is represented by a pointing abscess or parulis. Herpes zoster also produces pustules that eventually ulcerate and cause intense pain. See the discussions under "Localized Gingival Lesions" (Figs. 50.1 and 50.2), "Caries Progression" (Fig. 33.8), and "Vesiculobullous Lesions" (Figs. 84.1–84.4) for examples of diseases that produce pustules.

Bulla (Figs. 11.5 and 11.6) is a fluid-filled blister greater than 1 cm in size. A bulla develops from the accumulation of fluid in the epidermal-dermis junction or a split in the epidermis. Accordingly, the surface is smooth and dome shaped and easily ruptured by the slightest of trauma. On the skin, they are commonly associated with burns, frictional trauma, and contact dermatitis and typically appear clear pink to red. When they occur as multiples and because of their size, bullae often represent a more severe disease than do conditions associated with vesicles. Intraoral and extraoral bullae are commonly seen in pemphigus, pemphigoid, Stevens-Johnson syndrome, and epidermolysis bullosa. These conditions are discussed under "Vesiculobullous Lesions" (Figs. 86.1–86.8).

Cyst (Figs. 11.7 and 11.8) is a closed sac lined by the epithelium (known as the capsule) located in the dermis, subcutaneous tissue, or bone. A cyst results from entrapment of epithelium or remnants of epithelium that grow to produce a cavity (the cavity portion is known as the lumen). Cysts range in diameter from a few millimeters to several centimeters. Aspiration of a cyst may or may not yield luminal fluid, depending on the nature of the cyst. Cysts that contain clear fluid appear pink to blue, whereas keratin-filled cysts often appear yellow or creamy white. Some of the many types of oral cysts are dermoid cysts, eruption cysts, implantation cysts, incisive canal cysts, lymphoepithelial cysts, mucus retention cysts, nasoalveolar cysts, radicular cysts, odontogenic keratocyst, dentigerous cyst, and the lateral periodontal cyst. Figure 11.8 demonstrates a gingival cyst, which is a peripheral variant of the lateral periodontal cyst. Bone cysts and conditions that resemble bone cysts are discussed under "Radiolucencies of the Jaws" (Figs. 36.1–39.8).

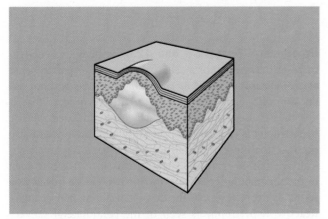

Fig. 11.1. Vesicle: small fluid-filled skin elevation.

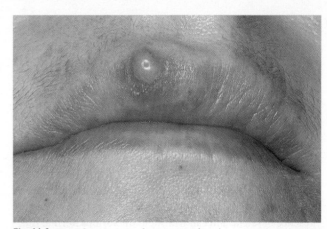

Fig. 11.2. Vesicle: recurrent herpes simplex.

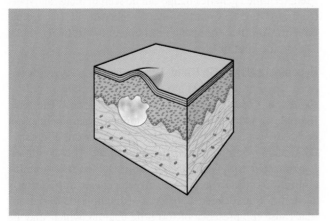

Fig. 11.3. Pustule: vesicle filled with purulent exudate.

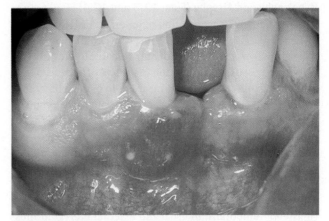

Fig. 11.4. Pustule: pointing periodontal abscess.

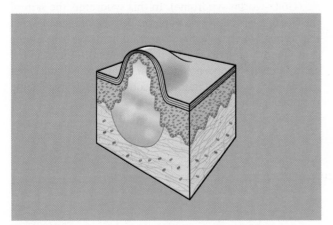

Fig. 11.5. Bulla: large fluid-filled mucocutaneous elevation.

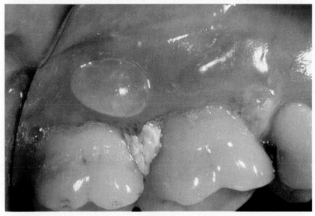

Fig. 11.6. Bulla: bullous lichen planus—a rare finding.

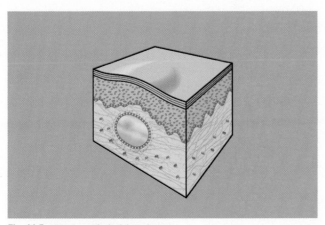

Fig. 11.7. Cyst: epithelial-lined cavity.

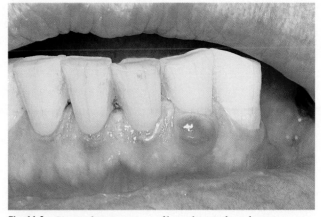

Fig. 11.8. Gingival cyst: variant of lateral periodontal cyst.

Normal (Figs. 12.1 and 12.2) implies an anatomic site or tissue that lacks significant deviation from the average. In other words, **normal** agrees with the regular established characteristics of appearance and function for the representative population. Appearance includes color, shape, size, topography or architecture, consistency, and temperature; histologically, it also includes characteristics seen on stained tissue specimens. Normal function implies the cells, tissue, or organs are performing as they should. For example, normal oral mucosa appears light pinkish in color, is usually moist because of the presence of saliva, and can withstand the various normal functions of the mouth without injury or other abnormal change.

Hypotrophy and Atrophy (Figs. 12.3 and 12.4) Hypotrophy is the progressive degeneration of an organ or tissue caused by *loss in cell size*. The condition results when there is incomplete growth or maintenance of nutrition to a tissue or organ. Hypotrophy causes a diminution in the size of a tissue, organ, or part. **Atrophy** is similar in meaning to hypotrophy but is reserved for the degeneration of cells—often the result of persistent hypotrophy. Atrophy is also referred to as "wasting/withering away" or a decrease in size of a body organ or tissue that is due to disease, lack of nourishment, injury, or lack of use. Examples of atrophy follow. The oral mucosa may become thinned when atrophic candidiasis develops. Muscles, such as the tongue or the muscles of mastication (masseter, temporalis, internal and external pterygoid muscles), may become atrophic as a result of disuse (disuse atrophy); muscle disuse may follow a loss of motor innervation that is due to trauma or following a stroke. Following the extraction of one, several, or all of the teeth, the alveolar bone of the mandible and/or maxilla will usually atrophy (diminish in size), providing less support for prostheses or sufficient bone for an implant. Continued atrophy of the alveolar bone results in impingement on vital strictures, such as the mental nerve or the maxillary sinus.

Hypertrophy (Figs. 12.5 and 12.6) implies the enlargement or overgrowth of a cell, tissue, organ, or part because of an *increase in size of its constituents or cells* without cell division. **Hypertrophy** may be a reactive process that is due to increased function or is genetically induced. Muscle hypertrophy is typically seen in body building but can also occur in the muscles of mastication in persons who chronically clench or grind their teeth (bruxism). It is also seen in the mandibular condyle, which may increase in size as a result of hypertrophic arthritic or developmental changes. Reactive hypertrophy is seen in the contralateral salivary gland following the removal of the opposite salivary gland. Predetermined genetic change can be seen in bilateral hypertrophy of the coronoid process occurring in susceptible patients. Another example is seen in hemifacial hypertrophy as described in this text.

Hypoplasia (Figs. 12.7 and 12.8) refers to an underdeveloped tissue or organ that has *decreased in number of cells or the amount of substance they produce or secrete*. The term **hypoplasia** is used when there is underdevelopment of an organ or tissue such that it fails to reach its full adult size. One dental example is enamel hypoplasia. This condition is associated with insufficient amount of enamel or mineralization within the enamel. Amelogenesis imperfecta is a condition associated with several hypoplastic variations that cause the presence of too little enamel, which may be smooth or pitted. Another example is focal dermal hypoplasia (Goltz-Gorlin syndrome). In this syndrome, the skin of the face appears depressed in places because of hypoplasia of the dermis, which is the tissue layer immediately beneath the skin. Condylar hypoplasia is a third example. In this case, the condyle of the temporomandibular joint is small and often deformed as a result of trauma or congenital defects affecting the cartilaginous growth center.

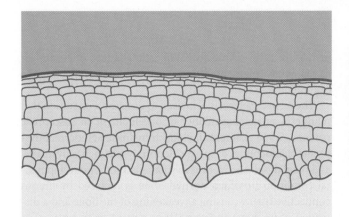

Fig. 12.1. Normal: appearance, number, size, architecture.

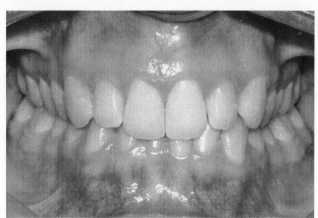

Fig. 12.2. Normal: soft tissues, gingiva, teeth, occlusion.

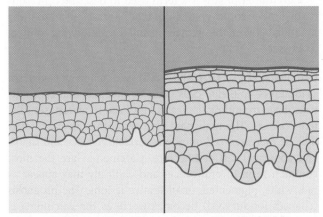

Fig. 12.3. Atrophy: decreased size of cells (*left*), normal (*right*).

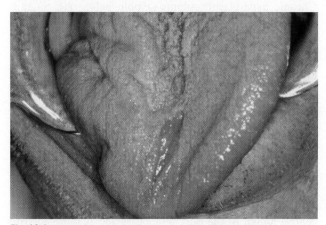

Fig. 12.4. Atrophy: poststroke; tongue muscles atrophied.

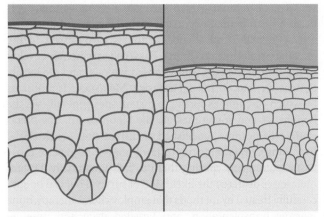

Fig. 12.5. Hypertrophy: increased size of cells (*left*), normal (*right*).

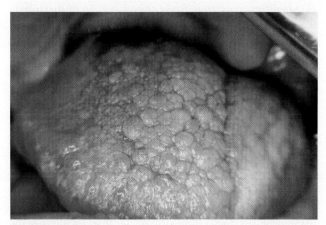

Fig. 12.6. Hypertrophy: tongue in facial hemihypertrophy.

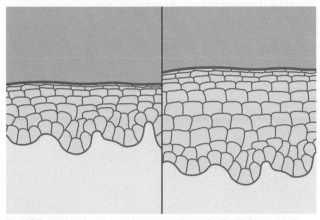

Fig. 12.7. Hypoplasia: decreased number of cells (*left*), normal (*right*).

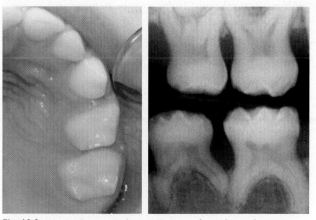

Fig. 12.8. Hypoplasia: amelogenesis imperfecta; hypoplastic enamel.

Hyperplasia (Figs. 13.1 and 13.2) is an *increase in the number of normal cells* in a tissue or organ that results in increased volume or size of the tissue or organ. The term implies there is an abnormal multiplication of cells that are normal in appearance, arrangement, and architecture. Hyperplasia is usually a reactive process secondary to some stimulus or growth factors. Puberty is a physiological stimulus that increases the size of the breast and gonadal tissue. In the oral cavity, inflammatory papillary hyperplasia is a reactive tissue growth that develops beneath a denture. Clinically, this condition produces numerous papillary growths on the palate that represent squamous epithelium increased in size. Chronic hyperplastic pulpitis (a pulp polyp; Fig. 33.2) is another example of this condition.

Metaplasia (Figs. 13.3 and 13.4) is the *replacement of one adult cell type with that of another adult cell type* not normal for that tissue. Metaplasia often occurs as a form of adaptation to a stressful environment. One of the more common examples is the metaplastic change of respiratory columnar epithelium to squamous epithelium in response to the chronic irritation of cigarette smoking. In another example, necrotizing sialometaplasia, there is squamous (epithelial) metaplasia of the cells lining the ducts of accessory salivary glands of the posterior palate as a result of ischemic necrosis. This condition shows the following: the normal central lumen of the duct disappears and is replaced with cells that appear like small clusters of epithelium within the surrounding connective tissue. Another type of metaplasia is seen in scar tissue, which begins as dense connective tissue but undergoes metaplastic change to become calcified. Atherosclerotic plaque or blood clots (thrombi) within blood vessels can undergo metaplastic change and calcify.

Dysplasia (Figs. 13.5 and 13.6) means disordered growth and loss of the normal maturation of cells. Dysplasia implies an alteration in the size, shape, and architectural organization of adult cells in tissue (oral mucosa). These changes are often considered premalignant; however, dysplasia does not necessarily progress to cancer. The specific cellular changes seen in epithelial dysplasia include (1) an expansion of immature cells (that display prominent nucleoli, nuclear pleomorphism, hyperchromatic nuclei that are abnormally large for the size of the cell, increased and abnormal mitosis, multinucleation) and (2) decrease in number and location of mature cells. Clinically, dysplastic changes often appear as red, white, pigmented, and ulcerative lesions affecting the oral mucosa.

The term dysplasia is also used to describe a condition that manifests as an abnormality of development in susceptible persons. Some examples include anhydrotic ectodermal dysplasia, cleidocranial dysplasia, dentin dysplasia, hip dysplasia, and renal dysplasia. Fibrous dysplasia is another developmental condition in which normal bone is replaced by fibrous connective tissue, causing a weakening of the bone and a distortion of its shape and size. These patients may have endocrine gland problems and café au lait brown spots on the skin.

Carcinoma in situ is a term used to describe cancerous tissue limited to the epithelium that has not spread past the junction between the epithelium and the underlying connective tissue.

Carcinoma (Figs. 13.7 and 13.8) is a malignant neoplasm made up of epithelial cells (skin or mucosa) that can infiltrate the surrounding tissues and give rise to metastases (distant lesions). The malignant changes seen with carcinoma include increased cell numbers, variable cell size and shape, and abnormal cell architecture. Carcinomas are the most common form of oral cancer and clinically may appear as red, white, pigmented, or ulcerative lesions. The prognosis (chances for survival) becomes worse as the carcinoma is located farther back in the mouth. The most common type of carcinoma is squamous cell carcinoma; other types include verrucous carcinoma, often seen on the gingiva; mucoepidermoid carcinoma, occurring in the major and accessory salivary glands; and adenocarcinomas as observed in the maxillary sinus mucous lining. Basal cell carcinomas develop in the skin of the face (sun-exposed regions) and are locally destructive, but do not metastasize. Metastasis is a process by which carcinomas spread to distant sites generally via the lymphatics and sometimes via the bloodstream. The metastatic cells become established at distant sites—such as the liver, lungs, brain, kidneys, or jaw bones—and replace those tissues, ultimately causing them to fail functionally. Distant metastases decrease the likelihood of survival but can be successfully treated by methods that employ chemotherapy, bone marrow transplantation, and targeted drug and immune therapy. For carcinomas, early recognition and biopsy followed by timely initiation of treatment can be lifesaving.

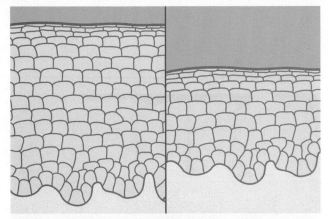

Fig. 13.1. Hyperplasia: increased number of cells (*left*), normal (*right*).

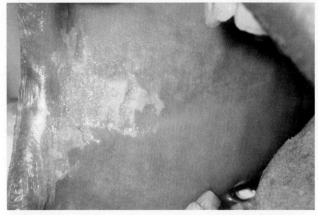

Fig. 13.2. Hyperplasia of surface cells as a result of cheek biting.

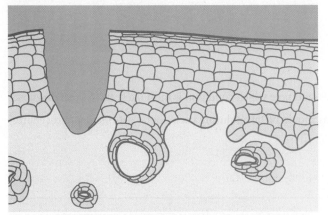

Fig. 13.3. Metaplasia: altered cell type, number, and architecture (*left*), normal (*right*).

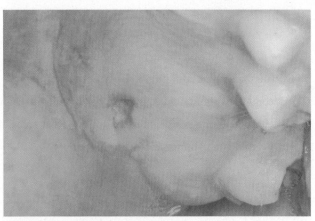

Fig. 13.4. Sialometaplasia: minor salivary gland duct cells altered.

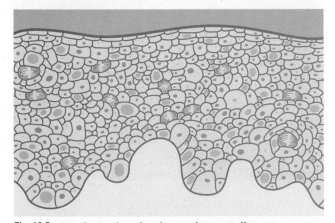

Fig. 13.5. Dysplasia: altered and premalignant cells.

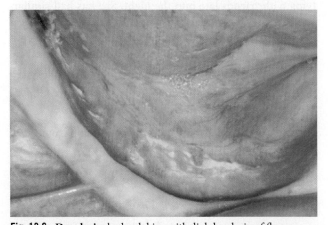

Fig. 13.6. Dysplasia: leukoplakia; epithelial dysplasia of floor.

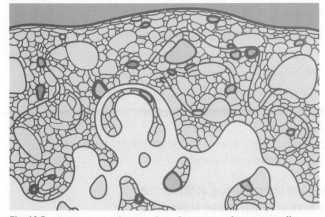

Fig. 13.7. Carcinoma: abnormal, malignant, and invasive cells.

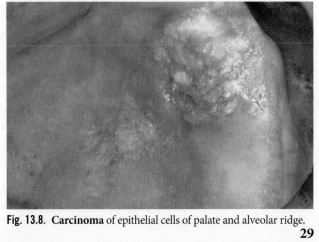

Fig. 13.8. Carcinoma of epithelial cells of palate and alveolar ridge.

CASE STUDIES

CASE 6. (FIG. 13.9)

This 53-year-old woman came to the dental clinic because of burning, painful gingiva of several months duration. An incisional biopsy was performed, and during the initial incision, the gingiva began to slough.

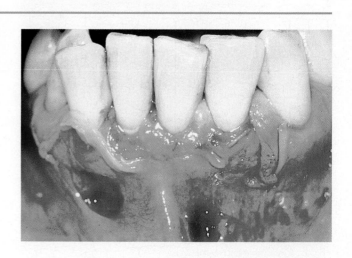

1. Describe the clinical findings.

2. Which term best describes this lesion?
   A. Fissure
   B. Vesicle
   C. Bulla
   D. Erosion

3. Is this a normal finding, a variant of normal, or disease?

4. How is this condition different from an ulcer?

5. Do you expect this condition to be symptomatic?

6. List conditions you should consider in the differential diagnosis, and note which condition is most likely the correct diagnosis.

7. Once this condition is brought under control, what precautions should be taken during periodontal debridement procedures?

8. How would you communicate with this patient?

CASE 7. (FIG. 13.10)

This young lady presents to your dental office with a sore tongue. She claims the lesion appeared 3 days ago, after partying with friends late into the night. She has had similar-appearing lesions under her tongue in the past, but this is the biggest lesion she has ever had. She is taking birth control pills and no other prescription medications. Her medical history form has no positive entries for any systemic diseases.

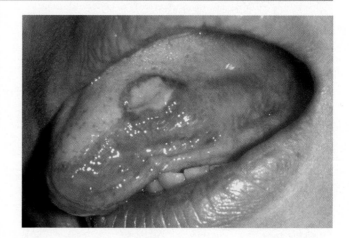

1. Describe the clinical findings. Include mention of the size, shape, color, surface, borders, and location.

2. How can you determine the size of the lesion from the findings presented?

3. What diagnostic and descriptive term best describes this lesion?

4. Do you expect this condition to be symptomatic? Why?

5. Is this a normal finding, a variant of normal, or disease?

6. True or false: This condition can be caused by subgingival calculus.

7. List conditions you should consider in the differential diagnosis for this condition, and note which condition is most likely the correct diagnosis.

8. What clinical features would help distinguish the conditions you listed in the differential diagnosis?

9. Which of the following should be considered with respect to periodontal maintenance therapy?
   A. It is okay to clean her teeth, as long as oral hygiene measures and food avoidance is discussed.
   B. It is okay to clean her teeth, just provide care to the contralateral side.
   C. Therapy should be provided in the affected quadrant because there is likely a cause-and-effect phenomenon.
   D. Therapy should be delayed until healing occurs and the patient is more comfortable.

Additional cases to enhance your learning and understanding of this section are available Online through the book's Navigate 2 Advantage Access site.

Oral Conditions Affecting Infants and Children

Objectives:

- Define and describe the clinical appearance of common oral conditions of infants and children.
- Recognize the causes and clinical features of these conditions.
- Use the diagnostic process to distinguish similar-appearing oral anomalies of infants and children.
- Describe the consequences of disease progression with respect to these conditions.
- Be knowledgeable of appropriate treatments for common oral conditions of infants and children.
- Identify conditions discussed in this section that require the attention of the dentist and/or affect the delivery of dental care.

Commissural Lip Pits (Fig. 14.1) are dimplelike invaginations of the corner of the lips. They may be unilateral or bilateral but tend to occur on the vermilion portion of the lip. They are generally less than 4 mm in diameter, and exploration of the pits yields a sealed depression. **Commissural lip pits** represent failure of fusion of the embryonic maxillary and mandibular processes. The pits occur more frequently in males than in females, and prevalence is about 1% to 8% of the population. The condition can be developmental or associated with an **autosomal dominant** (inherited) **pattern of transmission**. No treatment is required.

Paramedian Lip Pits (Fig. 14.2) are congenital depressions that occur in the mandibular lip, most often on either side of the midline. They develop when the lateral sulci of the embryonic mandibular arch fail to regress during the 6th week in utero. **Paramedian lip pits** are more often bilateral, symmetric depressions with raised, rounded borders. However, single pits and unilateral pits have been described. Inspection reveals a sealed depression that may express mucin. Paramedian lip pits are often inherited as an autosomal dominant trait in combination with cleft lip or cleft palate and hypodontia. When these features occur together, the condition is called **van der Woude syndrome**. The gene responsible for lip pits shows **variable penetrance**. That is, some patients who carry the gene may have a minor or submucosal cleft palate or no visible cleft, yet pass the full syndrome on to their children. Paramedian lip pits require no treatment unless they are of esthetic concern. Clinicians should inquire about affected family members and examine them for cleft lip and palate.

Cleft Lip (Figs. 14.3 and 14.4) is the result of a disturbance of lip development in utero. The upper lip is most commonly affected. **Cleft lip** results when the medial nasal process fails to fuse with the lateral portions of the maxillary process of the first branchial (pharyngeal) arch. Fusion normally occurs during the 6th and 7th weeks of embryonic development.

Cleft lip occurs in about 1 in 900 births and more often in Asians and Native American persons than in Caucasians. The condition occurs more in males than females and is more severe in males. About 85% of cleft lips are unilateral and nonmidline; 15% are bilateral. Midline cleft lip results from failure of fusion of the right and left medial nasal processes and is rare.

The severity of cleft lip varies. A small cleft that does not involve the nose is called an **incomplete cleft**; these sometimes appear as a small notch in the lip. A **complete cleft lip** involves the nasal structures in 45% of cases and is often associated with cleft palate. Cleft lip and palate can result from expression of abnormal patterning genes that are transmitted by autosomal dominant and recessive inheritance, as well as X-linked inheritance. To date, there are about 400 inherited syndromes associated with cleft lip or palate. Drugs taken during pregnancy (alcohol, tobacco smoke [nicotine], antiseizure drugs) increase the risk of clefts. Low intake of vitamin B (folic acid) is also contributory; therefore, folic acid supplements are recommended during pregnancy.

Cleft Palate (Figs. 14.5–14.8) The palate develops from the primary and secondary palate. The (anterior) primary palate is formed by fusion of the right and left medial nasal processes. It is a small triangular mass that encompasses bone, connective tissue, labial and palatal epithelium, and the four incisor tooth buds. The (posterior) secondary palate is formed by fusion of the palatine processes or shelves of the maxillary process. Palatal fusion is initiated during the 8th week in utero by expansion of the mandible; this permits the tongue to drop down and allows the palatal processes to grow inward. The palatal shelves merge with the primary palate, and fusion progresses posteriorly. Except for the soft palate and uvula, fusion of the palate is generally completed by the 12th week of gestation.

Disruption in palatal fusion leads to clefting. A **cleft palate** can involve the soft palate only; the hard palate only; the hard and soft palates; or the hard and soft palates, alveolus, and lip. Cleft palate without lip involvement occurs in about 30% of cases.

Bifid Uvula (Fig. 14.5) is a minor cleft of the posterior soft palate. It occurs more commonly in Asian and Native American persons; the overall incidence is about 1 in 250 people. A **submucosal palatal cleft** may occur with **bifid uvula**. It develops when the muscles of the soft palate are clefted, but the surface mucosa is intact. The clefted region is notched. An **incomplete cleft palate** is a small break in the hard or soft palate that permits communication between the oral and nasal cavities. A **complete cleft palate** extends forward to include the incisive foramen. The triad of cleft palate, micrognathia (small jaw) and retrognathia of the mandible, and glossoptosis (posterior displacement of the tongue) is called **Pierre Robin syndrome**. This condition is characterized by respiratory and swallowing difficulties.

Cleft lip and palate are often associated with cleft alveolus, malpositioned and missing teeth (or hypodontia, most commonly the lateral incisor), and occasionally supernumerary teeth. Cleft palate causes feeding and speech impairment and prominent malocclusion. Treatment involves a multidisciplinary team consisting of a pediatrician, pediatric dentist, oral and plastic surgeon, orthodontist, and speech therapist. Surgical lip closure is generally accomplished early in the infant's life (after 18 months), whereas cleft palate may require several surgical procedures because of growth plate considerations.

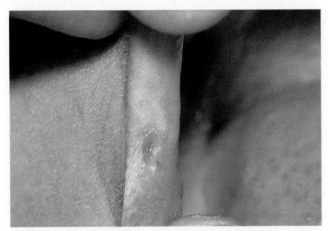

Fig. 14.1. **Commissural lip pits:** depression at commissure.

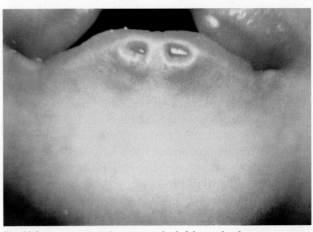

Fig. 14.2. **Paramedian lip pits:** with cleft lip and palate.

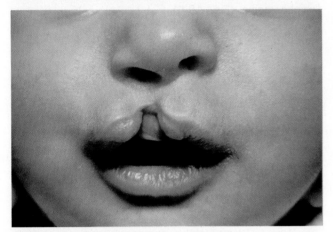

Fig. 14.3. **Incomplete cleft lip:** rare midline type.

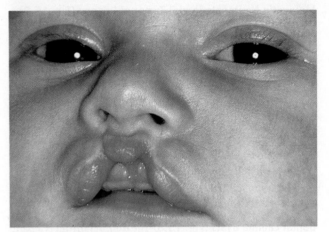

Fig. 14.4. **Bilateral cleft lip.**

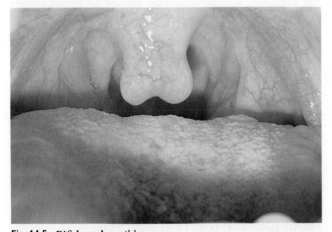

Fig. 14.5. **Bifid uvula:** mild case.

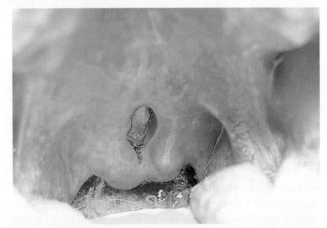

Fig. 14.6. **Bifid uvula:** more severe case.

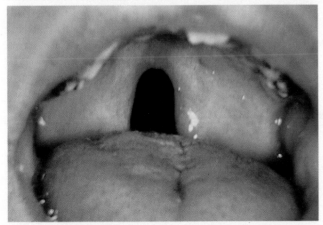

Fig. 14.7. **Cleft soft palate.**

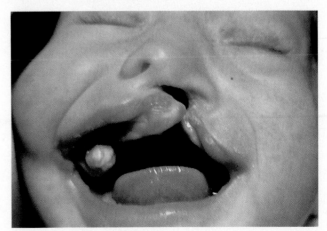

Fig. 14.8. **Cleft lip and cleft palate.**

33

Congenital Epulis (Fig. 15.1) is a benign, soft tissue growth arising exclusively in newborns from the edentulous alveolar ridge or palate. The **congenital epulis** develops most commonly in the anterior maxilla and is 10 times more likely to occur in females than in males. The lesion is a soft, pink fleshy growth that is compressible. The surface has prominent telangiectasis, and the base is either pedunculated (stalklike) or sessile (broad). Lesions can be several centimeters in diameter and should be excised. Recurrence is unlikely. Histologically, numerous granular cells are seen. Multiple lesions are present in 10% of cases.

Melanotic Neuroectodermal Tumor of Infancy (Fig. 15.2) is a rare benign tumor of neural crest cell origin that involves the head and neck region of infants. It typically appears as a rapidly growing mass in the anterior maxilla during the first year of life. It shows no sex predilection and begins as a small pink or red-purple nodule that resembles an eruption cyst. Radiographs usually show localized and irregular destruction of underlying alveolar bone and a primary tooth bud floating in a soft tissue mass. Urinary levels of vanilmandelic acid are elevated in conjunction with this tumor. Treatment is conservative excision. Histologic examination often shows melanin pigmentation. Recurrence and metastasis are rarely documented complications.

Dental Lamina Cysts (Fig. 15.3) The **dental lamina** is a band of epithelial tissue seen in histologic sections of a developing tooth (see Fig. 16.1). Remnants of the dental lamina that do not develop into a tooth bud may degenerate to form dental lamina (inclusion) cysts. These cysts are classified according to clinical location. **Gingival cysts of the newborn** are tiny keratin-filled cysts. They are often multiple and whitish and usually resolve when the tooth erupts. **Palatal cysts of the newborn** can be either Epstein pearls or Bohn nodules. **Epstein pearls** arise from epithelial inclusions that become entrapped at the median palatal raphe during fusion of opposing embryonic palatal shelves. **Bohn nodules** arise from remnants of minor salivary glands. The pearls and nodules are usually small, firm, asymptomatic, and whitish. They may occur in small groups anywhere in the hard palate. Most resolve spontaneously after several weeks, but may be incised to promote healing.

Natal Teeth (Fig. 15.4) are teeth that are present at birth or erupt within 30 days of birth. They occur in about 1 in 3,000 births. They often consist of cornified and calcific material, do not have roots, and are mobile. However, many **natal teeth** simply represent premature eruption of the primary teeth. The most common natal teeth are the mandibular central incisors; the mandible is affected 10 times more often than the maxilla. Natal teeth have been reported to cause ulcers of the ventral tongue (**Riga-Fede disease**) that result from irritation during nursing. In this case, smoothing of the incisal edge or extraction may be needed.

Eruption Cyst (Gingival Eruption Cyst, Eruption Hematoma) (Fig. 15.5) is a soft tissue cyst surrounding the crown of an unerupted tooth. It is a variant of the dentigerous cyst. Children younger than 10 years of age are most commonly affected. The **eruption cyst** appears as a small, dome-shaped, translucent swelling overlying an erupting primary tooth. The cyst is lined by odontogenic epithelium and is filled with blood or serum. The presence of blood casts a red, brown, or blue-gray appearance to the cyst. No treatment is necessary because the erupting tooth eventually breaks the cystic membrane. Incising the lesion and allowing the fluid to drain can relieve symptoms.

Lymphangioma (Fig. 15.6) is a benign malformation of lymphatic vessels that can be congenital or acquired. By definition, a **congenital lymphangioma** is present at birth. The tongue, alveolar ridge, and labial mucosa are common locations. Less commonly, the parotid gland and floor of mouth are affected. There is a 2:1 predilection for males, and 5% of African American neonates have one or more **alveolar lymphangiomas**. A lymphangioma typically produces a swelling that is asymptomatic, compressible, and negative on diascopy. When superficial, the swelling is composed of single or multiple discrete papulonodules that may be pink or dark red-blue. Deep-seated tumors produce diffuse swellings with no alteration in tissue color unless hemorrhage occurs. Large lymphangiomas of the neck are called **cystic hygromas**. Intraoral lymphangiomas may regress spontaneously, but persistent lesions should be excised or intralesionally injected with sclerosing solution.

Thrush (Candidiasis, Moniliasis) (Fig. 15.7), or **acute pseudomembranous candidiasis**, is a type of candidiasis (fungal infection) of mucosal membranes caused by *Candida albicans*. Lesions appear as milky white curds on the oral mucosa, primarily the buccal mucosa, palate, and tongue. The curds are easily wiped off, leaving a red, raw, painful surface. Newborns often acquire the infection from the mother's vaginal canal during birth and show clinical signs of **thrush** within the first few weeks of life. Fever and gastrointestinal irritation may accompany the disorder. Treatment consists of topically applied antifungal agents.

Parulis (Gum Boil) (Fig. 15.8) is an inflammatory response to a chronic bacterial infection of a nonvital tooth. It occurs most commonly in children when a pulpal infection spreads beyond the furcation of a posterior tooth and drains through a sinus tract to the surface. The **parulis** appears as a small, raised, fluctuant yellow-to-red boil that arises near the mucogingival junction of the affected tooth. Pressure to the area results in discharge of pus from the center of the lesion. Most cases are asymptomatic; however, palpation of the tooth or surrounding structures may elicit pain. The condition resolves when the infection is eliminated. Failure to eliminate the infection in a primary tooth can affect the development of the succedaneous (permanent) tooth.

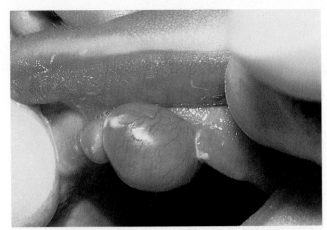

Fig. 15.1. Congenital epulis of the newborn: a pink nodule.

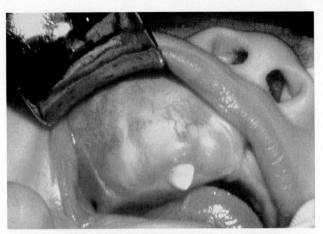

Fig. 15.2. Melanotic neuroectodermal tumor of infancy.

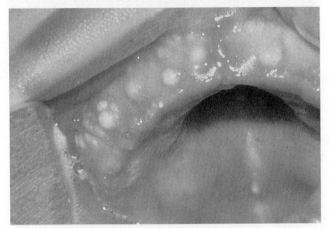

Fig. 15.3. Dental lamina cysts and Epstein pearl.

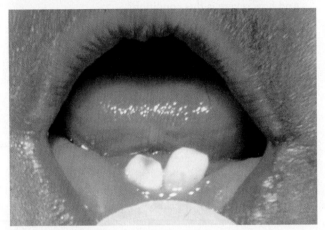

Fig. 15.4. Natal teeth: mandibular incisors in a newborn.

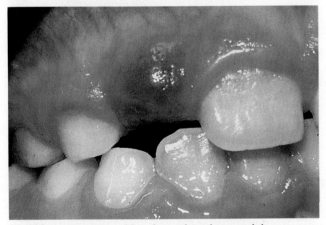

Fig. 15.5. Eruption cyst: blue, dome-shaped cyst nodule.

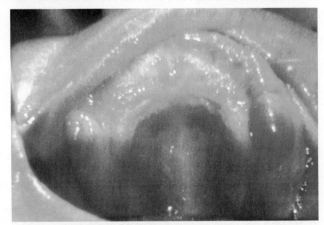

Fig. 15.6. Congenital lymphangioma.

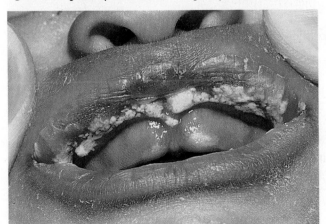

Fig. 15.7. Thrush caused by *Candida albicans*.

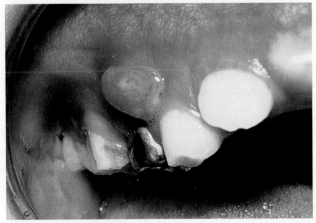

Fig. 15.8. Parulis: nonvital primary first molar.

3

CASE STUDIES

CASE 11. (FIG. 15.9)

This 26-year-old woman presents with the condition shown in the clinical image. The condition has been present since childhood. She is interested in speaking with the dentist about surgical correction.

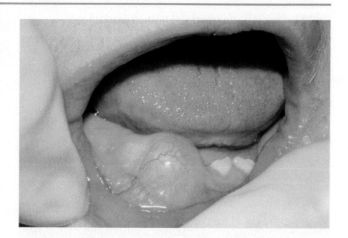

1. Describe the clinical findings.

2. Do you expect to see similar findings in the upper lip or any defects in the upper lip?

3. Is this a normal finding, a variant of normal, or disease? And how severe is this condition?

4. What is the cause of this condition?

5. Do you expect this condition to be symptomatic?

6. List conditions you should consider in the differential diagnosis, and note which condition is most likely the correct diagnosis.

7. What are the treatment options for this condition?

8. If this patient is seen by a dental hygienist, what should the hygienist communicate to the dentist regarding her interest in correction of this defect?

CASE 12. (FIG. 15.10)

A young woman brings her child to the dental office for the first time. The child has a noticeable growth within the mouth. The mother claims that the growth first presented several days ago but has been getting bigger every day. She is concerned that her child is now feeding less, and this entity may be a tumor. The adjacent teeth do not seem to be affected.

1. Describe the clinical findings, and explain why it appears translucent.

2. How old is the patient?

3. Is this a normal finding, a variant of normal, or disease? And how severe is this condition?

4. What is the cause of this condition?

5. Do you expect this condition to be symptomatic?

6. List conditions you should consider in the differential diagnosis for this condition, and note which condition is most likely the correct diagnosis.

7. What are the treatment options for this condition?

8. How would you communicate this to the child's mother?

Additional cases to enhance your learning and understanding of this section are available Online through the book's Navigate 2 Advantage Access site.

Tooth Development and Dental Anomalies

Objectives:

- Understand tooth development.
- Define and describe the clinical appearance of common alterations in tooth morphology, number, structure, color, and position.
- Identify common dental (tooth and root) anomalies.
- Recognize the causes and clinical features of these conditions.
- Distinguish clinical and radiographic appearances of similar-appearing dental anomalies.
- Define and describe the clinical and radiographic appearance of the different types of root resorption.
- Describe consequences of disease progression with respect to dental anomalies.
- Recommend appropriate treatments for dental (tooth and root) anomalies.
- Identify conditions discussed in this section that require the attention of the dentist and/or affect the delivery of dental care.

In the figure legends, * denotes the same patient.

Tooth Development (Odontogenesis) (Figs. 16.1–16.3) Teeth develop from "tooth germs" or "tooth buds." The term "tooth bud" is used because they bud from the overlying epithelium early in life. The **primary or deciduous teeth** begin their formation about the fifth week of life as an embryo. Formation occurs in stages: (1) epithelium budding (**bud stage**), called the **primary dental lamina**; (2) proliferation of the dental lamina (**cap stage**); and (3) differentiation into three components: the enamel organ, the dental papilla, and the dental follicle that surrounds the developing tooth (**bell stage**). Of note, the enamel organ is derived from the epithelium (ectoderm), whereas the dental papilla and follicle are derived from the surrounding connective tissue (mesoderm).

As the tooth develops, the layer just below the enamel organ differentiates into **odontoblasts**, and the cells of the enamel organ differentiate into **ameloblasts**. The odontoblasts begin producing dentin first, then the ameloblasts begin producing enamel. As more and more enamel and dentin are deposited, the distance between the ameloblasts and odontoblasts increases. Next, mineralization occurs at the cusp tips and spreads downward. The production of dentin (**dentinogenesis**) and of enamel (**amelogenesis**) is accompanied by maturation and elongation of the dental papilla, which is now called the **dental pulp**. The root of the tooth composed of pulp, dentin, and cementum does not develop until after crown formation is complete. This process involves the formation of cementum (**cementogenesis**) from an epithelial structure known as **Hertwig epithelial root sheath**. The root sheath shapes the root by budding off, which triggers the production of dentin and cementum. Cementum is laid down on top of the dentin by cementoblasts. The cementum serves to anchor the tooth to the bone through its contact with periodontal fibers.

Tooth Eruption (Figs. 16.3 and 16.4) Teeth erupt as a result of processes controlled by the dental follicle, which includes the developing and elongating root, the cementum, periodontal ligament, and adjacent alveolar bone. Although the process is not well understood, crown formation and some root development are required for normal eruption to begin. In fact, one half of the root must be developed before the tooth approaches the oral epithelium. As a general rule, two-thirds root development is seen before the tooth penetrates the oral epithelium. And, at least three fourths of the root develops before the tooth occludes with the opposing tooth. During the pre-eruptive phase, the radiographic appearance of the tooth bud (also called a **tooth crypt**) is a well-circumscribed radiolucency a few millimeters below the crest of the alveolar ridge (Fig. 16.3 left white arrow). As mineralization/calcification occurs, the cusps and eventually the entire crown of the tooth become radiopaque within the tooth crypt (yellow arrow). Teeth are genetically programmed to erupt axially toward the occlusal plane. However, the available space, location of neighboring teeth, and environmental factors, such as trauma, can influence the root shape and final position within the mouth. **Delayed eruption** is seen when root length exceeds crown length and the tooth crown is not yet erupted into the mouth. An impacted tooth is often judged to have lost its eruptive potential when the root apex is closed.

Primary Tooth and Permanent Tooth Eruption (Figs. 16.2–16.5) The primary (deciduous) teeth typically erupt between 6 months and 2 years of age. The teeth generally erupt into good alignment because space is not an issue. The permanent or **succedaneous teeth** begin erupting around age 6 years and continue to erupt (a new tooth at a time) annually through about age 12. Generally, eruption in girls occurs earlier than in boys. Third molars, if present, generally erupt around late adolescence. Permanent teeth resorb the primary tooth roots upon eruption and can encounter difficulties during eruption due to space issues or the location of erupted teeth. Sometimes, the primary roots are not fully resorbed, and a **retained root tip** of a primary molar can result. A retained root tip appears as a small, narrow radiopacity, most commonly in the interproximal bone between the posterior teeth (see Fig. 34.7). A periodontal ligament space can often be seen surrounding a retained root tip.

Eruption Sequestrum (Fig. 16.6) is a small fragment of nonviable bone overlying the site of an erupting tooth. It occurs most often when a molar erupts and the overlying bone separates instead of being resorbed. In this case, it is seen below the erupting maxillary third molar. An **eruption sequestrum** causes mild discomfort and can be seen clinically as a small bony spicule. They are easily removed, often with a hemostat.

Impacted Teeth (Figs. 16.7 and 16.8) are teeth that do not erupt into the mouth. About 15% to 20% of the population experiences one or more **impacted teeth**. The most common impacted teeth are third molars. The next most frequently impacted tooth is the maxillary canine, followed by mandibular premolars and supernumerary teeth. The most common cause of impaction is lack of space (obstruction), early extraction of a primary tooth, and abnormal position of the tooth germ. Genetic syndromes or metabolic conditions also can be contributory. Features that help determine an impacted tooth include delayed eruption (tooth remains below the alveolar ridge) and full root development.

Complications associated with impacted permanent teeth include migration, tooth resorption, and formation of a dentigerous cyst (Figs. 36.2 and 36.3) or odontogenic tumor (Figs. 39.8B and 40.3). Cysts or tumors can generally be ruled out if the follicle is not enlarged (remains less than 2 mm from the crown), and the follicle surrounds only the crown—it is not expanding to include the root.

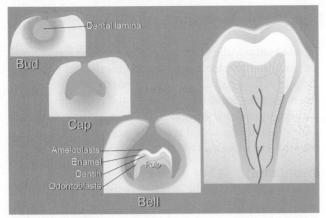

Fig. 16.1. Tooth development.

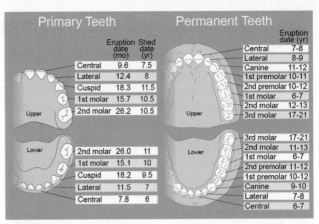

Fig. 16.2. Tooth eruption chart.

Primary Teeth	Eruption date (mo)	Shed date (yr)
Upper		
Central	9.6	7.5
Lateral	12.4	8
Cuspid	18.3	11.5
1st molar	15.7	10.5
2nd molar	26.2	10.5
Lower		
2nd molar	26.0	11
1st molar	15.1	10
Cuspid	18.2	9.5
Lateral	11.5	7
Central	7.8	6

Permanent Teeth	Eruption date (yr)
Upper	
Central	7-8
Lateral	8-9
Canine	11-12
1st premolar	10-11
2nd premolar	10-12
1st molar	6-7
2nd molar	12-13
3rd molar	17-21
Lower	
3rd molar	17-21
2nd molar	11-13
1st molar	6-7
2nd premolar	11-12
1st premolar	10-12
Canine	9-10
Lateral	7-8
Central	6-7

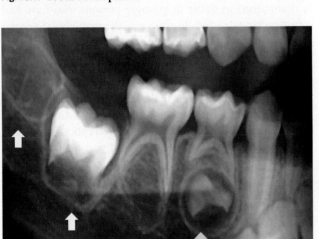

Fig. 16.3. Odontogenesis and tooth eruption. *Arrows* indicate different stages of development.

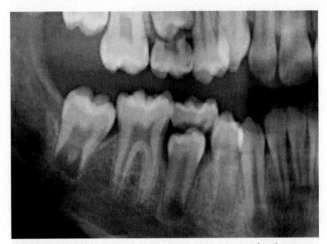

Fig. 16.4. Eruption of posterior teeth as lower roots develop.

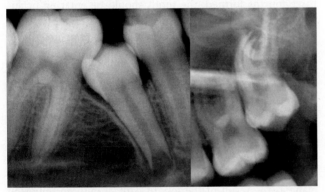

Fig. 16.5. Delayed eruption (two examples).

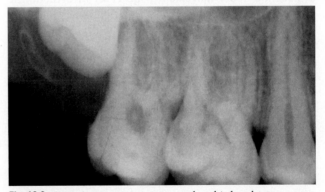

Fig. 16.6. Eruption sequestrum: coronal to third molar.

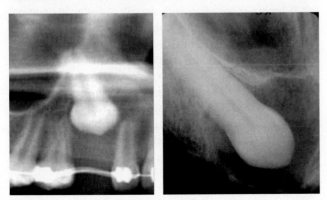

Fig. 16.7. Impacted canines (two examples).

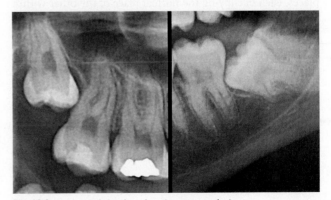

Fig. 16.8. Impacted third molars (two examples).

Rotated Teeth (Fig. 17.1) A rotated tooth is one that is altered in orientation in the dental arch. The amount varies, with severe cases reversing the buccal-lingual orientation of the tooth. Rotated teeth are often associated with crowding and malocclusion.

Axial Tilting (Fig. 17.1) All teeth have a normal axial inclination—the long axis tilt of a tooth. Anterior teeth have a normal, slightly outward axial inclination, which contributes to convex lip form and appropriate arch and facial profile. Teeth may be abnormally tilted inward or outward, as occurs with the maxillary incisors in class II, division 2 malocclusion (Fig. 4.8). Altered axial tilt is a sign of crowding, malocclusion habits, or periodontal disease.

Ectopic Eruption (Fig. 17.1) is one or more teeth erupting into an abnormal location outside the normal dental arch, usually because of lack of space. Ectopic eruption can result in overlapping or a double row of teeth. This frequently occurs when the primary teeth (especially mandibular incisors) are retained and the permanent successors erupt lingually. Similarly, one or more supernumerary teeth may erupt adjacent to the normal teeth and compete for the location (Figs. 20.1–20.4). Other causes of ectopic eruption include cysts or tumors that force an adjacent developing tooth to erupt in an abnormal place or syndromes (e.g., Treacher Collins syndrome) associated with small jaw formation. Some unusual ectopic eruption sites include the floor of the mouth, nose, sinus, and periocular region. Treatment often involves orthodontics and/or extraction.

Orthodontic Tooth Movement (Fig. 17.2) In orthodontic tooth movement, abnormally positioned teeth are brought into normal position. Teeth also can be moved into abnormal positions. In Figure 17.2, the first premolar has been extracted, and the canine and lateral have been positioned distally. This method can result in excellent alignment of the teeth but may flatten the appearance of the lower face. In Figure 17.2, mild resorption of several root apices has resulted from the orthodontic forces. The thickened lamina dura and prominent periodontal membrane space are suggestive of recent orthodontic movement or possible hyperocclusion.

Transposition (Fig. 17.3) occurs when two teeth exchange places, each occupying the normal place of the other within the dental arch. Transposition may occur idiopathically, or it may be a sign that a barrier to the normal path of eruption may have existed. Such patients should be examined radiographically. In this image, the maxillary canine and lateral incisor are transposed. An esthetic problem caused by transposition can be remedied by restorative procedures (e.g., veneers).

Translocation (Fig. 17.4) occurs when one tooth erupts into an abnormal location but remains within the dental arch.

In this example, the permanent lateral incisor was congenitally missing and the permanent canine did not encounter the root of the permanent lateral incisor to guide it in, so the canine erupted into the position of the lateral incisor and the primary canine was retained. The primary canine roots can resorb spontaneously and the tooth exfoliates. Alternatively, the primary canine may be retained for many years.

Distal Drift (Fig. 17.5) is distal movement of an erupted tooth or teeth within the dental arch as a result of a missing tooth. The normal forces of occlusion usually cause teeth adjacent to missing teeth to drift or tip mesially. Distal drift is more prone to occur in younger persons who have had a first molar extracted. In this case, the mandibular second premolar drifted distally into the position of the absent first molar; the first premolar and canine drifted distally, and interdental spacing is prominent.

Migration (Fig. 17.6) refers to the movement of an unerupted tooth into an abnormal position within the jaw. Migrated teeth usually do not erupt but can cause root resorption of adjacent teeth. Premolars are prone to migration, and some move into the ramus and other distant sites. In our example, a second premolar has migrated to the apical region of the first molar.

Partial (Delayed) Eruption (Fig. 17.6) occurs when a tooth erupts but not fully into occlusion. This may be caused by an impediment such as insufficient space. To assess eruption potential, root length is evaluated. For example, when root length is half complete (i.e., exceeds crown length), the tooth should be erupting through the gingiva. When the root is three-fourths formed, the tooth should be entering occlusion. When the apex has closed, eruption should be complete. Eruption potential is strongest during the first half of root development and diminishes as the apical half of root formation develops. Figure 17.6 is an example of delayed eruption where root length of the impacted second mandibular premolar exceeds crown length and eruption is delayed and impeded by the first molar. Orthodontic traction of this migrated tooth is a treatment option.

Supraeruption (Extrusion) (Figs. 17.7 and 17.8) occurs when one or more teeth erupt passively beyond the occlusal plane as the result of the loss of contact with an opposing tooth. Both maxillary and mandibular teeth can supraerupt, but it occurs more often with maxillary teeth. Periodontal disease may accelerate the problem, but its absence cannot prevent it. Supraeruption contributes to poor interproximal contact, food impaction, periodontal defects, and root caries (Figs. 32.6 and 32.7). The extruded tooth can occlude with the opposite edentulous ridge, causing pain, an ulcer, or leukoplakia, and leave little space for a replacement tooth. Extruded teeth may need root canal therapy, crown lengthening, and a crown to re-establish a normal plane of occlusion before replacing its antagonist.

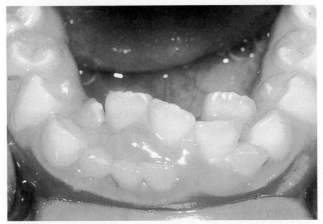

Fig. 17.1. Ectopic eruption, axial tilting, and rotated teeth.

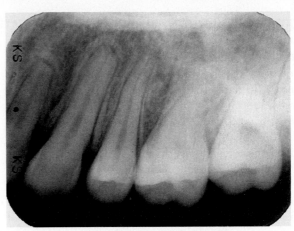

Fig. 17.2. Results of orthodontic tooth movement.

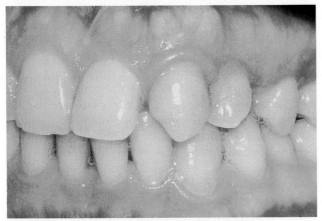

Fig. 17.3. Transposition of maxillary canine and lateral.

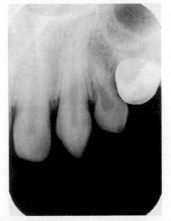

Fig. 17.4. Translocation of permanent canine.

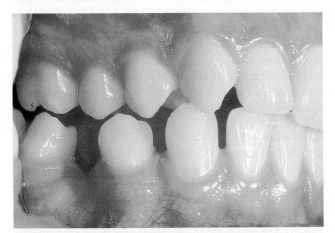

Fig. 17.5. Distal drift of mandibular premolar and canine.

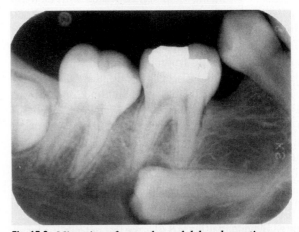

Fig. 17.6. Migration of premolar and delayed eruption.

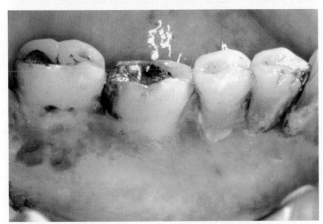

Fig. 17.7. Supraeruption of mandibular second molar.

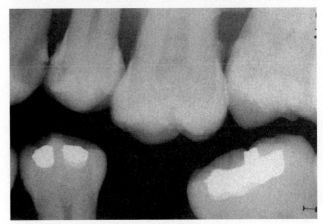

Fig. 17.8. Supraeruption of maxillary first molar.

ALTERATIONS IN TOOTH NUMBERS: HYPODONTIA

Hypodontia (Figs. 18.1–18.3) is the congenital absence of one or more teeth because of tooth **agenesis** (failure to develop). The term **oligodontia**, a subcategory of **hypodontia**, refers to six or more congenitally missing teeth. The term **anodontia** is reserved for the rare condition in which all teeth are absent. When teeth are missing, the patient must be carefully questioned to determine the reason for hypodontia. The healthcare provider should also count the number of teeth clinically and radiographically to confirm the condition. If teeth are missing because of extractions, the term **acquired hypodontia** is used. If teeth are missing because of lack of eruption, then the term **impaction** or **partial impaction** is used.

Tooth agenesis and hypodontia result from defects in genes involved in odontogenesis, often *MSX1, PAX9, EDA*, and *AXIN2*. Harmful environmental factors are also contributory. Hypodontia may involve any race, and the primary or permanent teeth; however, it is most common in the permanent dentition. About 5% of the population is affected; the prevalence is slightly greater in women than men. Because hypodontia is often inherited, several family members are usually missing the same tooth.

The most frequent congenitally missing teeth are the third molars, followed by mandibular second premolars, maxillary second premolars, and maxillary lateral incisors. Common clinical signs of hypodontia are prominent spacing between the teeth, overretained primary teeth, and **microdonts**.

Congenitally missing teeth are associated with **cleft lip** and **palate** and more than 100 syndromes, including Böök syndrome, chondroectodermal dysplasia (Ellis-van Creveld syndrome), ectodermal dysplasia, Down syndrome, Hajdu-Cheney (acro-osteolysis) syndrome, incontinentia pigmenti, otodental dysplasia, and Rieger syndrome. Radiation therapy to the head and neck of infants or children and rubella (measles) during pregnancy have also been implicated. Patients who are missing the central incisors, first molars, or several teeth and have no apparent reason for this finding should be evaluated for an inherited syndrome or one of the predisposing factors mentioned above. Early diagnosis helps ensure optimal patient management and can alert the clinician to similarly affected family members.

Acquired Hypodontia (Fig. 18.4) is the loss of teeth as a result of trauma or extractions. Falls, sport accidents, and motor vehicle accidents are the source of most traumatic cases, whereas periodontal disease, caries, and space requirements for orthodontia contribute to dental extractions and acquired hypodontia. Tooth loss produces excess space that may result in **drifting, tipping, rotation**, and **supraeruption** of adjacent or opposing teeth. In particular, splaying and spacing of the anterior teeth is an indirect result of loss of posterior teeth because of distribution of the occlusal load onto the remaining anterior teeth. In this condition, known as **posterior bite collapse**, the single-rooted anterior teeth are less able to handle the load and tilt anteriorly when the periodontal support is poor. **Acquired hypodontia** can produce alterations in occlusion and appearance that require surgical, orthodontic, periodontic, and prosthodontic therapy to restore function and esthetics. When all the teeth have been extracted, the condition is referred to as complete **edentulism**. In contrast, the term **anodontia** is used when all teeth are congenitally absent.

Ankylosis (Figs. 18.5 and 18.6) is often associated with **hypodontia**. It is defined as a tooth that demonstrates loss of the periodontal ligament and fusion of the cementum with the alveolar bone. **Ankylosis** most commonly occurs when a primary (second) mandibular molar fails to exfoliate, as a result of a missing permanent second premolar that fails to develop and erupt. It can also affect any tooth after trauma, transplantation, reimplantation, or chronic inflammation. An ankylosed tooth is often diagnosed during the mixed dentition and is typically in infraocclusion—submerged a few millimeters below the marginal ridges of adjacent teeth. Also, the adjacent teeth are often tipped toward the ankylosed tooth, and the opposing tooth may be supraerupted. Percussion of the ankylosed tooth produces a higher pitched or dulled sound compared with adjacent teeth. Ankylosed teeth often remain in the arch for many years and do not require extraction unless they become associated with advanced caries or periodontal disease. However, an ankylosed tooth may spontaneously exfoliate and create an edentulous space. Exfoliation is often preceded by tooth mobility, pocket formation, and radiographic changes (vertical bone defect). If an ankylosed tooth is maintained, a restoration (crown) may be required to achieve optimal occlusion and marginal ridge height.

Oligodontia (Figs. 18.7 and 18.8) refers to six or more congenitally missing teeth. Affected individuals typically have retained primary teeth and one or more erupted permanent teeth that are smaller than usual and show reduced and simplified shape (tapering). The condition causes difficulties in chewing, speech, and esthetic appearance. Early treatment is important for timely intervention. The edentulous space associated with missing teeth can be treated by closing the space orthodontically or prosthodontically using a bridge (Fig. 18.8) or implants. Patients and parents should be advised that since growth and development occur during childhood and adolescence, periodic re-evaluation of the patient is needed to ensure proper occlusion and esthetics are maintained as adulthood is reached.

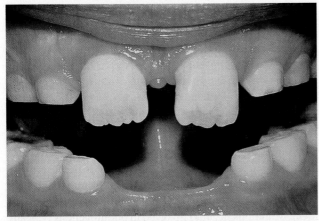

Fig. 18.1. Hypodontia: congenitally missing incisors.

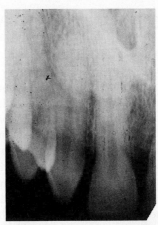

Fig. 18.2. Hypodontia: congenitally missing lateral incisor.*

4

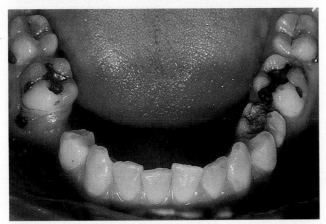

Fig. 18.3. Hypodontia: missing maxillary lateral incisor.*

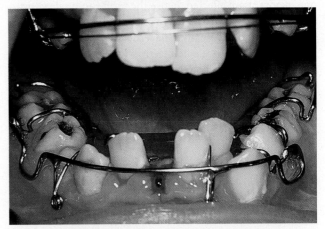

Fig. 18.4. Acquired hypodontia: for orthodontic space.

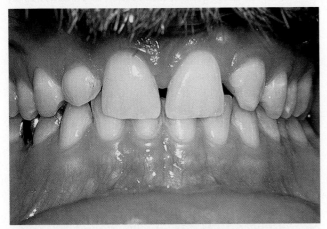

Fig. 18.5. Ankylosis: second primary molar.

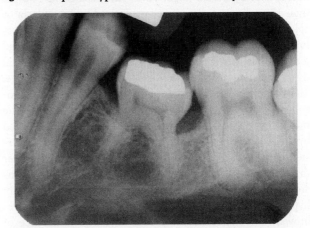

Fig. 18.6. Ankylosis: second primary molar.

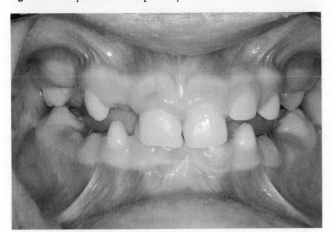

Fig. 18.7. Oligodontia: a 9-year-old, missing several teeth.*

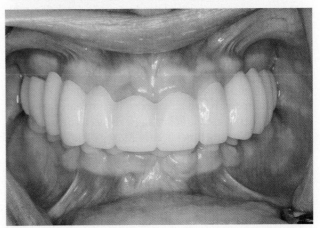

Fig. 18.8. Oligodontia: same patient as on left with prosthetic replacements.*

Regional Odontodysplasia (Ghost Teeth) (Figs. 19.1 and 19.2) is a rare developmental anomaly characterized by defective formation of the enamel, dentin, and pulp. Although most cases are considered idiopathic, changes in the vascular supply during tooth follicle growth and development appear contributory. Several cases have occurred in association with vascular and growth abnormalities (vascular nevi); other cases have occurred in patients with syndromes. Microscopically, the dentin is interglobular and diminished in amount, the enamel is abnormally thin and irregular, and the pulp is abnormally large and may contain pulp stones. Typically, several adjacent primary or permanent teeth in one quadrant are affected, hence the term **regional odontodysplasia**. The maxilla is more commonly involved. Affected teeth often fail to erupt or have delayed eruption. In the infrequent occurrence when teeth erupt, ghost teeth appear clinically as small yellow-brown crowns. The irregular coronal surface makes them susceptible to caries and rapid progression to the pulp, because enamel and dentin are thin and the pulp horns are enlarged. Children with this condition can have several painful malformed teeth with periapical inflammatory lesions and the need for tooth extractions. Radiographically, affected teeth are rather radiolucent, producing a ghostlike appearance. The demarcation between enamel and dentin is absent or is fuzzy, the pulp chambers are abnormally large, and root formation is minimal.

Ectodermal Dysplasia (Figs. 19.3–19.7) is a group of more than 150 inherited diseases characterized by hypoplasia or aplasia (underdevelopment or absence) of ectodermal structures, such as the hair, nails, skin, sebaceous glands, and teeth. In its best-known **hypohidrotic form**, **ectodermal dysplasia** demonstrates an X-linked recessive inheritance. This means that the defective gene located on the X chromosome is carried by the female and manifests clinically in the male. Less common forms of ectodermal dysplasia caused by autosomal dominant and autosomal recessive transmission have been reported in females who demonstrate fewer manifestations of the syndrome. About 1 in 50,000 persons are affected. Affected patients have fine, smooth dry skin; hypodontia, hypotrichosis (thin, sparse blonde hair and eyebrows), and hypohidrosis (partial or complete absence of sweat glands). Other signs include a depressed bridge of the nose, pronounced supraorbital ridges, periorbital skin with fine wrinkling and hyperpigmentation, ruddy complexion, midface hypoplasia resulting in protuberant lips, indistinct vermilion border, and varying degrees of xerostomia. Most patients have **oligodontia**, and the teeth that are present often are small, conical, and tapered. The canine is the tooth most commonly present, whereas incisors are generally missing. When present, molars show reduced coronal diameter. Anodontia sometimes occurs. Most patients do not perspire as a result of the reduced number of sweat glands and consequently suffer from heat intolerance; in infants, this may present as a fever of undetermined origin. Treatment of ectodermal dysplasia involves a team of healthcare providers, genetic counseling, the avoidance of heat, and the construction of partial dentures, full dentures, overdentures, and/or implants. Patients do well with prostheses even at a young age. However, new dentures must be reconstructed periodically as the jaws grow.

Syndromic Hypodontia (Fig. 19.8) There are many syndromes associated with hypodontia. This is because many genes that regulate the development and formation of teeth can be genetically altered or damaged during fetal development. Mutations in genes involved in odontogenesis typically involve the following genes: *MSX1, PAX9, EDA,* and *AXIN2.* Syndromes are often inherited by an autosomal dominant pattern; however, several syndromes are inherited by autosomal recessive or sex-linked patterns, and some can occur sporadically. A syndrome can display **variable expressivity**, meaning affected persons can have many or few features of the syndrome. When hypodontia occurs in conjunction with a syndrome, more than one tooth is typically missing. Because **syndromic hypodontia** is generally inherited, several family members typically are missing the same tooth. A partial list of syndromes associated with hypodontia is provided here.

Syndromes associated with hypodontia.		
Ankyloglossia superior	Böök	Cockayne
Coffin-Lowry	Cranio-oculo-dental	Crouzon
Down	Ectodermal dysplasia	Ehlers-Danlos
Ellis-van Creveld	Focal dermal hypoplasia	Freire-Maia
Fried	Frontometaphyseal dysplasia	Goldenhar
Gorlin	Gorlin-Chaudhry-Moss	Hallermann-Streiff
Hanhart	Hemifacial microsomia	Hurler
Hypoglossia-hypodactylia	Incontinentia pigmenti	Johanson-Blizzard
Lipoid proteinosis	Marshall-White	Melanoleukoderma
Oral-facial-digital, type 1	Otodental dysplasia	Pierre Robin
Progeria	Reiger	Robinson
Rothmund	Sturge-Weber	Tricho-dento-osseous
Turner	Van der Woude	Witkop
Wolf-Hirschhorn		

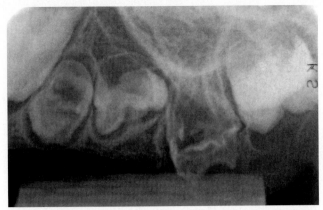

Fig. 19.1. **Regional odontodysplasia:** idiopathic.

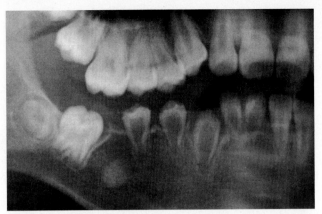

Fig. 19.2. **Regional odontodysplasia:** ghost teeth.*

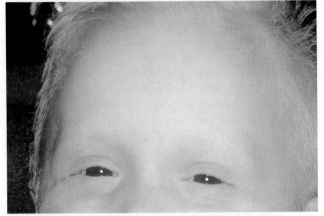

Fig. 19.3. **Hypohidrotic ectodermal dysplasia:** sparse hair.

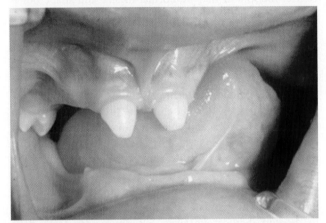

Fig. 19.4. **Hypohidrotic ectodermal dysplasia:** hypodontia.

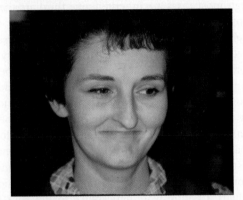

Fig. 19.5. **Ectodermal dysplasia.**

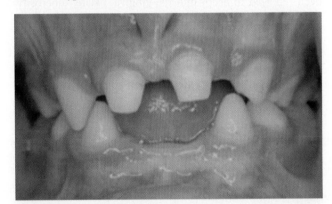

Fig. 19.6. **Ectodermal dysplasia:** same patient as on left.

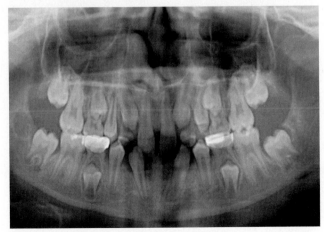

Fig. 19.7. **Ectodermal dysplasia:** a 10-year-old.

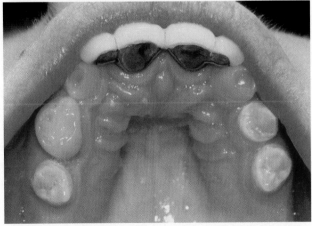

Fig. 19.8. **Tricho-dento-osseous syndrome:** a 17-year-old with missing teeth and pitted enamel.

Hyperdontia (Figs. 20.1–20.4) is the term for a dentition with an extra deciduous or permanent tooth; the additional tooth is termed supernumerary. Hyperdontia is associated with dysregulation of the RUNX family genes and focal overgrowth of the developing dental lamina. It occurs more often in the maxilla than in the mandible (8:1), more in males than females (2:1), more in permanent teeth than the primary dentition (1% to 3% of the population, compared with 0.5%), and more often unilaterally than bilaterally. The most common supernumerary tooth is the mesiodens, which is located, either erupted or impacted, between the maxillary central incisors. It may be normal in size and shape but is usually small with a short root and conically shaped crown that tapers incisally.

The second most common supernumerary tooth is the maxillary fourth molar, which can be fully developed or a microdont. When a fourth molar is buccal or lingual to the erupted third molar, the term paramolar is used. When the fourth molar is positioned behind the third molar, the term distomolar is used. Mandibular premolars are the third most common supernumerary teeth. They are usually malpositioned (ectopic eruption) because of late eruption into the arch.

Supernumerary teeth may fail to erupt or may erupt improperly. Those impacted in the jaw have the propensity to develop dentigerous cysts. Supernumerary teeth have been reported to erupt into the gingiva, palate, tuberosity, nasal cavity, and orbital rim. Space limitations in the arch often force the supernumerary tooth to fail to erupt or erupt buccally or lingually. Such teeth are often nonfunctional and may cause inflammation, food impaction, interference with tooth eruption, and esthetic and masticatory problems. In general, supernumerary teeth should be extracted to permit proper growth, development, and occlusion.

Supernumerary teeth develop as isolated occurrences but more frequently occur in several family members. The presence of several supernumerary teeth is associated with more than 15 syndromes, most commonly with cleidocranial dysplasia and Gardner syndrome. Accordingly, inherited syndromes should be ruled out when supernumerary teeth are present.

Cleidocranial Dysplasia (Figs. 20.5 and 20.6) is an autosomal dominant disorder affecting the face, skull, and clavicles linked to a defect in a gene known as *RUNX2*. This gene, also known as *CBFA1*, maps to chromosome 6 and controls bone and tooth formation. Most cases are inherited; however, as many as 40% result from spontaneous mutation. The syndrome affects women and men equally and is usually discovered during childhood or early adolescence.

Cleidocranial dysplasia is characterized by defective ossification of the clavicles and cranium together with oral and sometimes long bone disturbances. Prominent features include delayed closure of the frontal, parietal, and occipital fontanelles of the skull, short stature, prominent frontal eminences with bossing, small paranasal sinuses, an underdeveloped/depressed maxilla with a high narrow palate, and relative prognathism of the mandible. The head appears large compared with the short body, the neck appears long, and the shoulders appear narrow and drooping. The clavicles may be absent or underdeveloped, permitting hypermobility of the shoulders, whereby patients can bring their shoulders together in front of the chest.

The oral changes are dramatic, particularly as seen on a panoramic image. These findings can lead to early diagnosis. The most prominent features are numerous unerupted supernumerary teeth, especially in the premolar and molar areas, and delayed eruption of the permanent teeth. The maxilla is underdeveloped, resulting in a usually high-arched, narrow, and sometimes clefted palate. There is prolonged retention of the primary teeth. The permanent teeth are often short rooted and lack cellular (secondary) cementum, which may contribute to the defective eruption pattern. Treatment is complex and complicated by the fact that extraction of the primary teeth does not guarantee eruption of the secondary dentition. Surgical exposure of unerupted teeth and orthodontic and possibly prosthodontic therapy are required to produce a functional and aesthetic occlusion.

Gardner Syndrome (Figs. 20.7 and 20.8) is an autosomal dominant condition caused by a mutation in the adenomatous polyposis coli (*APC*) gene on chromosome 5. Although most cases are inherited, one third are the result of spontaneous mutations. It affects 1 in 15,000 persons. Gardner syndrome has prominent orofacial features characterized by hyperdontia, impacted supernumerary teeth, odontomas, and jaw osteomas that develop by puberty. In addition, patients have several epidermal cysts, dermoid tumors, and intestinal polyps. The osteomas occur most frequently in the craniofacial skeleton, especially in the mandible, mandibular angle, and paranasal sinuses. However, osteomas of the long bones are possible. Radiographs often demonstrate several supernumerary teeth, many odontomas, numerous round osteomas, and multiple diffuse enostoses that impart a cotton-wool appearance to the jaws. When superficial in the skin, these slow-growing tumors are palpable rock-hard nodules. The skin cysts (epidermoid, dermoid, or sebaceous) are smooth-surfaced lumps. Many soft tissue tumors (lipomas, fibromas, leiomyomas, desmoid tumors, and thyroid tumors/cancer) may accompany this disorder.

The most serious consideration of Gardner syndrome is the presence of multiple polyps that affect the colorectal mucosa. These intestinal polyps have an extremely high potential for malignant transformation, resulting in adenocarcinoma of the colon in 50% of patients by age 30 years and nearly 100% of patients by age 40 years. Early recognition of the orofacial manifestations necessitates prompt referral to a gastroenterologist and genetic counseling. Close annual colorectal examination is required; prophylactic colectomy is usually recommended. Facial osteoma may be surgically removed for aesthetic reasons.

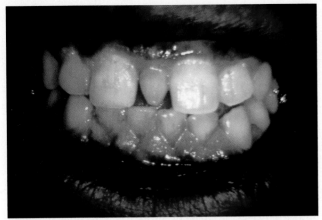

Fig. 20.1. Hyperdontia: erupted mesiodens in midline.

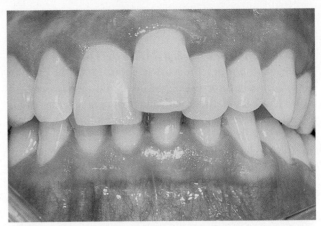

Fig. 20.2. Hyperdontia: extra maxillary lateral incisor.

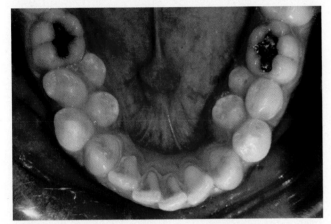

Fig. 20.3. Hyperdontia: supernumerary premolars.

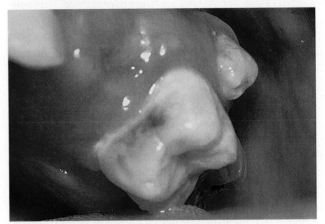

Fig. 20.4. Hyperdontia: buccal erupted paramolar.

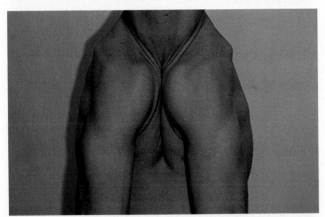

Fig. 20.5. Cleidocranial dysplasia: absent clavicles.

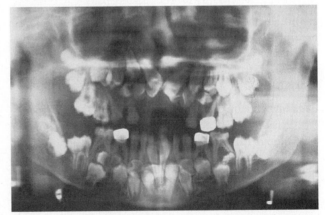

Fig. 20.6. Cleidocranial dysplasia: retained primary teeth.

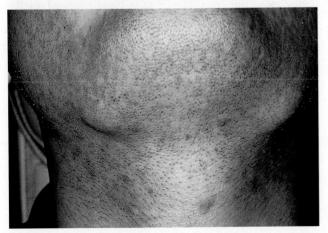

Fig. 20.7. Gardner syndrome: mandibular osteomas.

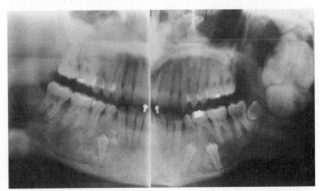

Fig. 20.8. Gardner syndrome: osteomas, supernumerary teeth.

ALTERATIONS IN TOOTH MORPHOLOGY

Microdontia (Figs. 21.1 and 21.2) refers to teeth that are smaller than normal. It occurs in about 1% of the population. **Microdontia** is usually bilateral and often associated with a familial trait (inherited) and hypodontia. It may occur as an isolated finding, a relative condition, or in a generalized pattern. The most common form occurs as an isolated finding involving one permanent tooth, usually the permanent maxillary lateral incisor. The term **peg lateral** is often used to describe this variant because the tooth is cone or peg shaped. Third molars are the second most frequently affected teeth. When microdontia occurs in a generalized pattern, it may be relative to the size of the jaws—that is, the teeth are normal in size, but the jaws are larger than normal. True **generalized microdontia** is rare and occurs when the jaws are normal in size and the actual tooth size is small. Generalized microdontia may be associated with pituitary dwarfism or an inherited syndrome. Cancer treatments (chemotherapy and radiation therapy) during tooth development are also causative. True microdonts should be distinguished from retained primary teeth.

Macrodontia (Fig. 21.3) is the opposite of microdontia and refers to an abnormal increase in tooth size. It is less common than microdontia. **Macrodontia** may affect one, several, or, rarely, all teeth. It is usually a relative phenomenon. It is more often seen in incisors and mandibular third molars and in a developmental condition known as **hemihypertrophy**, in which the affected side, including the teeth, is larger than the unaffected side. Single or even paired enlarged teeth are infrequently affected by **fusion** or **gemination** and may be clinically referred to as macrodonts until a more specific condition is determined from the radiographs. True **generalized macrodontia** is rare and may be seen in pituitary gigantism.

Dens Invaginatus (Dens in Dente) (Fig. 21.4) is a deep surface invagination of the crown or root lined by enamel. It is a common developmental anomaly that occurs in about 1% of the population. **Dens in dente** is so named because radiographically it resembles a tooth within a tooth. The condition develops embryologically when enamel grows inward (invaginates) into the coronal pulp chamber beginning at the lingual pit. It can extend a few or several millimeters in an apical direction. The condition is usually bilateral and may be relatively mild or severe with several invaginations in one tooth. The maxillary lateral incisors are most frequently affected, followed by the maxillary central incisors, mesiodens, cuspids, mandibular lateral incisors, and, rarely, a posterior tooth. The associated lingual pit is prone to caries, leading to early pulpitis and periapical inflammation. These pits require prophylactic placement of sealants. Radiographically, teardrop or bulb-shaped layers of enamel and possibly dentin extend apically toward or past the cementoenamel junction. The presence of caries may not be evident; however, a periapical radiolucency, such as a **globulomaxillary cyst**, alerts the practitioner to the loss of tooth vitality and the need for root canal therapy.

Accessory Cusps

Cusp of Carabelli is an extra cusp located about halfway down the lingual surface of the mesiolingual cusp of maxillary molars, usually the first permanent molar; however, in Figure 64.6, it is seen on the second molar. Primary molars may rarely be affected. It is usually bilateral. It is common in Caucasians and rare in Asians. There is often an associated groove between the **cusp of Carabelli** and the lingual surface of the tooth. This groove is prone to the development of stain and caries. When oral hygiene is fair and the diet is high in sugar, sealants are recommended.

Dens Evaginatus (Leong Tubercle) (Fig. 21.5) is less common than dens invaginatus and is usually classified as an **accessory cusp**. It consists of a small dome-shaped elevation emanating from the central groove of the occlusal surface or the lingual ridge of a buccal cusp of a permanent posterior tooth. **Dens evaginatus** occurs almost exclusively in mandibular premolars. It is especially common in persons of Asian descent. It is a feature of the **shovel-shaped incisor syndrome** common in Native Americans (see Fig. 23.8). The evaginated tubercle consists of enamel, dentin, and a slender but prominent pulp chamber. Pathologic pulp exposure may occur following fracture, attrition or iatrogenically during tooth preparation.

Protostylid (Fig. 21.6) is an **accessory** (extra) **cusp** on the buccal surface of a tooth; the mesiobuccal cusp of a molar is most commonly affected. *Premolarization* is a term used to describe affected canines, and *molarization* is used for affected premolars. An accessory cusp on molars is sometimes termed a *paramolar cusp*. The condition should be distinguished from the term **paramolar**, which is used to describe a small supernumerary tooth that develops lingual or buccal to a molar.

Talon Cusp (Figs. 21.7 and 21.8) (dens evaginatus) is a rare accessory cusp on an anterior tooth that results in a markedly enlarged lingual cingulum. It occurs more commonly in permanent maxillary incisors. Its name originates from the resemblance to a three-pronged eagle's talon. The **talon cusp** can interfere with occlusion. Also, the presence of a deep developmental groove can lead to lingual caries. Accordingly, the fissure should be prophylactically treated with a sealant or frequently treated with remineralization solutions/varnish. This condition may be an incidental finding or may be seen in association with the Rubinstein-Taybi syndrome, characterized by mental retardation, digital and facial anomalies, delayed or incomplete descent of the testes, and bone age below the 50th percentile.

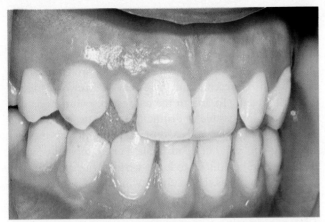

Fig. 21.1. Microdontia: peg lateral incisor.

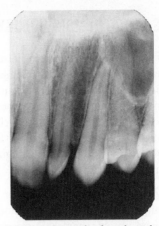

Fig. 21.2. Microdontia: radiograph of peg lateral incisor.

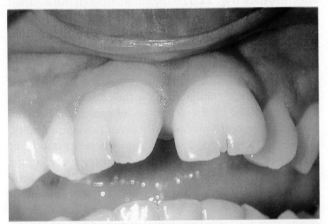

Fig. 21.3. Macrodontia: bilateral gemination.

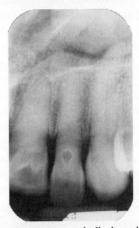

Fig. 21.4. Dens invaginatus: tear or bulb shaped.

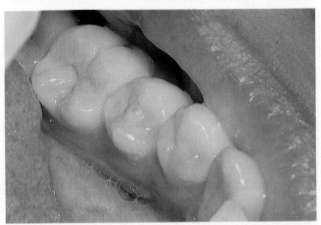

Fig. 21.5. Accessory cusp: dens evaginatus occlusal no. 20.

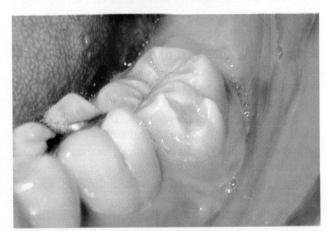

Fig. 21.6. Accessory cusp: protostylid on buccal second molar.

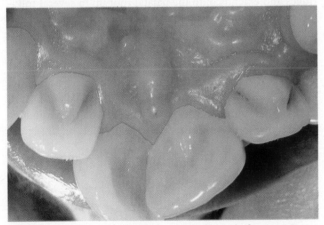

Fig. 21.7. Accessory cusps: talon cusps on lingual of incisors.*

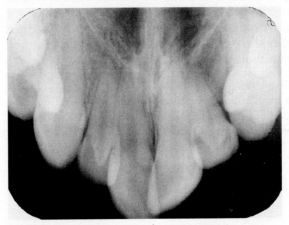

Fig. 21.8. Talon cusps: image of patient in 21.7.*

49

Introduction (Fig. 22.1) Fusion, gemination, twinning, and concrescence are developmental anomalies explained on this page. Figure 22.1 illustrates the essential differences among these similar conditions. It is important to note that sometimes, gemination and fusion are clinically indistinguishable. Questioning the patient about tooth loss and serial radiographs may be necessary to distinguish these conditions from supernumerary teeth.

Fusion (Figs. 22.2 and 22.5) occurs when two separate tooth buds attempt to join. The fused portion usually consists of dentin and, rarely, enamel. **Fusion** occurs in less than 1% of the population and may be familial. The primary teeth are affected about five times more frequently than the permanent teeth. Bilateral presentations are about 10 times less common than unilateral examples. The incisors are the most commonly involved teeth. One distinguishing feature is the number of teeth; when the fused teeth are counted as one, then there is one fewer tooth than normal. This leads to another feature: excess interproximal space. An exception occurs when a tooth from the normal dentition fuses with an adjacent supernumerary tooth, creating the appearance of gemination. Fused teeth, like geminated teeth, have a linear groove along the labial or lingual surface and a notch at the incisal edge where the two teeth fused. Radiographically, fused teeth are more likely to have two separate pulp chambers and root canal spaces. However, variations occur, depending on the degree of fusion present. Fused primary teeth are often followed by hypodontia of the succeeding permanent teeth.

Gemination (Figs. 22.3–22.5) occurs when a single tooth bud attempts to divide into two teeth, but the division is incomplete. It occurs in less than 1% of the population, may be familial, and involves the primary teeth about five times more often than the permanent teeth. The most commonly involved teeth are the primary mandibular incisors and the permanent maxillary incisors. Bilateral gemination is rare. Clinically, the most difficult problem is to distinguish gemination and fusion. Because **gemination** involves a single tooth bud, the patient will have a normal number of teeth; however, the affected tooth will appear enlarged (**macrodont**), and crowding is evident. The crown may be normal in appearance, or it may have a notch at the incisal edge or a groove on the labial or lingual surface. Radiographically, a geminated tooth often has a single enlarged pulp chamber, an enlarged root, and an enlarged or bifid crown. However, other variations are possible.

Twinning (Figs. 22.6 and 20.2) is the complete division of a single tooth bud. The condition is considered very rare. The divided teeth are seen as completely separate with no connection to each other except that each tends to be a mirror image of the other. They are often smaller than usual and could be described as **microdonts**. When the teeth are counted, an extra tooth is present, and there may be crowding of the remaining teeth. To add to the confusion, **twinning** is difficult if not impossible to distinguish from two microdonts (a peg lateral and a microdontic supernumerary incisor) involving two separate tooth buds. For example, in Figure 20.2, it would be difficult to know whether the supernumerary lateral incisor is the result of twinning of a single tooth bud or whether it developed from an extra tooth bud that erupted.

Concrescence (Fig. 22.7) is the union between two adjacent teeth along the root surfaces by cementum. **Concrescence** results from environmental or developmental factors after root formation is complete. Contributing factors include crowding during tooth development, inflammation due to infection, or trauma in which the interdental alveolar bone is resorbed. These conditions allow the adjacent tooth roots to become fused by the deposition of cementum between them. Concrescence may occur between two normal teeth, between a normal tooth and a supernumerary tooth, or between two supernumeraries. **True concrescence** occurs during the completion of tooth development and is seen most commonly between the second and third molars in the maxilla owing to lack of space. **Acquired concrescence** occurs after the teeth have completed development but are joined by hypercementosis associated with chronic inflammation (often pulpal inflammation of one of the teeth) in the region. Concrescence is important in orthodontics and tooth extraction. For example, when concrescence affects a third and second molar, extraction of the third molar can result in movement of the concrescenced second molar. It may not be possible to surgically separate such teeth.

Palatogingival Groove (Fig. 22.8) is an important developmental defect and risk factor for periodontal disease. It occurs in 1% to 9% of the population, most commonly in persons of Chinese or East Indian descent, although it can be detected in other populations. The most frequently affected tooth is the maxillary lateral incisor, followed by the maxillary central incisor. The **palatogingival groove** begins at the junction of the cingulum and one of the lateral marginal ridges and extends onto the palatal root up to several millimeters. This groove is a frequent site of an unsuspected periodontal defect because cementum fails to cover the groove and the periodontal ligament fails to attach to this portion of the root. The periodontal defect is detected with a periodontal probe as part of the routine periodontal examination; then, the groove is detected by probing the palatal aspect of the root adjacent to the defect. When present, the periodontal prognosis is diminished.

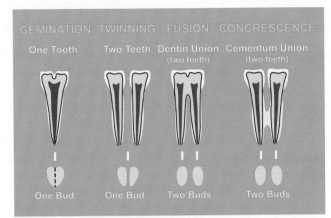

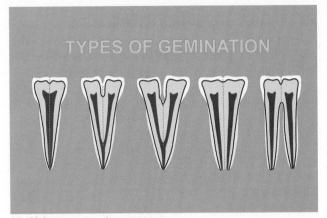

Fig. 22.1. Gemination, twinning, fusion, and concrescence.

Fig. 22.2. Variants of gemination.

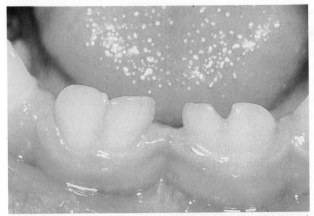

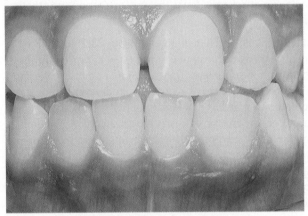

Fig. 22.3. **Fusion:** union of two teeth by dentin or enamel; bilateral.

Fig. 22.4. **Gemination:** a divided lower lateral incisor.

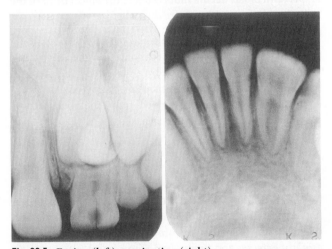

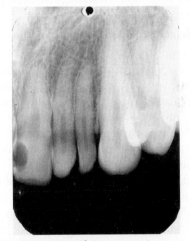

Fig. 22.5. **Fusion (left), gemination (right).**

Fig. 22.6. **Twinning:** extra tooth is a twin.

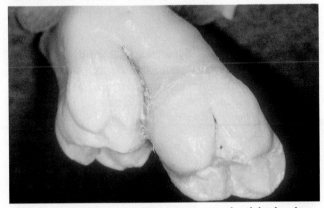

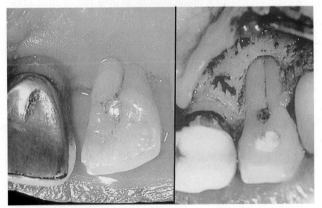

Fig. 22.7. **Concrescence:** Fused cementum second and third molars.

Fig. 22.8. **Palatogingival groove** and associated periodontal defect.

ALTERATIONS IN TOOTH MORPHOLOGY

Supernumerary Roots (Fig. 23.1) are developmental extra roots. Any tooth may be affected. The normal number of roots is one in incisors, canines, mandibular premolars, and maxillary second premolars, two in maxillary first premolars and mandibular molars, and three in maxillary molars. **Supernumerary roots** occur more frequently in permanent third molars, mandibular canines, and premolars. Mandibular molars are affected in 1% of Caucasians, 20% of persons of Mongolian extraction, and as many as 44% among Aleuts. Radiographically, extra roots can be suspected when the root canal space abruptly diminishes in size and bifurcates into two separate canals. Supernumerary roots can affect root canal therapy, extraction, prosthetics, and orthodontics.

Ectopic Enamel: Enamel Pearl (Figs. 23.2 and 23.3) is small pearl-like deposit of enamel, often at or slightly above the furcation of molars. They are more common in Asians, Malaysians, and Native Americans and seven times more common in maxillary molars. In upper molars, they usually locate on the mesial or distal root surface; in mandibular molars, they occur on the buccal or lingual surface. **Enamel pearls** are dome shaped, 1 to 2 mm in size, and rarely multiple. They do not contain pulp tissue. They may contribute to chronic periodontal inflammation and may hinder periodontal instrumentation. In Figure 23.3, the pearl moves opposite to the x-ray beam location; thus, the pearl is on the palatal surface of the tooth. Radiologically, false pearls occur in lower molars (see Fig. 6.7).

Ectopic Enamel: Cervical Enamel Extensions (Fig. 23.4) occur at the midbuccal cementoenamel junction of molars and consist of a V-shaped, smooth, or roughened extension of the buccal enamel extending toward the furcation area. They are more common in persons of Asian descent and are less frequent in Caucasians. Mandibular molars are involved more often than maxillary molars, with the first, second, and third molars affected in descending order of frequency. The **cervical enamel extension** is difficult to see in radiographs but may be detected with an explorer or periodontal probe. Cervical enamel extensions may be rough or smooth, are associated with periodontal pocket formation and furcation involvement, and with an inflammatory cyst known as the **buccal bifurcation cyst** (Figs. 36.5 and 36.6). This cyst is a radiolucent area delineated by a thin radiopaque crescent-shaped line superimposed on the buccal root, sometimes extending distally. The occlusal view shows the tooth is displaced lingually. Cystic complications tend to develop in children and adolescents.

Dilaceration (Figs. 23.5 and 28.5) is a sharp bend in a root—or less frequently, the crown of a tooth—usually greater than 20 degrees. It is common when crowding, trauma, adjacent bony lesions, or orthodontic traction occurs. Teeth often involved are molars, premolars, and maxillary lateral incisor roots. The bend in the root can be in any direction, but it is often toward the distal, distobuccal, or distolingual. When the **dilaceration** is buccal or lingual, radiographically, it appears as a bull's-eye, with the center representing the pulp canal. Dilaceration can complicate root canal therapy, orthodontics, and exodontia. Another example is shown in Figure 28.5.

Bulbous Root (Figs. 23.5 and 34.8) is a developmental variation in root morphology in which the normal apical taper is replaced by localized widening of the root. This condition is genetically determined rather than a response to local factors. The bulbous appearance is the result of increased amount of dentin—not cementum. Teeth with a **bulbous root** are more difficult to extract.

Hypercementosis (Fig. 23.6) is the excessive deposition of secondary cementum on the root(s) of any tooth. It occurs in association with local factors (supraeruption, apical periodontal infection, occlusal trauma) and systemic conditions (Paget disease, toxic thyroid goiter, acromegaly, pituitary gigantism). In a German study of 22,000 patients, the incidence of **hypercementosis** was 2%. In that study, mandibular molars, second premolars, and first premolars were the most commonly affected in descending order of frequency, and mandibular teeth were affected twice as often as maxillary. Radiographically, the root outline is enlarged and delineated by the periodontal membrane space and lamina dura. Hypercementosis occurs more often at the apical third of the root; it makes extraction more difficult.

Taurodontism (Fig. 23.7) (bull-like teeth with large body [crown] and short legs [roots]) is a condition affecting a multirooted tooth or teeth caused by a defective gene involved in odontogenesis. **Taurodontism** is characterized by an elongated and rectangular-shaped pulp chamber, disproportionately short roots, and a lack of constriction at the cementoenamel junction. Permanent teeth are affected more often than primary teeth and molars more than premolars. The incidence ranges from 0.5% to 5%. Severity is classified as **hypotaurodont** (mild), **mesotaurodont** (moderate), and **hypertaurodont** (severe). It occurs in association with inherited conditions including **Down, Mohr, Klinefelter, and tricho-dento-osseous syndromes**; some cases of **amelogenesis imperfecta**; and in children who receive antineoplastic treatment. Taurodonts are treated as normal, although the pulp floor and furcation are deeper, and the pulp space morphology affects root canal therapy.

Shovel-Shaped Incisor Syndrome (Fig. 23.8) is inherited and seen in Native Americans, Eskimos, and Hispanics. The main features are prominent marginal (shovel-shaped) ridges especially in the anterior teeth, accentuated lingual pits in maxillary incisors, and markedly shortened roots, especially the premolars; dens evaginatus in the lower premolars; and class VI caries at cusp tips. Patients are prone to class III and lingual pit caries in maxillary incisors.

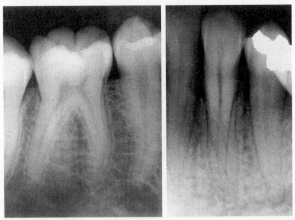

Fig. 23.1. Supernumerary root: first molar (**left**), canine (**right**).

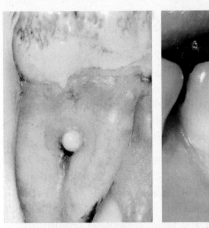

Fig. 23.2. Ectopic enamel: enamel pearls at furcation.

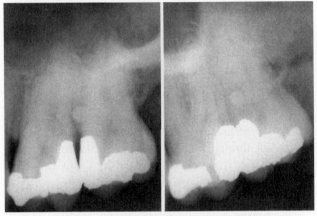

Fig. 23.3. Enamel pearl: palatal surface and perio defect.

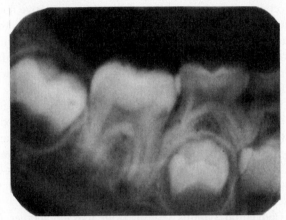

Fig. 23.4. Cervical enamel extension: first molar, bifurcation cyst.

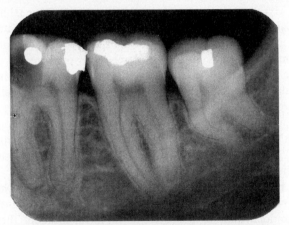

Fig. 23.5. Dilaceration third molar; bulbous root first molar.

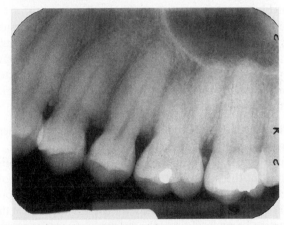

Fig. 23.6. Hypercementosis: premolars.

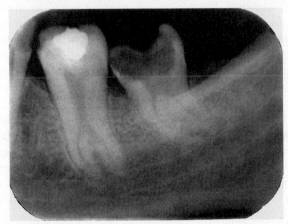

Fig. 23.7. Taurodontism: hypertaurodont.

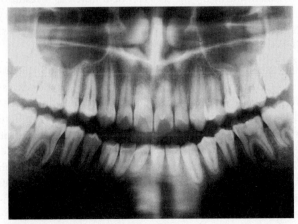

Fig. 23.8. Shovel-shaped incisor syndrome.

ALTERATIONS IN TOOTH STRUCTURE AND COLOR

Enamel Hypoplasia (Figs. 24.1–24.8) is incomplete or defective formation of the organic enamel matrix of primary or permanent teeth as a result of factors that affect ameloblast function. Two types of **enamel hypoplasia** exist: one caused by environmental factors and the other caused by hereditary factors termed **amelogenesis imperfecta**.

Enamel Hypoplasia: Environmental Types (Figs. 24.1–24.3)

Environmental factors that can cause enamel hypoplasia include **nutritional deficiencies** of vitamins A, C, and D; **infections** (i.e., measles, chickenpox, scarlet fever) that result in **exanthema** (fever and rash); **congenital syphilis**; hypocalcemia; birth injury; congenital Rh hemolytic disease; local infection or trauma; ingestion of chemicals (excessive fluoride); therapeutic radiation to the jaws at a young age; and idiopathic causes. The location of the defect in the enamel dates the disturbance, as seen in Figure 24.1. Enamel formation starts incisally and proceeds cervically; thus, the defects in Figure 24.2 occurred near age 3 years.

Fever-related enamel hypoplasia may occur in teeth undergoing mineralization during high fever. Thus, maxillary and mandibular teeth are affected equally. Defects vary from a horizontal white line, pits, or a groove on the crown if the fever is brief to severe malformations owing to lack of enamel. Mildly affected areas appear whitish; more severe cases are darker yellow to brown (Fig. 24.2).

Congenital syphilis (spread from infected mother to unborn infant) results in clinical abnormalities such as **Hutchinson triad**, consisting of interstitial keratitis of the cornea resulting in blurred vision; inner ear defects, resulting in hearing loss; and enamel hypoplasia of the central incisors, called **Hutchison incisors**. Affected incisors taper like a screwdriver with a notch on the incisal edge. Affected molars have supernumerary cusps and resemble mulberries (**mulberry molars**).

Turner Tooth (Fig. 24.3)

Turner Tooth (Fig. 24.3) is an enamel defect of a permanent tooth caused by inflammation involving, or trauma to, a primary tooth. The resulting damage insults the developing enamel of the permanent tooth. Premolars are commonly affected teeth, often the result of damage by an abscessed primary molar (Fig. 15.8). Typically, the abscess is located at the furcation immediately over the developing premolar crown. Permanent maxillary incisors can be affected as a result of an abscess or trauma—from a fall that intrudes the primary incisors. A **Turner tooth** may have a white, yellow, or brown spot or a more severe enamel defect.

Fluorosis or Mottled Enamel (Fig. 26.4)

Fluorosis or Mottled Enamel (Fig. 26.4) is caused by ingestion of high levels of fluoride in the drinking water or excessively prescribed fluoride during tooth development. The ideal concentration in water is about 0.7 to 1 part per million (ppm). Levels greater than 1.5 ppm can induce **fluorosis**. The severity increases with increasing concentrations of fluoride. Mild cases of fluorosis produce chalky white areas or small pits in enamel on several teeth; moderate to severe cases produce symmetrical yellow to dark brown spots or horizontal bands in both arches. In severely affected teeth, the enamel is soft and can fracture or wear off. Although all teeth can be affected, mandibular incisors are the least affected. Discoloration increases after eruption and can be removed by bleaching or covered with composites.

Amelogenesis Imperfecta (Figs. 24.4–24.8)

Amelogenesis Imperfecta (Figs. 24.4–24.8) is a group of inherited disorders characterized by a defect in one of the three stages of enamel formation (matrix formation, mineralization, and maturation). It affects the primary and permanent dentitions. **Amelogenesis imperfecta** is divided into four main types (hypoplastic, hypomature, hypocalcified, and hypomaturation/hypoplasia with taurodontism) and 15 subtypes according to clinical, histologic, radiographic, and genetic features. Autosomal dominant forms are linked to defects in enamelin and a gene on chromosome 4. Some X-linked recessive forms exhibit mutations in the gene encoding amelogenin.

Hypoplastic amelogenesis imperfecta (type I), the most common form, is caused by a reduction in the amount of enamel matrix secreted—the first stage of enamel formation. The enamel that forms is thin and well mineralized and does not chip. There are seven subtypes referred to alphabetically as type I A through G; four are autosomal dominant, two autosomal recessive, and one X-linked dominant. Clinically, the enamel demonstrates variable patterns, including generalized or localized pinpoint pitting that is most prominent on buccal surfaces, to smooth and rough changes with white to yellow-brown tapered teeth.

Hypomaturation amelogenesis imperfecta (type II) has quantitatively normal amounts of enamel, but the matrix is immature, so the enamel is soft, discolored, and poorly mineralized; thus, a dental explorer under pressure will pit the enamel surface. In this type, the enamel appears chalky, rough, grooved, and discolored. Fracturing of the enamel is common. In its milder form, snow-capped teeth appear; in more severe cases, teeth can resemble crown preparations, with excessive interdental spacing. There are four subtypes II, A through D, with autosomal and X-linked recessive inheritance.

Hypocalcified amelogenesis imperfecta (type III) has normal enamel matrix, but undergoes no significant mineralization, resulting in a severe defect in calcification. There are two subtypes, A (autosomal dominant) and B (autosomal recessive). Developing and erupting teeth are normal in shape, with normal enamel thickness, but with unusual honey-brown color. Soon after eruption, the brown enamel undergoes severe chipping, leaving a roughened, brown dentinal surface with some enamel remaining, especially at the gingival margin. An anterior open bite is often present as a result of loss of posterior vertical dimension.

Hypomaturation/hypoplastic amelogenesis imperfecta (type IV) has features of hypomature and hypoplastic subtypes A and B. The teeth exhibit yellowish to opaque mottling, buccal pitting, attrition, large pulp chambers, and varying degrees of taurodontism. Both subtypes are seen in the **tricho-dento-osseous syndrome** (brittle nails and sclerotic bone).

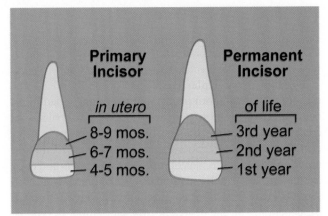

Fig. 24.1. **Enamel formation in teeth**.

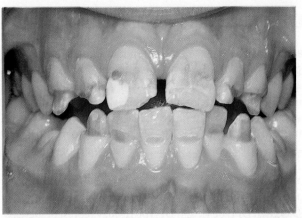

Fig. 24.2. **Enamel hypoplasia:** white and brown enamel defects.

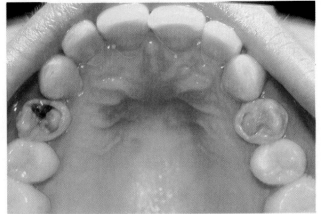

Fig. 24.3. **Turner teeth:** both maxillary first premolars.

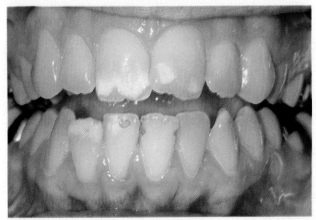

Fig. 24.4. **Amelogenesis imperfecta type IIC:** snow capped.

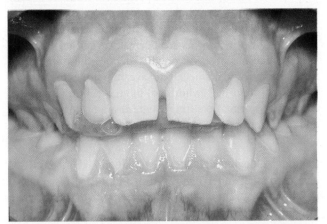

Fig. 24.5. **Amelogenesis imperfecta, type ID:** tapered incisors.

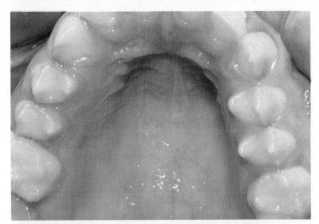

Fig. 24.6. **Amelogenesis imperfecta type ID:** lack of enamel.

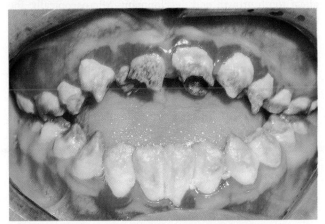

Fig. 24.7. **Amelogenesis imperfecta type IIIB:** open bite.*

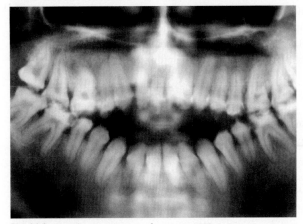

Fig. 24.8. **Amelogenesis imperfecta type IIIB.***

Dentinogenesis Imperfecta (Hereditary Opalescent Dentin; Figs. 25.1–25.3) and Dentin Dysplasia (Figs. 25.4–25.7) are two similar **autosomal dominant disorders** that involve abnormal dentin development of the primary and permanent teeth. For decades, they have been categorized as separate entities using the Shields classification scheme, which was based on clinical, radiographic, and histologic findings. This scheme recognizes three types of **dentinogenesis imperfecta (DI types I, II, and III)** and two types of **dentin dysplasia (DD types I and II)**. Genetic findings, however, suggest that DD type II, DI type II, and DI type III may represent increasing levels of severity of a single disease; thus, we might expect in the near future a transition from the Shields classification system to a newer genetic-based system that uses the gene defect to help classify these disorders. Until then, the Shields system is presented.

DI occurs in about 1 in 8,000 newborns. **DI type I** is the dental feature of **osteogenesis imperfecta**, a systemic condition involving bone fragility, blue sclerae, joint laxity, and hearing impairment. It is caused by defects in genes encoding type I collagen (COL1A1 or COL1A2). This results in variable levels of defective collagen in bone and dentin. **DI type II** results from a defect in a gene that regulates dentin sialophosphoprotein (DSPP) production—the major noncollagenous proteins of dentin. DI type II has similar dentinal features as DI type I but has no bone component. **DI type III**—also known as Brandywine isolate and first described in isolated triracial groups from southern Maryland—also results from an inherited defect in DSPP production. It is described as a variable presentation of DI type II and appears clinically similar to DI types I and II or may show slightly more severe features (see below).

All three types of DI produce misshapen and disoriented dentin tubules. The primary teeth are more severely affected than permanent teeth, with the last erupting teeth affected least. Affected teeth look clinically normal when they first erupt but shortly thereafter become discolored, amber to gray-brown, or opalescent. The enamel flakes away from the underlying defective, weak, and soft dentin, resulting in fissuring and significant attrition. Radiographs often show bulbous crowns, short tapered roots, and progressive obliteration of the root canal. A less common feature is **shell teeth**, which have extremely thin dentin and dramatically enlarged pulps; this feature was first described with DI type III. DI teeth, especially primary teeth, are more susceptible to decay, root fractures, and multiple pulp exposures.

Dentin dysplasia (DD) is less common than DI. It is a rare autosomal dominant disorder characterized by dentin disorganization, pulp chamber narrowing, pulp stones, shortened roots, and numerous periapical radiolucencies. There are two types: type I radicular DD and type II coronal DD. The cause of type I is not known, but DD type II (like DI type II and type III) is caused by a defect in DSPP.

DD type I (radicular dysplasia) primarily affects the roots of teeth, with both primary and permanent dentitions being affected. The crowns of the teeth appear normal in size, consistency, and shape, but may be slightly amber or translucent. Extremely short roots are characteristic and can cause eruption delays, tooth malalignment, mobile teeth, and early exfoliation after minor trauma. O'Carroll's classification (Fig. 25.4) divides DD type I into four subgroups (a through d), depending on the degree of root shortening. In type Ia, the roots are almost nonexistent **rootless teeth** (Fig. 25.5A). In types Ib and Ic, there is progressively more root formation; the pulp chambers are nearly obliterated and exhibit one or several thin horizontal radiolucent lines. In type Id, root length is normal; however, large pulp stones are prominent (Fig. 25.5B). DD types Ia, b, and c characteristically develop spontaneous periapical radiolucencies in noncarious teeth. These develop from ingress of bacteria through microscopic threads of pulpal remnants or from a periodontal defect associated with the shortened roots.

Type II (coronal) DD is less common than type I and affects the primary and permanent teeth. The primary teeth have features of DI type II (an amber, translucent appearance). Radiographically, the crowns are bulbous, the roots are thin and tapered, and there is early obliteration of the pulp spaces, exactly like DI. The permanent teeth are usually of normal shape, form, and color; however, the pulp chambers show thistle-tube deformity and pulp stones (Fig. 25.6). Histologically, the crowns are normal, except at the pulpal third, which has areas of globular dentin; the roots are of normal length and diameter but have pulp stones in the canal spaces and abnormal (whorls of) tubular dentin. Tooth loss is unlikely, as the roots in DD type II are of normal length and diameter and are not associated with spontaneous periapical lesions.

Regional Odontodysplasia (Ghost Teeth) (Fig. 25.8) is also discussed under Figures 19.1 and 19.2. This unusual developmental anomaly is characterized by malformed underdeveloped teeth in one quadrant of the mouth. The condition is associated with local and systemic factors that affect tooth growth and development. Microscopically, the affected teeth are characterized by disrupted calcification (thin and abnormal enamel, interglobular dentin, abnormally large pulp chambers with pulp stones, and minimal root). Radiographically, affected teeth are rather radiolucent, producing a ghostlike appearance. Clinically, ghost teeth are often carious and painful and often display delayed eruption (remain impacted). This figure is typical and from a patient with focal dermal hypoplasia (**Goltz syndrome**).

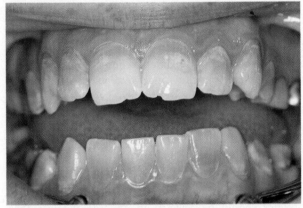

Fig. 25.1. Dentinogenesis imperfecta Shields type I: enamel chipping.

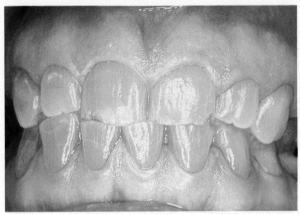

Fig. 25.2. Dentinogenesis imperfecta Shields type II: amber.

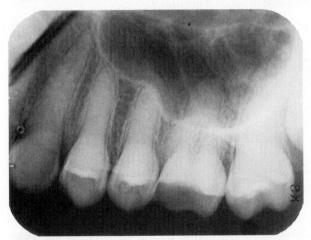

Fig. 25.3. Dentinogenesis imperfecta: obliterated pulps.

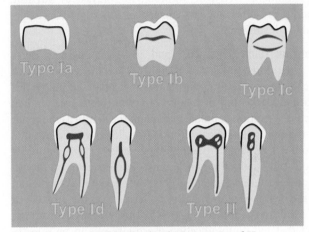

Fig. 25.4. Features of dentin dysplasia types I and II.

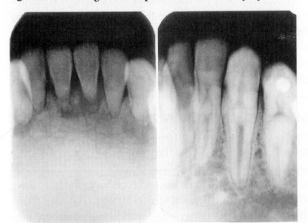

Fig. 25.5. Dentin dysplasia: type Ia (left); type Id (right).

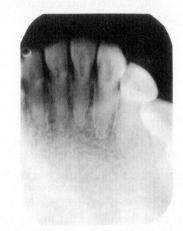

Fig. 25.6. Dentin dysplasia type II: thistle-shaped pulps.*

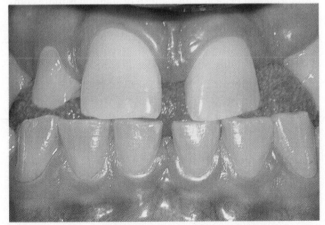

Fig. 25.7. Dentin dysplasia type II: clinical appearance.*

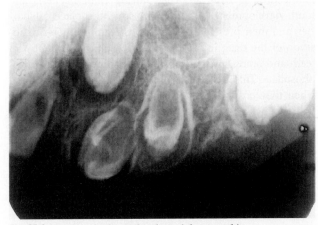

Fig. 25.8. Regional odontodysplasia (ghost teeth).

ALTERATIONS IN TOOTH COLOR

Intrinsic Discoloration (Staining; Figs. 26.1–26.4) is a permanent change in tooth color resulting from genetic or acquired factors that interfere with odontogenesis or allow stains to be incorporated into tooth structure. Genetic processes that alter tooth structure and color include amelogenesis and dentinogenesis imperfecta and dentin dysplasia. Acquired causes of **intrinsic staining** include restorations, trauma, and infections that cause loss of tooth vitality, intake of specific drugs (such as tetracycline and ciprofloxacin) and chemicals (such as excess fluoride), and certain disease states (hepatitis, biliary disease, erythroblastosis fetalis, and porphyria) that occur during periods of tooth development. **Extrinsic staining**, in contrast to intrinsic staining, results from dark substances adhering to the external tooth surface.

Nonvital Tooth (Figs. 26.1 and 26.2) is a common cause of a discolored or dark tooth. In this case, the teeth are dark (yellow-brown to gray-purple) because of loss of pulpal fluids and darkening of dentin. **Nonvital teeth** also darken from the rupture of pulpal blood into the dentin as the result of trauma, necrosis, or infection (e.g., leprosy). If death of a tooth occurs rapidly (within a few weeks), a pink to purple tooth can result. The typical pink discolored nonvital tooth shows greater discoloration along the neck of the crown than at the incisal edge and has been referred to as the **pink tooth of Mummery** (also see Fig. 29.7). This term arises from the fact that the mummification process results in pink teeth. Concurrent signs of nonvital teeth include fractured incisal edges, vertical fracture lines, deep caries, or large restorations. Amalgam restorations may contribute to tooth discoloration (in which a gray-blue hue seen) either by reducing the translucency of the tooth or by uptaking metallic particles into open dentinal tubules.

Tetracycline Staining (Fig. 26.3) The tetracyclines are a group of bacteriostatic antibiotics that inhibit protein synthesis of certain bacteria. These drugs are used to treat skin and periodontal infections as well as chlamydial, certain rickettsial, and penicillin-resistant gonococcal infections. Embryos, infants, and children who receive tetracyclines are prone to develop varying degrees of permanent tooth discoloration. This is more likely to occur during long-term use and repeated short-term courses and is directly related to the dose of drug absorbed during embryogenesis and tooth development. Tetracyclines cross the placental barrier, and their presence in the bloodstream promotes deposition of the drug in the developing enamel and dentin of teeth and bones in the form of tetracycline-calcium orthophosphate. This complex causes teeth to become discolored when they erupt and are exposed to sun (i.e., ultraviolet) light. The discoloration is generalized and bandlike if the drug was administered in courses; prolonged use produces a more homogeneous appearance. The discoloration appears (least) light yellow with oxytetracycline (Terramycin); yellow with **tetracycline** (Achromycin); or green to dark gray with the synthetic tetracycline minocycline. Chlortetracycline (Aureomycin), which is no longer available in oral form, is well known for its ability to produce gray-brown staining. Doxycycline is the least discoloring and appears to cause no staining when used in short courses in children. The diagnosis is confirmed by using an ultraviolet light, which makes the teeth fluoresce bright yellow. Adults receiving long-term tetracycline therapy have been reported to acquire tetracycline staining in permanent teeth. Accordingly, alternative antibiotics should be selected in children younger than 8 years of age, and long-term tetracycline treatment should be avoided in adults if possible.

Fluorosis (Fig. 26.4) is a disturbance of the developing enamel that is caused by excess levels of fluoride in the blood and plasma. The optimal fluoride concentration in drinking water is between 0.7 and 1 ppm. At this level, fluoride is incorporated into the enamel matrix and adds hardness and caries resistance. At levels greater than 1.2 ppm, there is increased risk for **fluorosis**. Blood levels are directly related to the level of fluoride ingested in water; excess levels can be acquired from drinking well water (endemic fluorosis) or from excessive water treatment. At elevated fluoride levels, ameloblasts are affected during the apposition of enamel and produce deficient organic matrix. At high levels, interference of the calcification process occurs. Mild fluorosis produces isolated, lusterless, whitish opaque spots in enamel. These spots occurring near the incisal edge and cusp tips are called **snow caps**. Moderate to severe fluorosis is characterized by generalized (symmetrically bilateral) defects ranging from several yellow to brown spots to numerous pitted enamel and mottled dark brown-white spots. In the severe form, crown morphology can be grossly altered. Maxillary incisors are more often affected than mandibular incisors.

Extrinsic Staining (Figs. 26.5–26.8) results from the adherence of colored material or bacteria to tooth enamel. Most **extrinsic stains** localize in the gingival third of the tooth above the gingival collar, where bacteria accumulate and absorb stain. **Chromogenic bacteria** produce green to brown stains in this region. These stains result from the interaction of bacteria with ferric sulfide and iron in the saliva and gingival crevicular fluid and the precipitation of chromogens into the dental pellicle. This pattern of staining is more common in children and patients with poor oral hygiene and gingivitis, where frequent bleeding from the gums results in breakdown of hemoglobin into green pigment (biliverdin). Colored fluids, such as coffee, tea, and chlorhexidine, and inhaled tobacco smoke can cause brown to black stains. These stains appear darkest in the gingival third of the tooth. Calculus and caries also discolor teeth. Calculus appears greenish black when subgingival, or tan when supragingival. Caries darkens the tooth; however, unlike stains, caries causes loss of tooth structure.

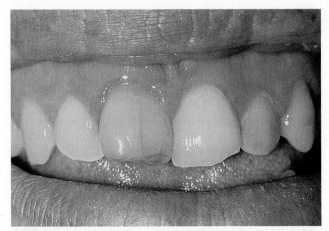

Fig. 26.1. **Intrinsic staining:** nonvital right central.

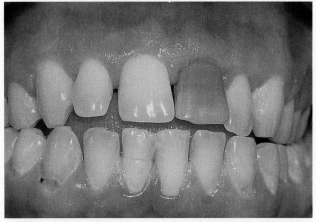

Fig. 26.2. **Intrinsic staining:** pink tooth of Mummery.

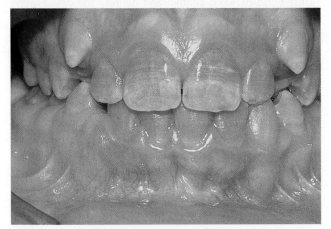

Fig. 26.3. **Intrinsic staining:** tetracycline staining.

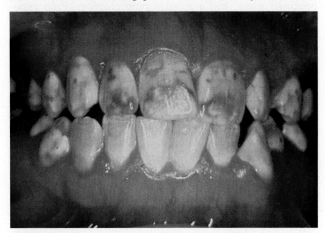

Fig. 26.4. **Intrinsic staining:** moderate to severe fluorosis.

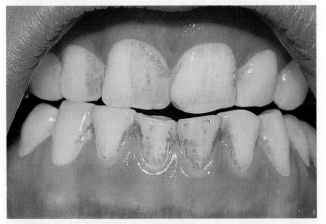

Fig. 26.5. **Extrinsic staining:** chlorhexidine staining.

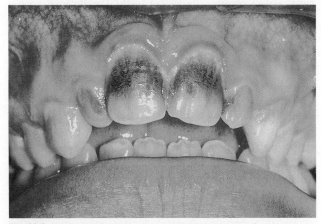

Fig. 26.6. **Extrinsic staining:** caused by chromogenic bacteria.

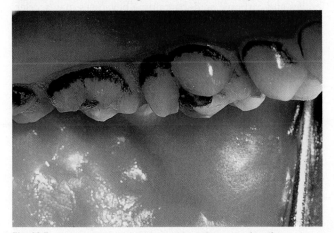

Fig. 26.7. **Extrinsic staining:** caused by tobacco and coffee.

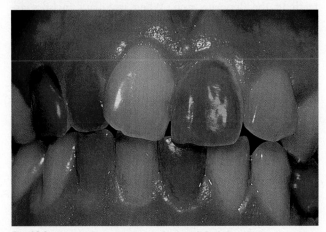

Fig. 26.8. **Extrinsic staining:** applied with holiday spirit.

4

ACQUIRED DEFECTS OF TEETH: NONCARIOUS LOSS OF TOOTH STRUCTURE

Attrition (Figs. 27.1 and 27.2) is considered a physiologic process—and is the wearing down and loss of occlusal, incisal, and interproximal tooth structure because of chronic tooth-to-tooth frictional contact. **Attrition** is seen most often in older adults, but the primary teeth of young children may also be affected. The condition is often generalized and accelerated by **bruxism** and abnormal use of selective teeth. Flattening of the incisal and occlusal surfaces, wear facets, and widened interproximal contact areas are common findings. Occlusal examination reveals a smooth and highly polished tooth surface that is broad and angled, the outline of the dentin-enamel junction, loss of the superior interproximal space, and a receded pulp chamber. Pulp exposure is rare, however, because the deposition of secondary dentin and pulpal recession occur concurrently with attrition. Affected teeth are generally not sensitive to hot, cold, or the explorer tine, but occasionally show areas of exposed root. Restoration of the teeth may be challenging because of acquired changes in vertical dimension.

Abrasion (Figs. 27.3–27.5) is the pathologic loss of tooth structure caused by abnormal and repetitive mechanical wear. Various agents can cause **abrasion**, but the most common form is **toothbrush abrasion**. It results from abrasive toothpastes being brushed against the teeth too frequently, with hard bristles, with improper technique, and with too much vigor. Toothbrush abrasion produces a rounded, saucer-shaped, or V-shaped notch in the cervical portion of the facial aspect of several adjacent teeth. The abraded area is usually shiny or polished and yellow (because of exposed dentin). The dentin is typically firm and noncarious, little plaque accumulation is present, and the marginal gingiva is healthy. Premolars opposite to the dominant hand are most often affected. Abraded teeth demonstrate dentinal sensitivity to hot, cold, or the explorer tine and are more susceptible to pulp exposure and tooth fracture.

Abrasive notching of the teeth also can be created by clasps of partial dentures or by factitial injury: pins or nails habitually held with the teeth, or a pipe stem persistently clamped between the teeth. Inappropriate use of toothpicks and dental floss can also abrade the interproximal regions of teeth. Porcelain restorations placed in occlusion often result in abrasion of the incisal and occlusal surfaces of unrestored teeth in the opposite arch. When maxillary incisors are restored with porcelain, the mandibular incisors are abraded at an upward and backward angle. Exposure to abrasive substances in the diet, chewing tobacco, powder cocaine, and long-term inhalation of sand, quartz, or silica can also promote abrasion, generally at the site of chronic exposure. For example, cocaine addiction can cause localized abrasion of the facial surface of maxillary anterior teeth when the drug is chronically rubbed against the gingiva and teeth.

Abrasion is a slow and chronic process, requiring many years before signs arise. Restoration of normal tooth contour may be unsuccessful in the long term if the patient does not alter the causative behavior.

Abfraction means *to break away* and is a term that has been used in dentistry to define the loss of tooth structure at or under the cementoenamel junction that is caused by abnormal tooth *flexure*. The condition is controversial, and current evidence suggests that it is a potential component of **cervical wear**. Past theories have suggested that the condition arises from eccentric and cyclic occlusal loading, which creates flexure and shearing stresses, and disruption of the bond between enamel and dentin. The defects have been described as a sharp, wedge-shaped loss of enamel and dentin along the cervical region of the facial aspect of a tooth, most commonly mandibular premolars. Clinicians should examine closely affected patients for occlusal causes of oblique stress loading on affected teeth and provide preventive and interventive therapies.

Erosion (Figs. 27.6–27.8) refers to the loss of tooth structure caused by chemicals such as dietary, gastric, or environmental acids that are placed in prolonged contact with the teeth. **Erosion** is exacerbated by hyposalivation and drugs that produce **xerostomia**, because loss of saliva reduces the buffering capacity of the oral cavity. The most commonly affected tooth surfaces are the labial and buccal surfaces.

The pattern of tooth erosion often indicates the causative agent or a particular habit. For example, sucking on lemons (citric acid) produces characteristic changes of the facial surfaces of the maxillary incisors. Horizontal ridges appear initially, followed by smooth, cupped-out, yellowish depressions. Eventually, the incisal edges thin and fracture. A similar erosive pattern may be seen in dedicated swimmers whose anterior teeth are chronically exposed to chlorinated swimming pools.

Erosion limited to the lingual surfaces of the maxillary teeth, especially the anteriors (**perimolysis**, also known as **perimylolysis**), indicates chronic regurgitation or vomiting caused by **bulimia, anorexia,** pregnancy, hiatal hernia, gastroesophageal reflux, or alcohol abuse. Affected posterior teeth have margins of occlusal amalgams raised above the eroded and adjacent enamel. Sensitivity of the exposed area is an early symptom. Excessive consumption of sweetened beverages and carbonic acid–containing beverages may accelerate the condition. Fluoride treatments for early erosions and restorations that cover exposed dentin for more extensive lesions are treatments of choice. Elimination of the causative habit or behavior modification is required for success. In cases of gastroesophageal reflux, the condition can be controlled by medications (antacids, H_2 histamine blockers, proton pump inhibitors) and use of sodium bicarbonate rinses after episodes of reflux.

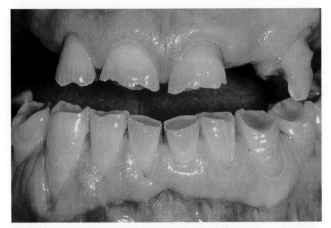

Fig. 27.1. Attrition: dentin exposure, enamel thinning.

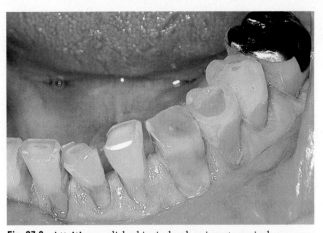

Fig. 27.2. Attrition: polished incisals; abrasion at cervical.

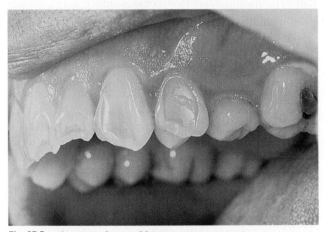

Fig. 27.3. Abrasion: worn by friction against porcelain.

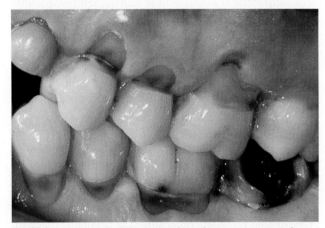

Fig. 27.4. Toothbrush abrasion: V-shaped grooves at cervical.

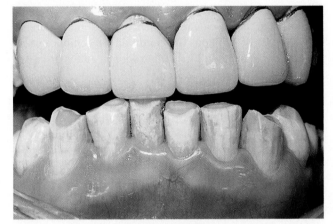

Fig. 27.5. Abrasion: from rubbing cocaine on gingiva.

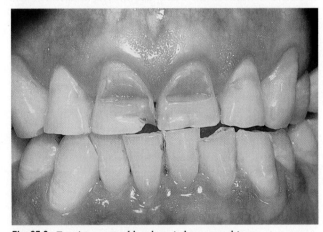

Fig. 27.6. Erosion: caused by chronic lemon sucking.

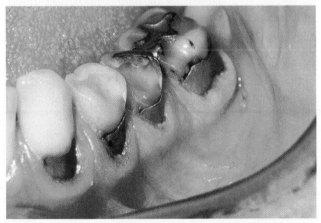

Fig. 27.7. Erosion: caused by intake of carbonated beverages.

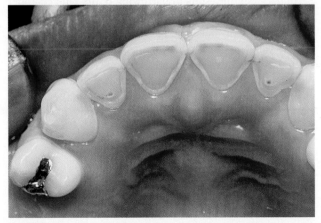

Fig. 27.8. Erosion: caused by chronic vomiting in bulimia.

ALTERATION IN PULP AND ROOT STRUCTURE

Pulp Calcification and Pulp Stones (Figs. 28.1–28.3)

Calcifications within the pulp are common occurrences—about 20% of the teeth are affected. There are three types of **pulp calcifications**: denticles, pulp stones, and diffuse linear calcifications. A **denticle** is a developmental anomaly believed to originate from the root sheath. Early in life, some unknown initiating event causes odontoblasts to deposit tubular dentin around a central nest of epithelium producing as a thimble-shaped structure, called a denticle. The central epithelium eventually undergoes sclerosis. The denticle generally forms in the root canal (below the crown) and is typically attached or embedded in the dentin.

A **pulp stone** is a collection of mineralized tissue within the pulp chamber of a tooth. They are classified as *true* or *false* pulp stones. A true pulp stone is composed of dentin and has dentinal tubules. It is more rare than the false pulp stone. A false pulp stone is a mineralized mass usually with a concentric or radial pattern lacking dentin and tubules. Both types produce round or ovoid structures that are easily seen on radiographs.

Most pulp stones develop as a part of the aging process or as a result of a pathologic event. Pulp stones are distinguished radiographically from denticles in that pulp stones are located within the crown of the tooth and the outline tends to conform with the pulp chamber, whereas denticles are located typically in a more apical position. Both denticles and pulp stones are frequently seen in conjunction with inherited conditions including dentin dysplasia, calcinosis universalis, and Ehlers-Danlos syndrome.

Diffuse linear calcifications are smaller than pulp stones and consist of fine, fibrillar irregular calcifications within the pulp. These calcifications tend to be multiple and parallel the course of the vasculature within the pulp. Because of their small size, they are not seen on radiographs.

Another calcification process that occurs within the pulp is **pulpal sclerosis**, which is often due to **secondary dentin formation**. Secondary dentin can be the result of a physiologic or pathologic process. Physiologic secondary dentin typically occurs with advancing age. Under these circumstances, attrition and abrasion cause secondary dentin to be deposited slowly in a regular pattern. In contrast, pathologic processes like caries or severe trauma cause the secondary dentin formation to be more rapid and disorganized. Secondary dentin results in narrowing of the pulp chamber and canal due to deposition of mineralized dentin (Fig. 28.3). This in turn can make the affected tooth darker in color, usually yellow to yellow-brown appearance. In some cases, secondary dentin formation can cause severe sclerosis and obliteration of the pulp canal. Not surprisingly, each of the calcification processes mentioned above can make the pulp canal more difficult to locate during endodontic therapy.

Variation in Root Canal Space (Fig. 28.4)

The number of root canal spaces present in a tooth tends to match the number of roots present. In other words, a single-rooted tooth typically has one root canal space, and double-rooted teeth typically have two root canal spaces. A variant of this occurs when the root canal space splits into one or more chambers. It is seen more commonly in posterior teeth and likely occurs in less than 10% of patients. Radiographically, splitting is evident by the loss in radiolucency of the canal as it progresses apically. In the examples shown in Fig. 28.4, the canals are very radiolucent at least halfway down the root, before the canal almost disappears—this is the split.

Dilaceration (Fig. 28.5)

is a sharp bend in a root that often results when the developing root encounters an interference with the path of eruption. This condition can complicate root canal therapy, orthodontics, and exodontia and is discussed under Fig. 23.5.

Fractured Root (Fig. 28.6)

is an injury produced by external force, often blunt trauma. In these instances, the root can be fractured at the apical third, in the middle of the root, or near the cementoenamel junction. When a root is fractured, the more common location is below the middle of the root. During the acute situation, there is typically bleeding, swelling, and pain. If the tooth is not treated, the fracture can result in necrosis of the pulp, displacement of the root fragment, or internal or external root resorption. Radiographically, **fractured roots** produce a radiolucent line that is 1 to 3 mm in width that traverses the root from mesial periodontal ligament space to the distal periodontal ligament space. Fractured roots often require tooth removal.

Root Shortening (Figs. 28.7 and 28.8)

Biological processes and environmental factors that can affect cementum, dentin, and pulpal development during the early years of life or can resorb mineralized root structure later in life can result in **root shortening**. External factors such as radiation therapy or chemotherapy are known causes of short spiky roots. Root shortening is also seen with dentin dysplasia, regional odontodysplasia, and hypoparathyroidism. Impacted teeth that are crowed against an adjacent tooth can resorb and shorten a root. Likewise, an inflammatory condition, such as periapical inflammation or periodontitis, can resorb roots making them short. Orthodontics can resorb roots, generally leaving the root blunted or rounded at the periapex. In addition, cysts and tumors can resorb roots, with the pattern of root shortening dependent on the location of the lesion and amount of osteoclastic activity it induces. The loss of the lamina dura is often the earliest sign of root shortening.

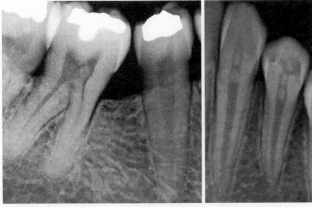

Fig. 28.1. **Pulp stones:** discrete in molar, premolars, and canine.

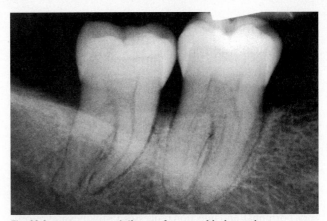

Fig. 28.2. **Pulp stones:** diffuse in first mandibular molar.

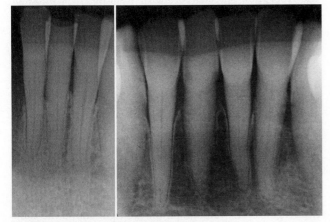

Fig. 28.3. **Pulp narrowing:** obliteration.

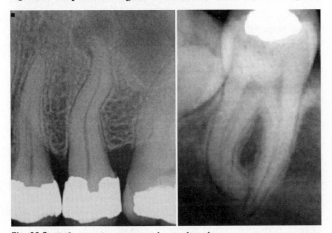

Fig. 28.4. **Root canal chambers:** splitting into two or more canals.

Fig. 28.5. **Dilacerations:** premolar and molar.

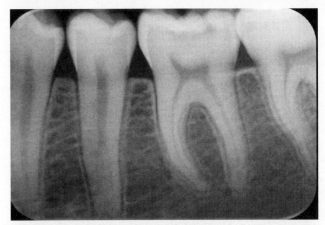

Fig. 28.6. **Diagonal root fracture:** periapical and indicated by *arrow* in cone-beam tomographic image.

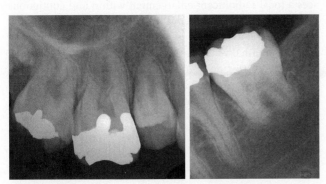

Fig. 28.7. **Root shortening:** due to radiation therapy.

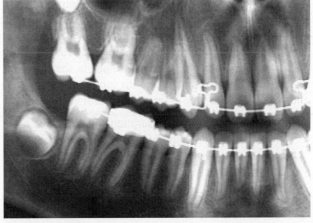

Fig. 28.8. **Root shortening:** due to orthodontics.

ALTERATION IN ROOT STRUCTURE: RESORPTION

Resorption (Figs. 29.1–29.8) is the loss of dental hard tissues, and it generally affects the root. The loss is caused by multinucleated **dentinoclasts** (cells similar to **osteoclasts**) that arise from within the pulp (i.e., internal resorption) or the periodontal ligament (external resorption). **Internal resorption** starts at the pulp-dentin interface and extends outward, destroying dentin. In contrast, **external resorption** is initiated at the outer surface, destroying cementum first, then extending inward through dentin toward the pulp. Resorption occurs most often after trauma and injury, but is also associated with inflammatory, hormonal, and infection processes. Cytokines and resorbing molecules are involved. Radiographs are generally required for the diagnosis. From a clinical perspective, resorption is classified as coronal, cervical, radicular, and periapical.

False Resorption (Fig. 29.1) is the loss of root structure by a clinical (not biological) process. Two examples are shown here. An **apicoectomy** (29.1A) is a procedure in which the apical tooth structure has been surgically removed to treat a nonvital tooth. The apex of a tooth is often reduced and flattened and filled with a gutta-percha or amalgam. A second example of **false external root resorption** (Fig. 29.1B) shows loss of cementum and dentin along the lateral surfaces of the roots in the cervical regions. This type of false resorption is iatrogenic (i.e., caused by the dentist, hygienist, or self-induced injury by the patient). In this case, the patient severely damaged her teeth from overzealous use of a curette, resulting in nonvitality of a central incisor.

External Resorption (Figs. 29.2–29.4) is much more common than internal resorption, and the causative factors that initiate the process are more varied. External resorption of primary tooth roots occurs physiologically both in association with the eruption of the permanent teeth and with retained primary teeth that have no permanent successor. The most common causes of external resorption include pressure on the tooth from various sources, such as excessive orthodontic or occlusal forces; tumors, cysts, and impacted teeth; following trauma or reimplantation of teeth; internal bleaching; inflammation of the pulp or periodontium; and idiopathic (when no obvious cause is present). Figure 29.2 shows an example of external resorption of primary tooth roots related to physiologic tooth eruption. Resorbed areas are not limited to root apices. With second molars, the resorption can affect the distal surface because of an erupting or impacted third molar, which is a sign of crowding of the permanent teeth. Figure 29.3 shows **inflammatory external resorption**. Here, the inflammation and infectious condition resorb dentin and replace it with inflamed granulation tissue in the periapical region. This occurs commonly with long-standing pulpitis and can continue as long as the pulp remains vital.

Orthodontic External Root Resorption (Fig. 29.4) is common when excess pressure is exerted on the teeth being moved orthodontically. Affected roots are shortened and flattened and may have the root apex shifted slightly mesially or distally.

Note: External root resorption can also occur following tooth **reimplantation or transplantation**. In addition, tumors and cysts can produce inflammatory periapical root resorption (Figs. 37.2–37.4). One of the more common cysts to cause external root resorption is the dentigerous cyst.

Cervical Resorption (Fig. 29.5) is a less common type of external root resorption. It begins on the external surface of the tooth in the cervical area without apparent cause. The resorption spreads coronally, resulting in a pink- or reddish-appearing crown because of enlarging vascular tissue within the crown. One or more teeth may be affected. This resorptive pattern is prone to be rapid and is also known as **invasive cervical resorption**. Treatment requires removal of the granulation tissue and then use of restorative materials.

Multiple Cervical Resorption of Hyperparathyroidism (Fig. 29.6) is a rare condition that begins at the cervical or apical region and may involve many or most of the teeth. Our example is a case reported by Hutton in 1985. The patient was a 22-year-old woman with secondary hyperparathyroidism associated with end-stage renal disease (Fig. 29.6A). Multiple teeth show idiopathic internal resorption in the cervical regions. The radiograph on the right shows the same patient 4 years after initiation of hemodialysis. The areas of root resorption have filled in presumably with an osteodentin or cementoid tissue. It is not known if the process began externally or internally.

Internal Resorption (Figs. 29.7 and 29.8) is usually initiated by chronic hyperplastic pulpitis; thus, pulp testing may produce variable results. There are two radiographic patterns of internal resorption, **inflammatory** and **metaplastic internal resorption**, and the crown or root of the tooth maybe affected. **Coronal internal resorption** can induce a pink tooth of Mummery, which occurs when inflammation produces a hyperplastic pulp that thins the internal elements of the crown, resulting in a pink appearance. Clinically, such teeth are weak and need endodontic therapy and a post and core. Coronal internal resorption may also be initiated by internal crown bleaching procedures done within endodontically treated teeth.

Internal root resorption begins in the root canal space (Fig. 29.8). Inflammation is contributory. In radiographs, one sees a focal radiolucent enlargement within and contiguous with the root canal space. The radiolucent area is typically round or oval and balloons beyond the pulp chamber space into the dentinal walls. Treatment is with calcium hydroxide and mineral trioxide aggregate pastes. If the resorptive process perforates the outside margin of the root, the tooth is often considered unrestorable.

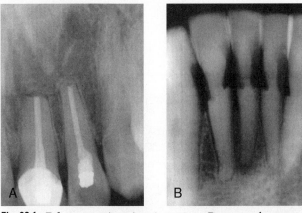

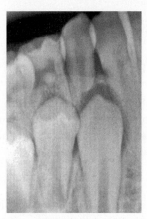

Fig. 29.1. **False resorption: A:** apicoectomy; **B:** curette damage.

Fig. 29.2. **External resorption:** physiologic associated with tooth eruption.

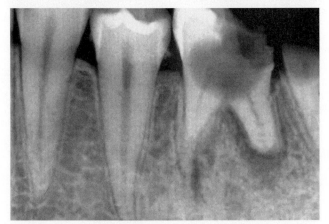

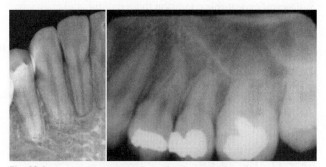

Fig. 29.3. **External resorption:** molar roots due to chronic periapical infection.

Fig. 29.4. **External resorption:** orthodontic induced.

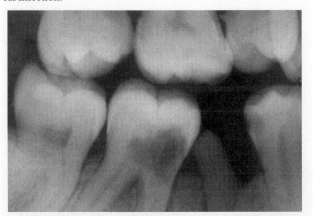

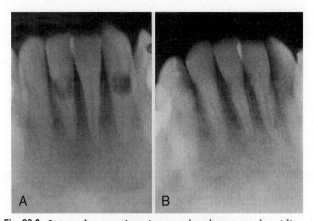

Fig. 29.5. **Cervical resorption:** invading first mandibular molar.

Fig. 29.6. **Internal resorption: A:** secondary hyperparathyroidism; **B:** healed 4 years later.

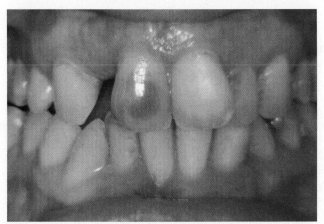

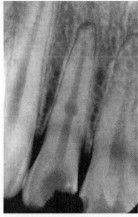

Fig. 29.7. **Internal resorption:** coronal; pink tooth of Mummery.

Fig. 29.8. **Internal root resorption:** inflammatory; note apical signs.

CASE STUDIES

CASE 16. (FIG. 29.9)

This 22-year-old woman presents with the condition shown in the clinical image. The condition has been present since she can remember but seems to be getting worse. She is interested in cosmetic dentistry.

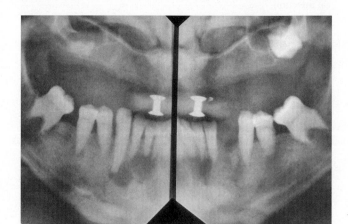

1. Describe the clinical findings in this quadrant.

2. What radiographic findings of this condition would you expect to see?

3. Is this a normal finding, a variant of normal, or disease? And how severe is this condition?

4. What is the cause of this condition?

5. Do you expect this condition to be painful, and if so, why?

6. List conditions you should consider in the differential diagnosis for this condition, and note which condition is most likely the correct diagnosis.

7. What are the treatment options for this condition?

8. Once the dentist has discussed the diagnosis with the patient, what additional information should be communicated by the hygienist to this patient about this condition?

CASE 17. (FIG. 29.10)

This 31-year-old man recently moved to your town and presents with the condition shown in the panoramic radiograph. He is interested in having his teeth cleaned and a new upper denture made. He is concerned about a couple of lower teeth that seem loose.

1. Describe the radiographic findings shown in this panoramic image. Divide your findings into tooth-related changes and bone-related changes, and note what seems unusual.

2. What most likely caused him to lose his maxillary teeth?

3. What color and contour changes do you expect to see during the clinical examination of the mandibular teeth?

4. Is this a normal finding, a variant of normal, or disease?

5. Do you expect this condition to be painful, and if so, why?

6. List three conditions that you should consider in the differential diagnosis for this condition, and note which condition is most likely the correct diagnosis.

7. What are the treatment options for this patient?

8. What should be communicated by the hygienist about this condition to the dentist?

Additional cases to enhance your learning and understanding of this section are available Online through the book's Navigate 2 Advantage Access site.

Dental Caries

Objectives:

- Identify the features of caries and their common locations.
- Define and recognize the different types of caries and their sequelae.
- Identify factors that make patients susceptible to caries.
- Use the diagnostic assessment process to distinguish caries, pulp polyp, and apical pathoses from similar-appearing oral conditions.
- Discuss caries prevention with a patient who has high risk for caries.
- Recommend appropriate treatments for the different types of caries and their sequelae.
- Identify conditions discussed in this section that (1) require the attention of the dentist and/or (2) affect the delivery of periodontal debridement and oral hygiene measures.

In the figure legends, *‡ denotes the same patient.

DENTAL CARIES

Caries (Figs. 30.1–30.8) Dental caries, or tooth decay, is an infectious disease—specifically, a bacterial infection that results in demineralization and damage to the mineralized structures of teeth. The process requires four components: dental plaque, diet, tooth structure, and time. The process begins with the accumulation of plaque biofilm that contains acid-producing bacteria (*Streptococcus mutans, Actinomyces viscosus, Lactobacillus species,* and *Streptococcus sanguis*). Plaque biofilm, when exposed to food substrates that contain fermentable carbohydrate, creates an environment for the bacteria to produce lactic acid. The acid causes electrochemical changes and the outflow of calcium and phosphate ions from the mineralized portion of the tooth. High consumption of, and repeated exposures to, sugary foods and starches is contributory to the carious demineralization and destruction of the organic matrix. In contrast, diets rich in dairy products, fish, meats, and polyphenols are caries preventive.

Demineralization caused by caries requires a drop in pH—a process triggered by exposure to sugary foods. Carbonated drinks are also contributory, because the acid in the soft drink lowers mouth pH rapidly. Enamel will begin to demineralize at pH 5.5 and below. Demineralization of dentin requires a drop in pH to 6.0. Saliva buffers the oral cavity and teeth and helps to keep the pH above 6. Thus, factors that stimulate saliva are protective against caries. Chewing sugarless gum that contains xylitol is anticaries, primarily because it uses a nonfermentable sugar and stimulates salivary flow.

A carious lesion begins as enamel decalcification that appears clinically as a chalky white spot, line, or fissure. The initial lesion is termed **incipient caries.** Incipient caries is defined as a small lesion (area of demineralization) limited to the enamel (Fig. 30.3). As the lesion matures, it destroys enamel and spreads laterally along the **dentinoenamel junction (DEJ)**, through the dentin. Clinicians should understand that once caries reaches the dentin, the process tends to go more rapidly since dentin is softer than enamel, and dentin requires less in drop in pH to demineralize. If left untreated, eventually, the demineralization can spread downward through the dentin toward the pulp and jeopardize the health of the pulp.

The classic clinical features of a carious lesion are (1) color change (chalky white, brown, or black discoloration), (2) loss of hard tissue (cavitation), and (3) stickiness to the explorer tine. The color change is caused by decalcification of enamel, exposure of dentin, and demineralization and staining of dentin. Classic symptoms of caries are sensitivity to sweets, hot, and cold. These symptoms are generally absent with incipient lesions. Larger lesions that invade the dentin permit ingress of fluids into exposed dentinal tubules. The hydrostatic (pressure) changes are sensed by pulpal nerves that transmit signals to the trigeminal sensory complex, which results in the perception of pain.

Two types of caries are classified according to location: fissural and smooth surface. **Fissural caries** is the most common form. It occurs most often in deep fissures in the chewing surfaces of the posterior teeth. **Smooth surface caries** occurs at places that are protected from plaque biofilm removal, such as just below the interproximal contact, at the gingival margin, and along the root surface. Caries is subdivided into six classes according to anatomic location. Class I caries is fissural; the remaining five classes are smooth surface caries.

Management of caries is most effective when risk factors (i.e., plaque biofilm; diet; number of initial, prior, and active caries; number of restorations; level of fluoride exposure and oral hygiene; patient compliance; number of exposed root surfaces; and salivary flow) are assessed, plaque biofilm is reduced, cariogenic bacteria are eliminated, tooth remineralization is enhanced, and teeth are repaired based on lesion size, location, and esthetic requirements. Remineralization is accomplished by applying topical fluoride and saturated calcium solutions.

Class I Caries (Figs. 30.4–30.8) **Class I caries** is decay affecting the occlusal surface of a posterior tooth. It arises when bacteria invade a central pit, deep occlusal groove, or fissure, remain sheltered for months, and produce acid dissolution of enamel. Destruction of enamel and dentin permits the carious groove to enlarge, darken, and become soft. A small class I carious lesion is the size of the tip of a sharpened lead pencil and may exist beneath a stained fissure. Larger lesions can encompass the entire occlusal surface, leaving only a shell of facial or lingual enamel and a symptomatic tooth. The permanent first molar is the tooth most commonly affected with class I caries. This is because (1) the first molar is the earliest erupting posterior tooth, (2) many children eat candy and sugary foods, and (3) good oral hygiene habits are often not yet established in children. Current guidelines are to detect carious lesions by visual inspection of a dry tooth, bitewing radiographs (for a radiolucent shadow in the dentin beneath the occlusal enamel), and minimal examination with an explorer. Additional supplementary methods available to clinicians include the use of electric, laser, and light-emitting devices for caries detection.

Class I caries that are incipient or small can be remineralized with fluoride varnish application and sealants. Larger lesions require restoration using composite materials or amalgam. Caries can also develop in the lingual pit of maxillary incisors (Fig. 30.7) and around existing restorations resulting in **recurrent caries** (see Fig. 30.8). Patients who have caries should be advised of what constitutes a cariogenic diet and how to change dietary habits.

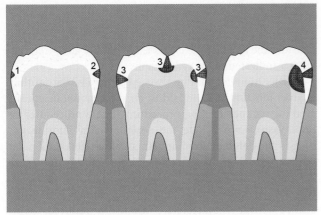

Fig. 30.1. Caries: stages of invasion illustrated.

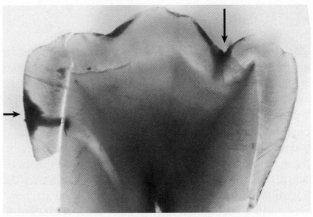

Fig. 30.2. Caries (*arrows*) invasion into dentin: histology.

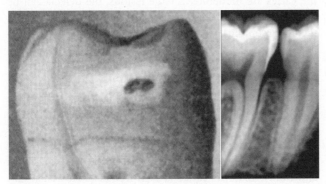

Fig. 30.3. Incipient caries.

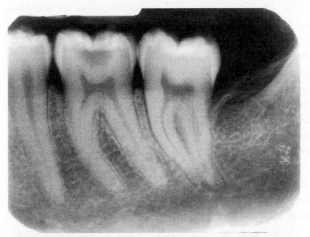

Fig. 30.4. Class I caries: below occlusal enamel first molar.

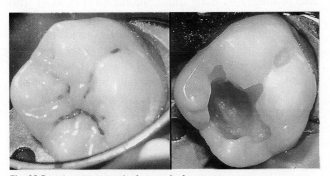

Fig. 30.5. Class I caries: before and after preparation.

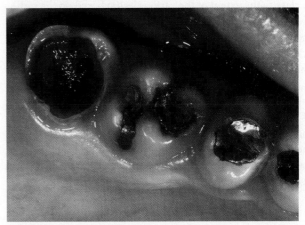

Fig. 30.6. Large class I caries: maxillary second molar.

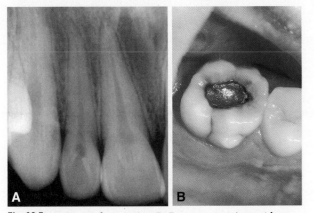

Fig. 30.7. A: Lingual pit caries. B: Recurrent caries: evident around restoration.

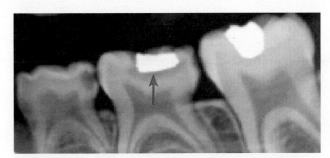

Fig. 30.8. Recurrent class I caries: primary mandibular second molar.

DENTAL CARIES

Class II Caries (Figs. 31.1–31.4) is a decay that affects the interproximal surface of a posterior tooth. These lesions are often difficult to identify clinically and require an astute eye; a clean, dry tooth surface; and a bitewing radiograph. One feature that may help in the clinical detection of class II caries is the appearance of decalcification (chalkiness or translucency) along the marginal ridge or a linear defect in the marginal ridge that is caused by hollowing of the subjacent dentin. Class II caries can occasionally be seen from the lingual or buccal aspect of the interproximal contact; however, small lesions would likely require tooth separation to see, or the use of radiographs.

The clinician is responsible for determining the presence and extent of a carious lesion. Since the class II caries lesion is difficult to assess by visual or tactile means, other methods should be employed. The most accepted method is by taking and viewing bitewing radiographs. The early incipient carious lesion appears as a triangular radiolucency in the enamel just below the contact point. The base of the triangle parallels the external aspect of the tooth, and the tip of the triangle points inward toward the dentin. As the lesion reaches dentin, it spreads along the DEJ and enlarges, making the lesion larger in the dentin than it is in the enamel. As the demineralization progresses, the caries advances toward the pulp and can cause death of the pulp. Of note, class II caries often occur in two adjacent teeth, so if a lesion is detected in one tooth, the adjacent tooth should be closely inspected.

Because caries is a progressive condition, it is important to classify the extent of the carious lesion based on the radiograph. A common classification scheme (see Fig. 30.1) uses the following categories: stage 0, no caries detected; stage 1, caries observed as a radiolucency in the outer half of the enamel; stage 2, caries observed as a radiolucency in the inner half of the enamel with no penetration of the DEJ; stage 3, caries observed as a radiolucency limited to the outer half of the dentin; and stage 4, caries observed as a radiolucency that extends more than halfway through the dentin toward the pulp. Use of a classification scheme is important for judging the severity of the caries and in helping to make clinical decisions regarding treatment. Also, clinicians should always consider the fact that the caries is often more advanced than what is indicated in the radiographs.

Small carious lesions that have not penetrated the dentino-enamel junction (i.e., limited to enamel) should be considered for remineralization procedures. These procedures are noninvasive and include the application of fluoride varnish to the demineralized area in an effort to reharden and remineralize the softened enamel. In moderate caries (stage 2, radiographic evidence of enamel penetration up to the DEJ without penetration into the dentin), remineralization can also be used if risk factors are minimal or reduced, lesions are closely monitored, and the patient is motivated to implement excellent oral hygiene. If several teeth are affected, custom-made fluoride trays and daily fluoride applications can be used to reduce the risk of caries progression. When the caries are moderate to large lesions, the defects can be restored with posterior composites, amalgam, transition metal (zirconium), or metal castings.

Class III Caries (Figs. 31.5–31.8) is a decay affecting the interproximal surface of an anterior tooth. Like class II interproximal caries, class III caries begins just below the contact point. Invasion results in triangular destruction of enamel and lateral spread into dentin. Interproximal caries (classes II and III) are common in persons who seldom floss their teeth and frequently consume sugar in beverages and candy. Class III caries is seen frequently in Asian and Native American persons who have prominent marginal ridges (shovel-shaped incisors). Class III caries is easier to diagnose than class II caries, because the interproximal space in anterior teeth is more readily visible. Class III lesions can also be diagnosed using transillumination (Fig. 31.6). This technique uses light applied from the facial or lingual side of the anterior teeth to demonstrate caries as a dark region within the enamel (or deeper) located below the interproximal contact point. Class III caries is more common in the maxillary incisors than the mandibular incisors. This is in part due to the position of the tongue and pooling of saliva around the mandibular incisors. Involvement of the mandibular incisors indicates high caries risk behavior.

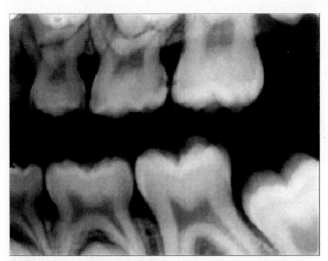

Fig. 31.1. **Interproximal class II caries:** maxillary molars.

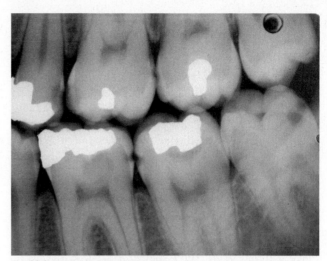

Fig. 31.2. **Class II caries:** posterior teeth.

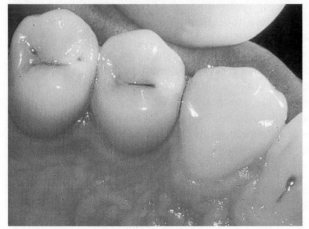

Fig. 31.3. **Caries: class II** mesial premolars.*

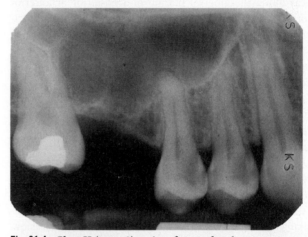

Fig. 31.4. **Class II (stage 3) caries of premolars.***

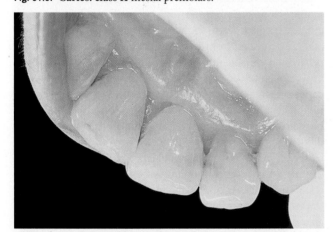

Fig. 31.5. **Class III caries:** between central and lateral.‡

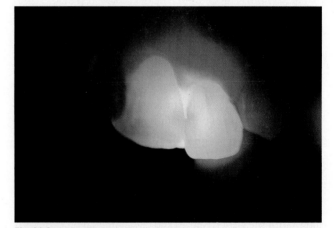

Fig. 31.6. **Transillumination:** demonstrates class III caries.‡

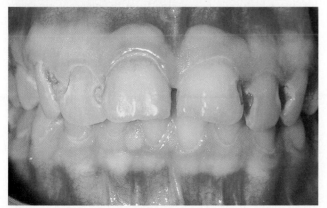

Fig. 31.7. **Class III caries:** centrals, laterals, and canines.

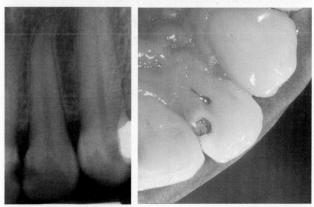

Fig. 31.8. **Class III caries:** lateral incisor.

Class IV Caries (Figs. 32.1 and 32.2) affects the interproximal surface and incisal line angle of an anterior tooth. It usually results when class III caries remains untreated, allowing the lesion to progress and undermine the dentin that supports the incisal line angle. As a result, loss of the enamel line angle occurs when the undermined enamel is traumatized by occlusion or chewing. **Class IV caries** is restored with bonded composite resins, providing excellent esthetics. Porcelain laminate veneers or zirconium restorations are also useful in select cases. Restorations have longer life spans when patients are educated about the causes of caries and make changes in behavior, and occlusal forces are minimized.

Class V Caries (Figs. 32.3 and 32.4) is characterized by decay along the gingival margin of a posterior or anterior tooth. Early signs of class V caries are chalky, white decalcification lines along the cervical portion of the tooth parallel to and just above the gingiva. Any dental plaque covering the lesion must be removed for adequate detection of the caries. With time, lesions enlarge mesially and distally, thereby producing an oval defect. As **class V caries** reaches interproximal regions, spread toward the contact point occurs, and the lesion becomes L-shaped. Patients with class V caries usually consume large amounts of sugary carbonated drinks, sip on such drinks for several hours during the day, or produce low amounts of saliva. Drugs and therapies that dry the mouth are contributing risk factors (see Figs. 94.1 and 94.2, **Meth Mouth**). Radiographically, class V caries should be distinguished from cervical burnout and toothbrush abrasion. In Figure 32.4, a typical class V lesion is present on the first premolar; the second premolar has recurrent decay beneath the amalgam restoration, and toothbrush abrasion is evident along the distal-cervical surface as a V-shaped radiolucent area. Smaller class V lesions can be treated with disking and fluoride varnish to remove either whitish or brownish stains without further treatment. Cavitated lesions require composite/glass ionomer resins or amalgam. Esthetic situations can require the use of porcelain-bonded laminate veneers.

Class VI Caries (Fig. 32.5) is characterized by decay of the incisal edge or cusp tip. This type of caries is uncommon but is more frequent in persons who chew sugary gums or consume sticky candy bars. Patients with low salivary flow are also predisposed to this type of caries. **Class VI caries**—along with the class III caries and class I lingual pit caries—is seen in the shovel-shaped incisor syndrome.

Root Caries (Figs. 32.6 and 32.7), also known as cemental caries, radicular caries, and senile caries, is decay that occurs on exposed root surfaces. It is detected more often on posterior teeth in older patients. The elderly are more commonly affected because they have increased prevalence of (1) gingival recession; (2) periodontal disease, altered interproximal contacts, and food impaction; and (3) hyposalivation. Root caries often starts at the cementoenamel junction on the interproximal surface and along the gingival margin of the root surface. Early on, it appears as a shallow, ill-defined, softened and discolored area that tends to extend more circumferentially than in depth. Examination with an explorer reveals a soft rubbery consistency. As the lesion progresses, the decay surrounds the root, leading to the crown fracturing off; this is called **amputation caries**. Progression is often fast because this region of the tooth has only a thin layer of enamel and dentin. Radiographically, root caries is seen in interproximal (buccal and lingual) areas below the cementoenamel junction, and although neither the contact point nor the enamel is involved, the caries can spread coronally under the enamel and deep toward the pulp. Root caries often recurs when root surfaces remain exposed, salivary flow remains low, and oral hygiene does not improve. Frequent prophylaxis and home daily applications of fluoride are often needed. Restorations are complicated by the fact that margins end on cementum, and often, there is little tooth structure remaining between the carious lesion and the pulp.

Recurrent Caries (Secondary Caries) (Fig. 32.8) is defined as decay within the immediate vicinity of a restoration. It may be a sign of high caries risk, poor oral hygiene, or a defective restoration. Recurrent caries begins at a failing (ditched or leaking) margin along the edge of a restoration. These defective margins are predisposed to the accumulation of bacteria and food and are protected from usual oral hygiene measures. Lesions progress at variable rates, appear stained or dark, and are soft to the touch of the explorer tine. Radiographically, recurrent caries presents in two ways. First, the decay may be seen as a radiolucent area beneath a restoration with or without a visibly defective margin beneath (see distal amalgam of the mandibular second premolar; Fig. 32.8). Second, the decay may be seen as one or several flame-shaped or arrow-shaped radiopaque areas occurring uniquely beneath an amalgam-type restorative material, with the point of the arrow directed toward or encroaching on the pulp. An associated radiolucent area is sometimes present as in this case. Spectroscopy studies have shown the radiopaque material represents softened dentin into which radiopaque zinc from the adjacent amalgam restoration has been leached. Recurrent caries are treated by removing the decay and repairing or replacing the restoration.

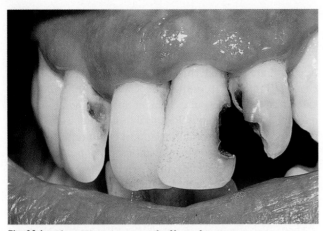

Fig. 32.1. Class IV caries: mesial of lateral incisor.

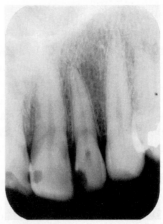

Fig. 32.2. Class IV caries: mesial of lateral; lingual caries.

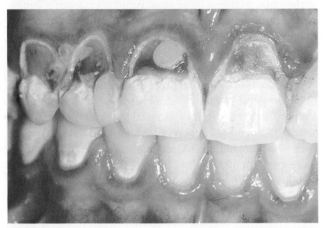

Fig. 32.3. Class V caries: maxillary anteriors.

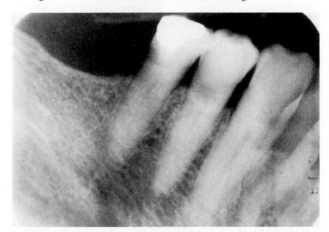

Fig. 32.4. Class V caries: first premolar.

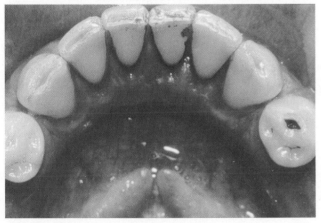

Fig. 32.5. Class VI caries: premolar cusp tip.

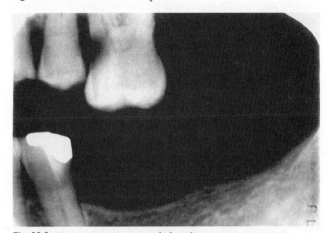

Fig. 32.6. Root caries: on extruded molar.

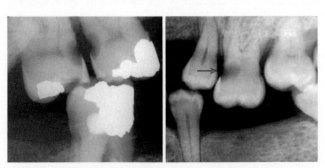

Fig. 32.7. Root caries: interproximal sites of molars.

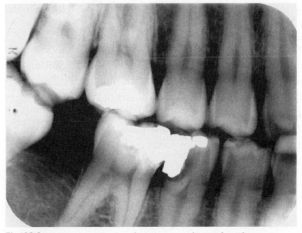

Fig. 32.8. Recurrent caries: lower premolar and molar.

73

DENTAL CARIES AND SEQUELAE

Caries Progression (Figs. 33.1–33.8) The invasion of caries may be a slow or fast process and may involve the pulp before the patient is aware of the lesion. In most cases, it takes several years for caries to reach the pulp. Some caries are particularly aggressive or have a unique cause. These caries have descriptive definitions. For example, **rampant caries** is a type of caries that develops at an extremely rapid pace in some children and young adults (see also "Meth Mouth," Fig. 94.1). **Radiation** or **amputation caries** occurs and progresses rapidly in patients who have received radiotherapy who lack the protective action of saliva. This caries appears along the gingival margin of teeth and can weaken teeth so severely that the crown fractures. **Root caries** has an appearance similar to that of radiation caries but is not associated with a history of radiation therapy. Rather, these patients usually have a history of xerostomia. Root caries progresses more slowly than radiation caries because xerostomia is less severe. **Nursing bottle caries** results from prolonged contact of primary teeth with sugar-containing liquids in the baby bottle in infants.

If caries is left untreated, the bacterial infection can progress through tooth dentin and produce pulpal inflammation. The initial stage of pulpal involvement, **reversible pulpitis**, is characterized by pulpal hyperemia and tooth sensitivity to hot and cold that dissipates when the temperature source is removed. Persistent pulpal inflammation produces irreversible changes, or **irreversible pulpitis**, in which the patient experiences spontaneous and persistent pain in the tooth after removal of the temperature source. Severe destruction of pulpal tissue from bacterial infection or interruption of the blood supply to the pulp produces a **nonvital pulp** and subsequent periapical changes (chronic periapical inflammation).

Prevention is the best way to reduce the incidence and progression of caries. Clinical examinations are provided at least twice a year to minimize the sequelae of caries. Bitewing radiographs should be taken at 6-month intervals in children if clinical caries is detected or the patient has a high risk for caries. Adults at high risk should receive bitewing radiographs annually. Sealants should be placed over deep fissures of posterior teeth in caries-susceptible youths. Remineralization products, such as fluoride, fluoride varnishes, and certain sugarless gums, are advocated to prevent caries. Pulp vitality should be tested when caries has invaded to or beyond 50% of the space between the DEJ and the pulp margin (stage 4 caries).

Pulp Polyp (Fig. 33.2) is an inflamed pulp resulting from chronic bacterial infection in which a red, nonpainful, soft tissue mass grows out of the affected pulp. Extensively carious primary molars and 6-year molars of young children are most frequently affected. Although the tooth is initially vital, the condition eventually erodes and results in nonvitality. Treatment is extraction or root canal therapy.

Periapical Inflammation (Figs. 33.4–33.6) and **apical periodontitis** are clinical terms used to describe the radiographic changes and clinical findings associated with inflammation extending from the pulp chamber into the adjacent periodontal ligament around the apical foramen of a chronically inflamed tooth. The condition is most commonly associated with pulpal degeneration (nonvital tooth) but may occur in vital teeth from occlusal trauma or constant and repetitive pressure placed on a tooth. Radiographs show a widening of the apical periodontal ligament space. The **chronic** form may be symptomatic or asymptomatic. In contrast, **acute periapical inflammation** is painful. Both conditions cause the apical periodontal ligament to be sensitive to percussion. Chronic periapical inflammation has chronic inflammatory cells at the periapex and often shows greater periradicular destruction of alveolar bone than acute periapical inflammation.

Periapical tissue produces three responses to the degradation products of a nonvital pulp: (1) a periapical granuloma, (2) a periapical cyst, or (3) an apical abscess. The granuloma and cyst originate from a nonvital tooth and both have a similar radiographic appearance (round radiolucency at the apex of a nonvital tooth), although the cyst tends to have more growth potential (i.e., larger). The distinction is made histologically. The **periapical granuloma**, the most common response, consists of an accumulation of granulation tissue, lymphocytes, plasma cells, histiocytes, and polymorphonuclear leukocytes (see Fig. 37.2). The **periapical cyst** arises from a pre-existing periapical granuloma when inflammation stimulates proliferation of periapical epithelial rests of Malassez (see Figs. 37.3–37.4). Regression of the inflammation occurs after root canal therapy in most cases.

Periapical (Apical) Abscess (Figs. 33.7 and 33.8) is the acute phase of an infection that spreads from a nonvital tooth through alveolar bone into the adjacent soft tissue. A **periapical abscess** is composed of neutrophils, macrophages, and necrotic debris. Clinical examination shows a red or reddish yellow, swollen nodule that is warm and fluctuant to the touch. The affected tooth is tender to percussion and slightly extruded and responds abnormally or not at all to heat, cold, and electric pulp testing. Radiographically, it appears as an irregular poorly defined periapical radiolucency without a radiopaque border. Abscesses can be drained by opening into the pulp chamber or incising the soft tissue swelling. An alternate treatment is tooth extraction, which provides an avenue for drainage. Antibiotics are used when the abscess is large and spreading, regional lymphadenopathy and fever are present, and drainage is not established. Penicillin VK is the antibiotic of choice. If the infection is unresponsive to penicillin or rapidly spreading, a bacterial culture and sensitivity should be obtained. Antibiotics are generally not needed if the affected tooth is extracted, adequate drainage is established, and the patient is otherwise healthy.

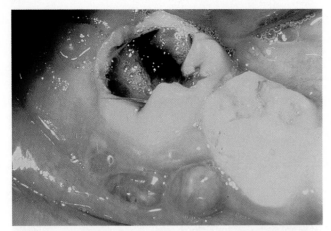

Fig. 33.1. **Extensive caries:** mandibular molar with parulis.

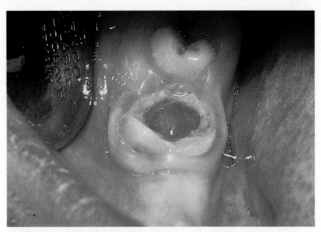

Fig. 33.2. **Pulp polyp:** red, exuberant mass arising from pulp.

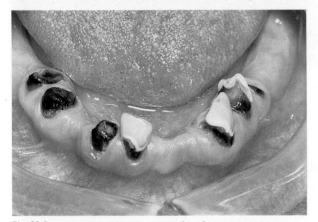

Fig. 33.3. **Rampant caries:** associated with xerostomia.

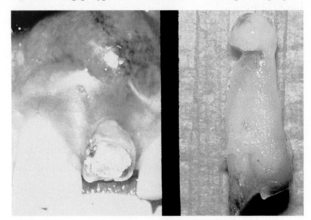

Fig. 33.4. **Periapical inflammation:** granuloma at apex.

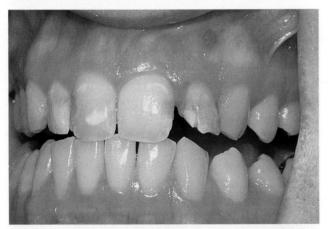

Fig. 33.5. **Periapical inflammation:** draining parulis from periapical inflammation of lateral incisor (tooth no. 10).*

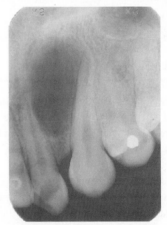

Fig. 33.6. **Periapical inflammation.***

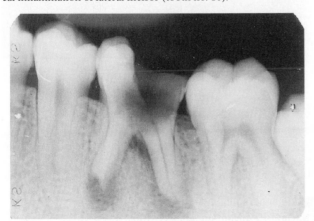

Fig. 33.7. **Caries, chronic periapical inflammation, abscess first molar.**‡

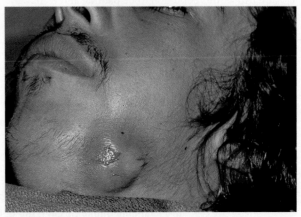

Fig. 33.8. **Abscess:** draining through mandible.‡

CASE 21. (FIG. 33.9)

This 14-year-old boy presents with this condition. He is unaware of the exact duration but remembers the tooth breaking off a few weeks ago. He has been chewing on the other side, but still little pieces seem to break off every few days. His mother wants to know what is going on, and can it be fixed?

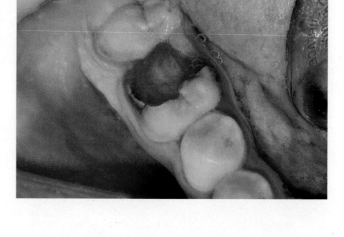

1. Describe the most prominent findings in this quadrant.

2. Is this a normal finding, a variant of normal, or disease?

3. Are caries evident in this quadrant? If so, which teeth have caries?

4. What could you do to make the clinical assessment more effective?

5. Which of the following actions should the dental hygienist consider first?
   A. Calculate his plaque score.
   B. Conduct a gingival index.
   C. Discuss with the dentist the need for x-rays.
   D. Recommend fluoride varnish.

6. The most likely diagnosis for the condition affecting the mandibular first molar is:
   A. Leukemic infiltrate
   B. Pyogenic granuloma
   C. Pulp polyp
   D. Irritation fibroma

7. Is the pulp vital?

8. What other features are apparent on the teeth in this quadrant, and what are they suggestive of?

CASE 22. (FIG. 33.10)

This young girl (Sally) presents with the condition shown in the clinical and radiographic image. She says that the inside of her mouth in this region has gotten larger during the last 2 days.

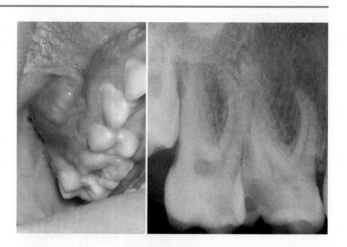

1. How old is this girl?

2. Describe the clinical findings in this quadrant, as well as the radiographic findings.

3. Is this a normal finding, a variant of normal, or disease?

4. Do you expect this condition to be painful, and if so, why?

5. The most likely diagnosis for the condition affecting the primary maxillary second molar is:
   A. Leukemic infiltrate
   B. Lipoma
   C. Pulp polyp
   D. Periapical abscess

6. Is this condition limited to the primary teeth?

7. What are the treatment options for this tooth?

8. How would you communicate with this patient and her parent?

Additional cases to enhance your learning and understanding of this section are available Online through the book's Navigate 2 Advantage Access site.

Radiopaque and Radiolucent Lesions of the Jaws

Objectives:

- Define and identify common radiolucent, radiopaque, and mixed lesions of the jaws.
- Describe the common radiographic appearance of these lesions of the jaws.
- Recognize the causes and clinical features of these conditions.
- Use the diagnostic assessment process to distinguish similar-appearing anomalies of the jaws.
- Describe the consequences of disease progression with respect to jaw cysts and tumors.
- Recommend appropriate treatments for these anomalies.
- Identify conditions discussed in this section that would affect the delivery of noninvasive and invasive dental procedures or need to be further evaluated by a specialist.

Exostoses are asymptomatic, bony outgrowths of the outer cortex of the mandible and maxilla. Specific types include mandibular tori, palatal tori, and reactive subpontine exostosis. The clinical and histologic features are discussed under "**Nodules**." All have a shell of cortical bone with various amounts of inner spongy (cancellous) bone. They occur on buccal, lingual, or crestal alveolar bone as rounded bony nodules. Exostoses appear as dense, round radiopacities; thus, they appear light on radiographs.

Mandibular Tori (Fig. 34.1) are exostoses on the lingual alveolar bone adjacent to the premolars and canines, and sometimes molars. They are developmental outgrowths that occur in 10% of the population. Most show a hereditary pattern. Sizes range from 0.5 to 1.5 cm in diameter; however, they can slowly increase in size throughout life (see Figs. 80.5 and 80.6). They appear as bilateral, focal, uniformly dense radiopacities with single or multiple lobes in the mandibular anterior and premolar periapical radiographs and occlusal and panoramic views. In periapical images, they are often superimposed on the roots of the teeth. The bosselated types appear as separate rounded or ovoid radiopacities with a smooth outline.

Palatal Tori (Fig. 34.2) are common bony hard masses that arise from the midline of the hard palate. These developmental and usually hereditary exostoses occur in 15% of the population, more often in women. Most appear as dome-shaped midline protuberances, but flat, nodular, spindle, and lobular variants exist (see Fig. 63.1). They consist of dense lamellar, cortical bone that can slowly increase in size. Typically, they are painless unless the overlying thin mucosa is traumatized. Radiographically, they appear as a focal, homogeneously dense radiopacity in the palatal region of maxillary anterior or posterior periapical radiographs and panoramic views. No treatment is required, unless desired for prosthetic reasons.

Osteoma (Figs. 34.3 and 34.4) is a benign tumor composed of compact or cancellous bone. These bony hard masses arise in limited locations restricted to the craniofacial skeleton and rarely appear within soft tissue. Most appear in the posterior mandible or condyle as bony hard masses that arise from a polypoid or sessile base. When they extend beyond the confines of the parent bone, they are termed **peripheral osteoma**. Those confined within bone are known as **central osteoma**. The site of origin may be **periosteal** (lining of the cortex) or **endosteal** (from cancellous bone). They are generally painless and slow growing. Radiographically, they appear as a sclerotic mass of the same density as cortex. The borders are smooth, well defined, and rounded. Histologically, they appear identical to tori and exostoses. Peripheral osteomas are often removed for cosmetic and/or prosthetic reasons.

Central osteomas usually are not removed unless there is extensive asymmetry or interference with function. Multiple osteomas may be a sign of **Gardner syndrome** (Figs. 20.7 and 20.8).

Reactive Subpontine (Hyperostosis) Exostosis (Fig. 34.5) is a reaction of crestal alveolar bone to the presence and occlusion of a mandibular fixed partial denture pontic. They occur in men twice as often as women, most after 40 years of age and most in the mandibular molar-premolar region within 10 years of prosthesis placement. They have mild growth potential and can enlarge beneath the pontic, causing the overlying tissue to become red or inflamed or even to dislodge the bridge. Radiographically, they appear as a conelike dense radiopacity or broad-based opacity that completely fills the edentulous space. The radiographic margin is smooth and well defined. A corticated margin may or may not be present. Regression occurs when the bridge is removed.

Retained Roots (Root Fragments or Root Tips) (Figs. 34.6 and 34.7) are remnants of roots of teeth that are retained in the alveolar bone. In children, root tips occur often in the premolar-molar region when a portion of the primary molar root fails to resorb and is retained after the primary tooth exfoliates. Primary molar root tips are often 1 to 4 mm in length and apically tapered. Treatment depends on location. If the primary tooth root tip can be removed easily, it is often recommended to be removed. However, very small, deeply located primary root tips can be left to resorb on their own.

Permanent tooth roots can also be retained but for different reasons. These root tips are usually observed when a tooth is traumatized (fractured) or the crown of the tooth is severely broken down due to caries. Single- or multirooted teeth can display retained roots. Characteristics of retained roots include a root-like structure with the density of dentin and a centrally located pulp chamber, variable size—but consistent in size with a root in that anatomic location—and tapering of the radiopacity in the apical direction. The periodontal ligament surrounds the outline of retained root(s); the lamina dura may or may not be evident.

Socket Sclerosis (Fig. 34.8) is an asymptomatic, reactive lesion that occurs after tooth extraction. It is commonly associated with systemic disease involving calcium metabolism (gastrointestinal [malabsorption] and kidney disease). Most cases occur in the mandible after 40 years of age. There is no sex or racial predilection. Radiographically it is characterized by (1) lack of resorption of the lamina dura, which usually resorbs 6 to 16 weeks after tooth extraction and (2) deposition of sclerotic bone within the confines of the socket. Multiple root sites may be affected. This condition does not require treatment, and the sclerosis persists after the systemic health issue resolves.

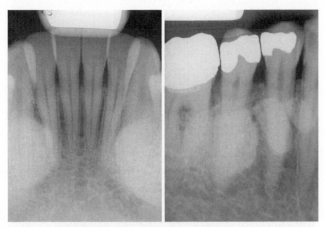

Fig. 34.1. **Mandibular tori:** typical locations.

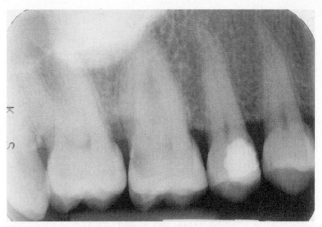

Fig. 34.2. **Palatal torus:** large rounded radiopacity.

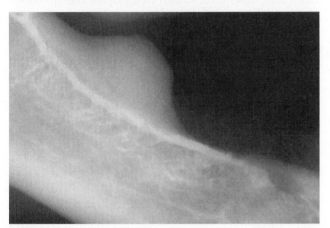

Fig. 34.3. **Osteoma:** posterior mandible; dense throughout.

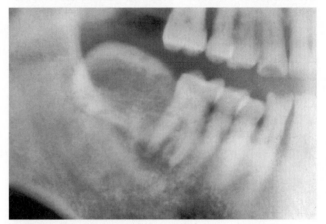

Fig. 34.4. **Osteoma:** posterior mandible; denser peripherally.

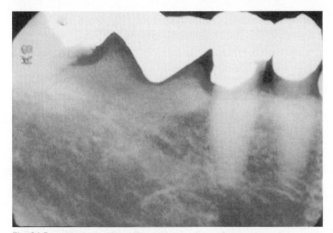

Fig. 34.5. **Reactive subpontine exostosis:** under pontic.

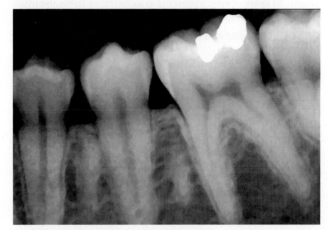

Fig. 34.6. **Primary molar root fragments.**

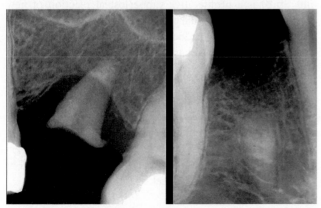

Fig. 34.7. **Retained root fragments.**

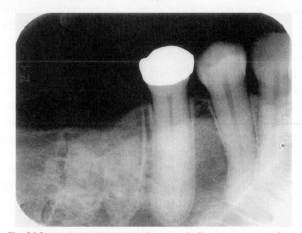

Fig. 34.8. **Socket sclerosis:** molar area; bulbous root premolar.

6

Idiopathic Osteosclerosis (Enostosis) (Fig. 35.1) is bone deposition within marrow spaces of the jaws. There is no racial or sex predilection and no inflammatory or infectious cause. Most lesions are in the mandible in the premolar-molar area. They appear as radiopaque densities or foci (55% of cases) at or near the apex of a tooth, in interradicular areas (28%), and distant to teeth (17%). When near teeth, the teeth are always vital (confirmed by vitality testing), and the apical periodontal membrane space is normal or rarely obliterated by the opaque bone. No treatment is required.

Condensing Osteitis (Figs. 35.2 and 35.3) is a proliferative reaction of dense bone deposited within marrow spaces of the jaws in response to pulpitis or pulpal necrosis. It is more common in persons younger than 20 years. Affected teeth are usually asymptomatic but are dying. Most lesions are in the mandibular molar region and appear as a densely radiopaque area (sclerotic bone) localized to the apex of a tooth root, with widening of the apical periodontal membrane space. Often, there is carious involvement of the pulp, or a large restoration or crown. Although the radiographic appearance is similar to periapical idiopathic osteosclerosis, the associated tooth is nonvital. Root canal therapy or extraction is recommended for the nonvital tooth. About 85% of cases regress, either partially or fully after therapy.

Cementoblastoma (Fig. 35.4) is a slow-growing benign neoplasm of cementum and cementoblasts seen usually between 10 and 30 years of age. It presents as a central radiopaque mass fused to the root of a tooth with an outer well-circumscribed, corticated circular radiolucency. The tooth is usually a vital permanent mandibular first molar or lower premolar. The lesion markedly attaches itself to the root apex, is expansile, and may cause pain. Root resorption is often present, or the root is obscured by the mass. Treatment involves surgical extraction of the tooth and attached lesion.

Osteoblastoma (Fig. 35.5) is a benign tumor of compact or cancellous bone that preferentially occurs in the spine, long bones, and small bones of hands and feet. Only about 15% appear in the skull and jaws. Jaw lesions are more common in the posterior mandible and more often appear in adolescent men. The lesion consists of plump proliferating osteoblasts and osteoid and well-vascularized connective tissue. The osteoid undergoes varying degrees of mineralization, and the mass measures generally more than 1.5 cm in diameter. Lesions appear as radiolucent, radiopaque, or radiolucent-radiopaque circular masses, located centrally within bone or arising from the cortex. Most are slow-growing round radiodensities that respond to conservative excision. Pain and swelling are common features. A small percentage display aggressive behavior.

Cemento-Osseous Dysplasia is a group of benign fibro-osseous lesions that are separated based on the extent of jaw involvement (i.e., **periapical, florid,** or **focal**). Each progresses through three radiographic stages: (1) an early osteoporotic phase (radiolucent), (2) a mixed radiolucent/radiopaque lesion, and (3) a radiopaque lesion surrounded by a thin radiolucent rim. Because this condition is progressive and exhibits both radiolucent and radiopaque features, we discuss this disease here on this page as well as in Unilocular Radiolucencies.

Periapical Cemento-Osseous Dysplasia (Periapical Cemental Dysplasia, Cementoma) (Figs. 39.1 and 39.2) is an asymptomatic fibro-osseous disorder that by definition associates with the apex of a tooth. It is seen almost uniquely in middle-aged black women. Lesions are mixed radiolucent/radiopaque, occur usually in multiples, and are associated with the apices of *vital* anterior mandibular teeth. Three distinct stages occur. In stage I, the alveolar bone demonstrates periapical radiolucencies. Stage II (cementoblastic stage) has circumscribed radiolucencies with small internal calcific spherules. In stage III (mature stage), lesions have a central radiopaque mass surrounded by a radiolucent border yielding a "target" appearance. The radiolucent border helps distinguish these lesions from an osteoma and fibrous dysplasia. Treatment is not required.

Focal cemento-osseous dysplasia is a type of cemento-osseous dysplasia that exhibits a single site of involvement. It typically produces one *target-like* mixed radiopaque-radiolucent lesion, less than 1.5 cm in diameter. It predominantly affects women and the posterior mandible. Treatment is not required.

Florid Cemento-Osseous Dysplasia (Fig. 35.6) is a diffuse variant of periapical cemental dysplasia that demonstrates multiple involvement of the apices of the posterior teeth in bilateral quadrants. It is found predominantly in middle-aged and older black women. Lesions progress through three stages (as described above), with the production of large cemental masses that coalesce. Lesions tend to grow inferiorly and laterally and coalesce after tooth extractions. Focal mild expansion is occasionally described, but pain is typically absent. Complications include the presence of simple bone cysts, infection, and discomfort. Trauma can induce ulcers and bony sequestration. Surgical intervention and antibiotics may speed healing.

Garre Osteomyelitis (Periostitis Ossificans) (Figs. 35.7 and 35.8) is a proliferative subperiosteal reaction of new bone that forms secondary to inflammation and infection. The most common jaw location is the posterior mandible in a young patient who has an infected tooth. Other causes include periodontal disease, bone fracture, an unerupted tooth, or tumor. This form of osteomyelitis classically produces mandibular swelling, facial asymmetry, and pain. Radiographically, the new bone is laid down in layers under the periosteum producing dense bone that if imaged at an oblique angle shows an *onion layer* appearance with fine perpendicular lines intersecting them. Treatment is removal of the source of infection and weeks of antibiotics.

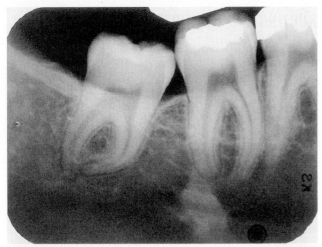

Fig. 35.1. **Idiopathic osteosclerosis:** vital second molar.

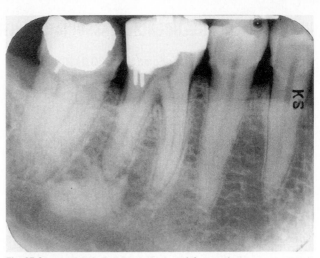

Fig. 35.2. **Condensing osteitis:** nonvital first molar.

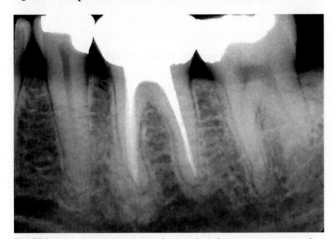

Fig. 35.3. **Condensing osteitis:** first molar after recent root canal therapy.

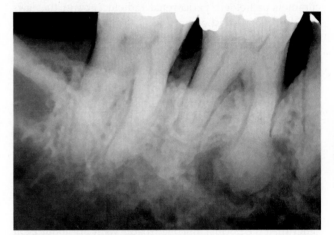

Fig. 35.4. **Cementoblastoma.**

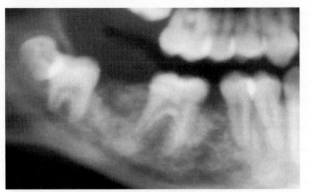

Fig. 35.5. **Osteoblastoma** surrounding mandibular first molar.

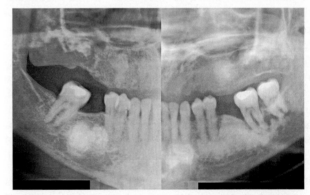

Fig. 35.6. **Florid cemento-osseous dysplasia:** all four quadrants affected.

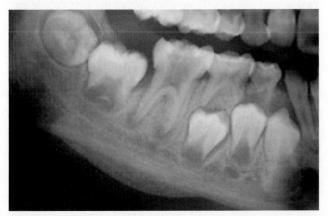

Fig. 35.7. **Garre osteomyelitis:** onion skin appearance.

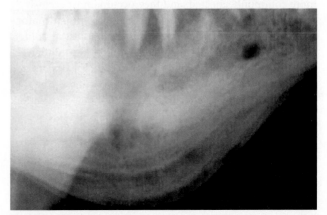

Fig. 35.8. **Garre osteomyelitis:** onion skin appearance.

Eruption Cyst (Eruption Hematoma) (Fig. 36.1) is a soft tissue cyst surrounding and overlying the crown of an unerupted tooth. It is a variant of the dentigerous cyst. Infants and young children under 10 years of age are most commonly affected (Fig. 15.5). It appears as a small, bluish, dome-shaped, translucent swelling on the gingiva overlying an erupting primary tooth. The **eruption cyst** is lined by odontogenic epithelium and is filled with blood or serum, which casts a red, brown, or blue-gray appearance to the cyst. No treatment is necessary because the erupting tooth eventually breaks the cystic membrane. Incising the lesion and allowing the fluid to drain can relieve symptoms.

Dentigerous (Follicular) Cyst (Figs. 36.2–36.4) is the most common pathologic pericoronal radiolucency in the jaws and the second most common jaw cyst after the periapical cyst. It arises from remnants of **reduced enamel epithelium** (sulcular epithelium) around the crown of an unerupted or impacted tooth. The remnants undergo cystic degeneration, and then, fluid accumulates within the central portion of the lesion. The **dentigerous cyst** occurs around erupting teeth; thus, the majority develop in persons under age 20 years. The dentigerous cyst classically consists of a well-corticated pericoronal radiolucency that is attached to the tooth at the cervical margin. It is called a **primordial cyst** when a tooth, typically a third molar, fails to develop; however, the cyst remains. Histologically, the dentigerous cyst appears similar to the normal follicular sac but produces a larger radiolucency than the normal follicular space. Many are about 2 cm in size but can expand to become very large and fill the body or ramus of the mandible. Most occur in the mandibular third molar region; however, maxillary dentigerous cysts are common. Most lesions are unicystic, but some are multilocular; and in the latter case, the locules tend to be large with the septa forming only partial cavities. The margins are well corticated unless infection is present, and buccal expansion is possible. The associated tooth may be displaced, unerupted, or impacted. The pressure of the cyst can resorb the roots of adjacent teeth. A dentigerous cyst can give rise to an **ameloblastoma, squamous cell carcinoma**, or **mucoepidermoid carcinoma**. Thus, tooth extraction and excision are essential.

Inflammatory Paradental Cyst (Figs. 36.5 and 36.6) is a variant odontogenic cyst that arises because of inflammation in the infected follicle around an erupting tooth. Males are more commonly affected, and they occur almost exclusively around an erupting mandibular molar. The **inflammatory paradental cyst** arises because of inflammation and proliferation of the follicular epithelium and remains firmly attached to the cementoenamel junction of the tooth. The mixed inflammatory infiltrate found in the wall lining of the cyst causes a hard bony swelling and localized bone destruction.

Symptoms include pain, swelling, and pus discharge and usually develop within 1 year of the expected eruption time of the affected tooth. If a third molar is affected, then trismus may also accompany the condition. When the condition is localized to the buccal region of a mandibular first or second molar, it is often termed a **buccal bifurcation cyst**. Radiographically, a 1- to 2-cm well-defined pericoronal unilocular radiolucency is seen below and above the CEJ of an erupting molar. The cyst is often displaced to one side, its margins are thin and sclerotic, and often, the crown of the affected tooth is tilted causing prominence of the lingual cusps. In the occlusal or cone-beam radiographic view, the root tips appear to be in close contact with the endosteal surface or even within the lingual cortex. A buccal periosteal reaction is seen in the majority of cases. Treatment is conservative cystectomy without extraction of the vital tooth.

Keratocystic Odontogenic Tumor (KCOT; Fig. 36.7) is a benign but destructive odontogenic tumor, previously called an **odontogenic keratocyst (OKC)**. This cystic neoplasm arises from remnants of the dental lamina and is defined by its histologic appearance. Most begin as a unilocular radiolucency in a location where a tooth (e.g., third molar) fails to develop. The molar region is the most common site and young men (10 to 30 years of age) are more frequently affected. Although many **KCOT** become multilocular radiolucencies, over time, they tend to remain asymptomatic. The margins are smooth, corticated, and often scalloped. Internally, some septa and a cloudy lumen (representing desquamated keratin) are seen. They have remarkable growth potential, and bony erosion tends to occur anteroposteriorly within the medullary bone. Histologically, the cystic epithelium is uniform, 8 to 10 cell layers thick, and **parakeratinized**. After excision, the recurrence rate is about 30%.

Nevoid Basal Cell Carcinoma Syndrome (Gorlin-Goltz Syndrome) (Fig. 36.8) This syndrome is transmitted by a single autosomal dominant gene; thus, male and females are affected equally. The syndrome is characterized by multiple jaw KCOTs, basal cell nevi on the skin, skeletal anomalies (bifid and other rib anomalies, hypertelorism), and soft tissue anomalies (prominent finger pads and palmar pitting of the hands). The skin nevoid lesions may be pink, pale brown, or dark brown and vary from 1 to 10 mm. The unilocular radiolucent jaw KCOTs develop during the first decade and peak during the second and third decades. They typically are bilateral, involving both jaws, and often displace teeth. The jaw tumors associated with this syndrome have a higher recurrence rate than solitary KCOTs and should be treated by complete removal. Periodic monitoring for the development of recurrent lesions is advised.

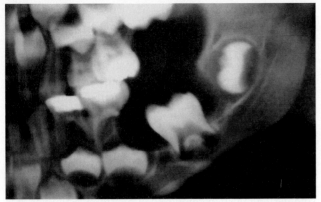

Fig. 36.1. Eruption cyst.

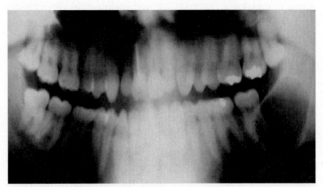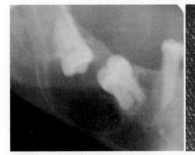

Fig. 36.2. Dentigerous cyst.

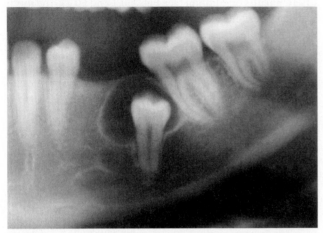

Fig. 36.3. **Dentigerous cyst** in mandibular premolar location.

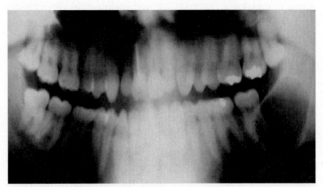

Fig. 36.4. **Primordial cyst** and missing third molar.

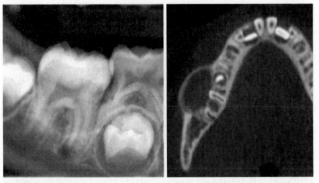

Fig. 36.5. Inflammatory paradental (buccal bifurcation cyst).

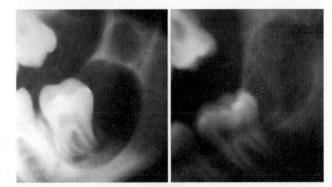

Fig. 36.6. Inflammatory paradental (buccal bifurcation cyst).

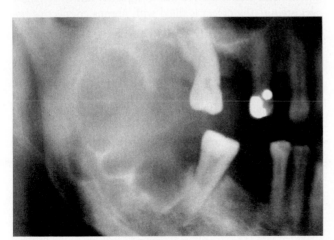

Fig. 36.7. **Keratocystic odontogenic tumor.**

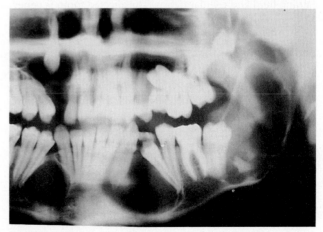

Fig. 36.8. **Nevoid basal cell carcinoma:** multiple OKCs.

6

Mental Foramen (Fig. 37.1) The mental foramen is a normal anatomic structure that should be distinguished from the pathologic radiolucencies discussed on this page.

Periapical Granuloma (Fig. 37.2) is a localized area of chronically inflamed granulation tissue that forms at the apex of a nonvital tooth. The process develops as bacteria, necrotic tissue, and toxins exit the pulp canal. The host sensing these toxins sets up an inflammatory defense reaction in an attempt to eliminate the noxious substances. There is no epithelial lining, but instead a fibrous connective tissue outer wall. The tooth often is asymptomatic and does not respond to vitality tests. However, the tooth can become painful or sensitive to pressure or percussion if the inflammatory reaction becomes acute. Note that the term **periapical granuloma** is generally reserved for the histological description of the tissue once the tooth is extracted and the associated inflammatory mass is examined under the microscope. In contrast, a periapical granuloma is often called **chronic apical periodontitis** when seen radiographically. The radiographic appearance is a well-circumscribed radiolucency of varying size—depending on its chronicity and the ability of the host to defend against the necrotic process. The associated tooth generally has a large carious lesion, a large restoration, or evidence of endodontic therapy. Early lesions show widening or slight thickening of the periodontal ligament space and loss of the lamina dura along the periapex of the root. Mature lesions tend to advance slowly upward along the root and expand uniformly in all directions producing a well-circumscribed circular periapical lesion that is 2 to 10 mm in size that lacks a radiopaque border.

Periapical Cyst (Figs. 37.3 and 37.4), also known as a **radicular cyst**, is the most common cyst of the jaws. It is a reaction to a nonvital tooth that results in the stimulation of an epithelial-lined inflammatory cavity at the site of the root apex. The epithelium that reacts arises from the root region and generally is from the rests of Malassez, which are remnants of Hertwig root sheath. As the lesion expands in size—typically at the periapex—the nutritional support for the inner cells diminishes resulting in central necrosis, thus forming an epithelial-lined cavity with the inner lumen containing fluid and cellular debris. The affected tooth is generally asymptomatic but can become tender or symptomatic if the area becomes acutely inflamed. Radiographically, a **periapical cyst** may be distinguished from a periapical granuloma. While both show loss of lamina dura and have the potential to enlarge, the periapical cyst tends to be larger (greater than 1 cm in diameter) and tends to have a thin radiopaque margin. On an occasion, a periapical cyst may occur lateral to the tooth root from inflammation exiting a lateral/accessory pulp canal. In this case, the entity is called a **lateral radicular cyst**. Treatment of the periapical granuloma and the periapical cyst requires elimination of the infection through root canal therapy or extraction. If extraction is performed, then the socket should be curetted to remove the granuloma or cyst.

Chronic Apical Abscess (Fig. 37.5) is a long-standing, low-grade inflammatory reaction that arises as a result of pulpal death. In contrast to the "acute" periapical abscess discussed under Figures 33.7 to 33.8, the chronic apical abscess is a smoldering infection composed of neutrophils and pus. It is often associated with a draining sinus tract, which is referred to as a **parulis** or gumboil (see Figs. 50.1 and 50.2). The tooth is typically asymptomatic, unless drainage is inadequate and pressure builds up. Radiographically, the chronic apical abscess produces a periapical radiolucency that can appear less dense than a granuloma or cyst. Also, the border can be a bit diffuse. These lesions heal after adequate root canal treatment.

Postextraction Socket (Fig. 37.6) is an easily recognized radiolucent region where a tooth root used to be. They appear on a radiograph during the first 12 months after a tooth is extracted. As the socket heals, the lamina dura disappears first (within about 6 weeks), and then, the area fills in with bone trabeculae and marrow. The lamina dura is generally seen as a feint rim around the radiolucent extraction site. In most instances, the extraction socket heals completely between 9 and 15 months; however, in cases of chronic kidney disease, the postextraction socket can persist.

Residual Cyst (Fig. 37.7A) is a remnant epithelial-lined cyst seen in an edentulous area after tooth extraction because some or all of the periapical cyst was left behind. The radiographic appearance is a round or oval well-circumscribed radiolucency several millimeters below the alveolar ridge, at an extraction site where the root apex used to be. The cyst is lined by squamous epithelium and appears similar histologically to the periapical cyst. Treatment is excision.

Apical Scar (Fibrous Scar or Fibrous Healing Defect) (Figs. 37.7B and 37.8) is a localized region where a periapical inflammatory lesion fails to heal completely due to damaged periosteum. The defect is filled with fibrous connective tissue and involves both the buccal and lingual cortical plates. A history of a surgical extraction, apicoectomy, injury, or bony fracture is common. The nonossified region is invariably asymptomatic and can occur at any age. Most defects are less than 5 mm in diameter. They appear as a well-circumscribed dark radiolucency with no evidence of trabeculation within the lesion. If the defect is associated with an extraction site, they generally appear punched-out with a well-defined margin in an edentulous area. No treatment is required.

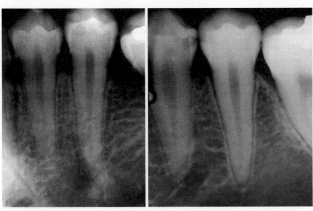

Fig. 37.1. **Mental foramen:** to be distinguished from periapical radiolucency.

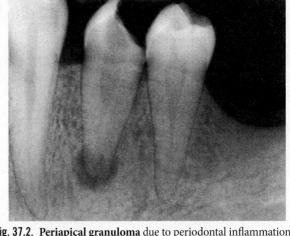

Fig. 37.2. **Periapical granuloma** due to periodontal inflammation.

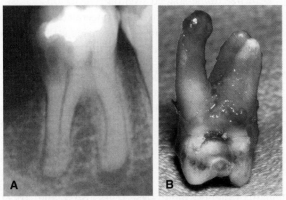

Fig. 37.3. **Periapical cyst** due to (A) pulpal disease and (B) fracture.

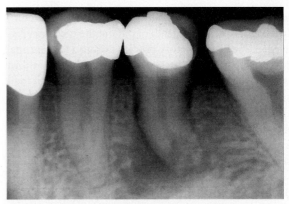

Fig. 37.4. **Periapical cyst** due to periodontal disease.

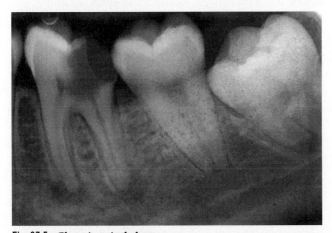

Fig. 37.5. **Chronic apical abscess.**

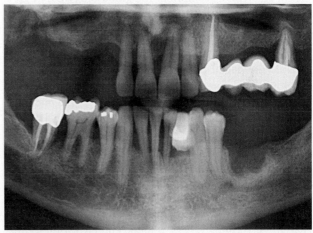

Fig. 37.6. **Molar extraction socket.**

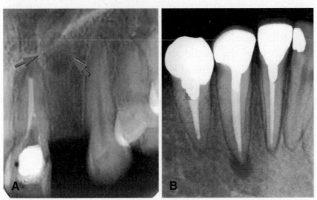

Fig. 37.7. A: Residual cyst. B: Apical/fibrous scar.

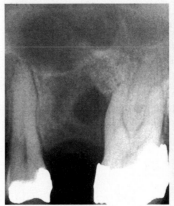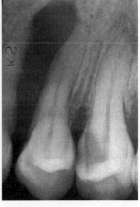

Fig. 37.8. **Fibrous healing defects.**

85

Interradicular unilocular radiolucencies are frequently inflammatory or neoplastic conditions that arise from the lateral aspects of teeth or the epithelial, mesenchymal, or osseous structures or remnants found between the teeth. The most common epithelial-associated condition found in the interradicular space is a **cyst**. These abnormal epithelial-lined saclike (often fluid-filled) pathologic cavities develop commonly in the jaws when epithelial remnants of developing or erupted teeth or embryonic structures undergo cystic degeneration. Jaw cysts tend to be asymptomatic and slow growing. They are classified as developmental, odontogenic, inflammatory, and pseudocysts (not epithelium lined) and appear as unilocular or multilocular radiolucencies. Multilocular types are aggressive and more likely to recur.

Globulomaxillary Cyst (Fig. 38.1) is a cyst that most commonly arises as a result of death of pulp of the maxillary lateral incisor. The inflammatory process exiting a lateral canal or periapex of the incisor results in a well-defined oval or pear-shaped radiolucency between the maxillary lateral incisor and maxillary canine. Close inspection will often show a lateral incisor with a dens in dente or a deep lingual pit with caries that has resulted in death of the incisor. This cyst produces a lesion about 1 cm in diameter that is interradicular, has well-defined border, and generally contacts the lower one third of the lateral root surface of the lateral incisor (also see Fig. 33.6). Larger lesions can cause divergence of the adjacent tooth roots. Endodontic treatment of the affected lateral incisor resolves the condition. The **globulomaxillary cyst** is no longer recognized as a separate entity; however, it does remain as a clinical descriptive term for a periapical cyst uniquely found in this location.

Lateral Periodontal Cyst (Fig. 38.2) is a small, well-defined developmental nonkeratinizing odontogenic cyst that develops lateral to a tooth root, commonly in the premolar-canine region. It arises from proliferation of epithelial rests of dental lamina and occurs mostly in the mandible in men between 40 and 70 years. The **lateral periodontal cyst** generally appears as a small (less than 5-mm) corticated radiolucency that contacts the mid- and coronal portion of the root. The adjacent teeth are vital. It has two variants: the **gingival cyst of the adult** and the botryoid lateral periodontal cyst (Fig. 40.1). The gingival cyst is found entirely within soft tissue (Fig. 11.8). Gingival and lateral periodontal cysts rarely recur after excision.

Median Mandibular Cyst (Fig. 38.3) is a clinical term that describes a rare odontogenic cyst uniquely located in the midline of the mandible, seen overlying the apices of the mandibular central incisors or between the roots of these teeth at the midline. It can develop from (1) an inflammatory cyst arising from a lateral accessory root canal, (2) an odontogenic keratocyst, (3) a lateral periodontal cyst, or (4) a residual cyst. The radiolucency it produces is variable in size

and can extend to encompass the posterior teeth. Treatment involves assessing for a nonvital mandibular incisor and endodontic therapy, or if all teeth test vital, biopsy to disclose the cause.

Incisive Canal Cyst (Nasopalatine Duct Cyst) (Fig. 38.4) is a developmental cyst arising from entrapped epithelium in the incisive canal. Radiographically, it produces a classic heart-shaped radiolucency that is at least 1 cm in diameter located between the roots of vital maxillary central incisors arising from within the incisive canal(s). It is described more under "**Swellings of the Palate**," Figures 63.3 and 63.4. A soft tissue variant of the incisive canal cyst is the **cyst of the incisive papilla** (Fig. 31.1). It occurs within the incisive papilla as a slow-growing, dome-shaped swelling. Occlusion against the lesion can cause it to appear red or ulcerated. Mastication-associated pain may be a symptom. Excision is the treatment of choice. Recurrence is rare.

Median Palatal Cyst (Fig. 38.5) is a clinical term that describes a well-defined posteriorly located nasopalatine duct cyst. The **median palatal cyst** is unilocular and evenly distributed in the midline of the palate. The cyst is lined with stratified squamous epithelium and has a fibrous connective tissue boundary. Treatment is removal and recurrence is rare.

Traumatic (Simple) Bone Cyst (Figs. 38.6 and 38.7) is an empty intrabony cavitation that affects the jaws or long bones. It is a pseudocyst, as it lacks an epithelial lining. It is believed to arise after trauma, although a history of trauma is not required. About 60% occur in males. The average age of detection is 18 years. Most are asymptomatic, occur in the mandible molar-premolar area, and are radiolucent with a scalloping superior radiopaque margin extending between the roots of the teeth. The inferior margin is usually rounded. Adjacent teeth are generally vital, and mild cortical expansion may occur. The mesiodistal dimension is usually wider than the superior-inferior. The simple bone cyst regresses spontaneously or after curettage.

Squamous Odontogenic Tumor (Fig. 38.8) is a benign but destructive odontogenic tumor thought to arise from proliferation of the epithelial rests of Malassez. The tumor can occur at any age and is characterized by islands of stratified squamous epithelium in a fibrous connective tissue stroma. Most show a well-defined unilocular and triangular or semicircular radiolucency in the alveolar bone between the roots of teeth. These tumors tend to grow slowly, displace tooth roots, destroy the crestal alveolar bone, and produce a thin sclerotic scalloping apical rim. Clinically, the adjacent teeth commonly are mobile, and there is gum swelling and moderate pain. Multifocal lesions have been described, and maxillary tumors tend to be more aggressive. Surgical removal is recommended.

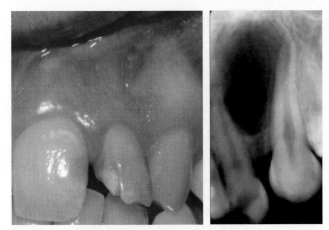

Fig. 38.1. Globulomaxillary cyst.

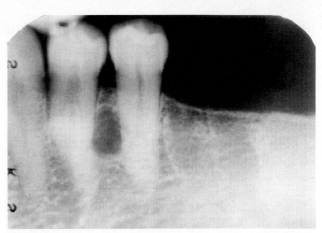

Fig. 38.2. Lateral periodontal cyst: common location and size.

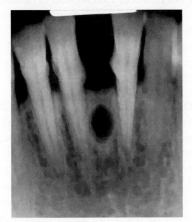

Fig. 38.3. Median mandibular cyst.

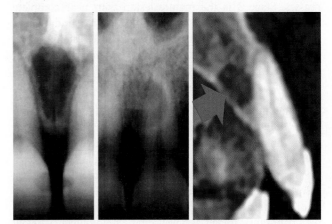

Fig. 38.4. Incisive canal cyst: Three different cases.

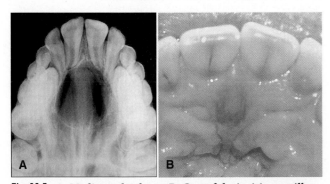

Fig. 38.5. A: Median palatal cyst. B: Cyst of the incisive papilla.

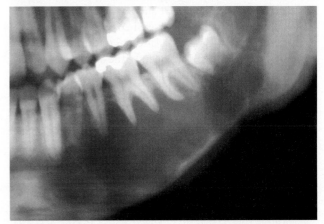

Fig. 38.6. Traumatic bone cyst.

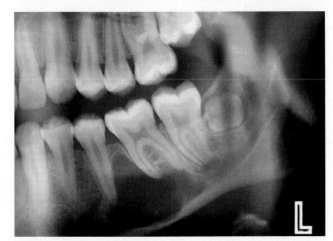

Fig. 38.7. Traumatic bone cyst.

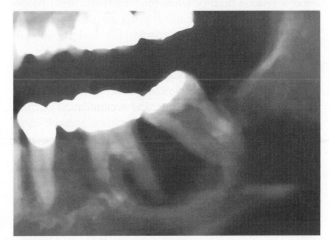

Fig. 38.8. Squamous odontogenic tumor.

6

87

Periapical Cemento-Osseous Dysplasia (Figs. 39.1 and 39.2)

is a benign fibro-osseous lesion resulting in cementum- and osseous-like deposition at and below the root apices of mandibular teeth. The condition is most common in black women over the age of 30 and only rarely affects maxillary teeth. Most cases of **periapical cemento-osseous dysplasia** involve the anterior mandibular teeth, which are asymptomatic and *vital upon pulp testing*. The condition generally produces multiple individual lesions and has three stages. The initial lesion (stage 1) produces well-defined radiolucencies at the apices of vital mandibular anterior teeth. Stage 2 produces well-circumscribed radiolucencies with internal cementoid masses. Stage 3 is the mature lesion with near complete mineralization centrally that is surrounded by a radiolucent border. Notably, a patient may demonstrate lesions in one or more stages, adjacent lesions may fuse, and some lesions can resolve completely over time, often after extractions. See Figure 35.6 for more information.

Submandibular Salivary Gland Depression (Stafne or Static Bone Defect) (Fig. 39.3)

is an asymptomatic depression in the lingual aspect of the mandible that accommodates the submandibular salivary gland. As the gland grows and presses against the adjacent bone, the cortex depresses or resorbs. Most **static bone defects** occur after age 40 years. Radiographically, the depression appears, most commonly on a panoramic image, as a well-defined radiolucency below the mandibular canal in the posterior region of the lower jaw between the second molar and angle region. The radiolucency is often round or oval, well corticated, and in close approximation to the mandibular canal or the lower cortical margin of the mandible. Infrequently, the depression extends above the mandibular canal or appears bilaterally. Lesions are not lined by epithelium (i.e., not a cyst), do not require treatment, and tend to remain stable in size.

Pseudoradiolucency of the Anterior Mandible (Fig. 39.4)

is the appearance, in a panoramic image, of an ill-defined radiolucency in the anterior portion of the mandible below the incisor roots. At first glance, the lucency may cause the clinician to believe there are nonvital teeth in the region. However, this is not the case. The **pseudoradiolucency** is caused by a prominent chin depression, or cleft, that produces a relative lucency when the panoramic beam passes through the region. Since this is just a variation of normal, no treatment is required. A periapical film and palpation of the region confirm that disease is not present.

Hematopoietic (Focal Osteoporotic) Bone Marrow Defect (Fig. 39.5)

is the accumulation of red and/or yellow marrow in a localized region of the jaw. The accumulation of marrow produces a radiolucency. The condition is much more common in females and typically is detected on radiographs after age 40. The most common site is the mandibular molar region above the mandibular canal, often in an edentulous area or at the site of previous surgery or injury. The **hematopoietic bone marrow defect** appears as a radiolucency, often less than 1.5 mm in diameter, that has a wavy thin sclerotic border. Wispy internal trabeculae are seen, but the overall density compared to the adjacent bone is much less.

Surgical Ciliated Cyst of the Maxilla (Fig. 39.6)

is a cyst that forms after surgery involving the maxillary sinus. Typically, a Caldwell-Luc operation was performed years earlier. It can be asymptomatic but often produces pain and swelling. Paresthesia is infrequent. Small maxillary lesions appear as a less than 1-cm round or oval radiolucency, above the roots of maxillary teeth and in close proximity with the maxillary sinus. Larger cysts may occupy most of the maxillary sinus and can have curved and thickened borders. Imaging with cone-beam computed tomography is helpful for identifying its anatomic location. Treatment is enucleation.

Cemento-Ossifying Fibroma (Fig. 39.7)

is a fibro-osseous lesion that develops during the third and fourth decades of life, with women being more often affected. Most are asymptomatic, with pain or bony enlargement being infrequent findings. The early lesion is typically a well-demarcated round radiolucency that appears in close approximation to the roots of teeth or periapical region. More than 70% occur in the mandible. As the lesion slowly matures, mineralized matrix is deposited (Fig. 37.7B), transitioning it from a unilocular radiolucency to one with radiopaque foci. The ossifying fibroma can become large, displace teeth and resorb roots. Treatment is complete enucleation.

Neural Sheath Tumor (Fig. 39.8A)

is rather rare and can be a neurilemmoma, schwannoma, neurofibroma, or neurofibromatosis. These tumors have proliferating neural tissue that collate in histologically distinct patterns. They may arise at any age in bone, within the inferior alveolar canal or subperiosteally. The most common site is the posterior mandible, below the roots of teeth. Pain, swelling, jaw expansion, and paresthesia are frequent complaints. Most are well-defined, dark radiolucencies that display a round, scalloped, and sclerotic rim. Adjacent root resorption is seen. Treatment is surgical excision.

Ameloblastoma (Fig. 39.8B) and Ameloblastic Fibroma

are odontogenic tumors that can appear as unilocular or multilocular radiolucencies and should be considered in a differential diagnosis when these types of radiolucencies are seen in patients 30 years or younger. The **ameloblastoma** is discussed under Figures 40.3 and 40.4. In comparison, the ameloblastic fibroma is a less aggressive tumor and occurs at a younger age, often between 10 and 20 years. The most common features are jaw swelling and a unilocular or multilocular radiolucency in the posterior region of the jaws in a child or adolescent.

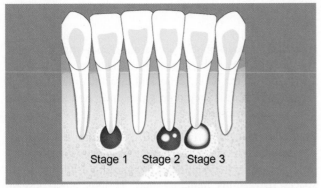

Fig. 39.1. **Periapical cemento-osseous dysplasia:** three stages.

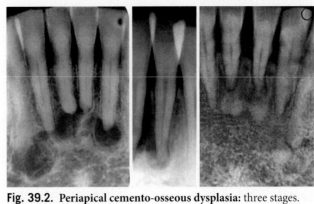

Fig. 39.2. **Periapical cemento-osseous dysplasia:** three stages.

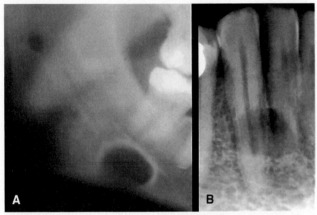

Fig. 39.3. **Submandibular (A) and sublingual (B) salivary gland depressions.**

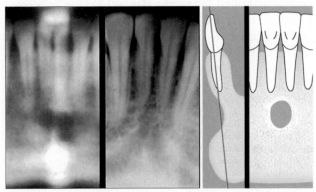

Fig. 39.4. **Pseudoradiolucency due to prominent chin cleft.**

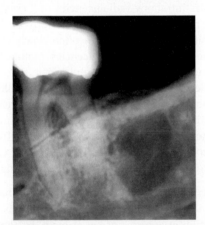

Fig. 39.5. **Hematopoietic bone marrow defect.**

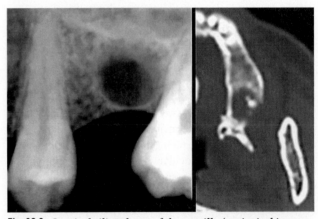

Fig. 39.6. **Surgical ciliated cyst of the maxilla (periapical image and CT image).**

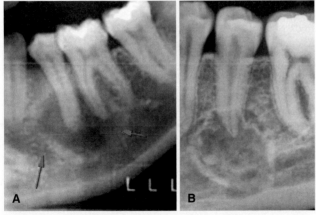

Fig. 39.7. **Ossifying fibroma:** early **(A)** and late **(B)** stage.

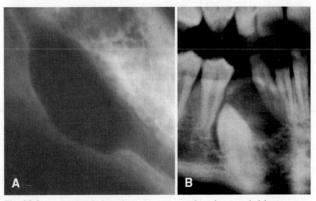

Fig. 39.8. **A: Neural sheath tumor. B: Unilocular ameloblastoma.**

6

Botryoid Lateral Periodontal Cyst (Fig. 40.1) is a multilocular variant of the lateral periodontal cyst. These lesions are previously mentioned under Figure 38.2. Radiographically, they appear between the root surfaces of the mandibular premolar and/or canine. Incisor involvement is rare. The **botryoid lateral periodontal cyst** has the following features: (1) more than one circular loculation each of varying size, (2) one locule located where the lateral periodontal cyst occurs, (3) resorption of lamina dura, (4) extension up to the alveolar ridge or below the root apices, and (5) locules becoming larger as the lesion advances apically. Treatment is enucleation, but recurrence is common, often years after excision.

Central Giant Cell Granuloma (Fig. 40.2) is an inflammatory lesion composed of multinucleated giant cells in a background of ovoid to spindle-shaped mesenchymal cells and well-vascularized connective tissue. Females are affected more often. The **central giant cell granuloma** can develop at both peripheral (soft tissue) and central (within bone) locations. Most begin in children and young adults as a well-defined unilocular radiolucency below the roots of teeth in the anterior segments of the jaws. In fact, nearly 75% are seen in the mandible anterior to the first molars and cross the midline. Mature lesions often become multilocular expansile radiolucencies with thin wispy trabeculae, a well-defined scalloped border that interdigitates between the roots of teeth, and thinning of the peripheral cortex. Lesions are slow growing and often displace teeth and resorb roots. They respond to surgical removal; however, about 20% recur.

Ameloblastoma (Figs. 40.3 and 40.4) is an aggressive and locally invasive tumor arising from odontogenic epithelium. It is the second most common odontogenic tumor and most are detected between 20 and 35 years of age. Men and women are equally affected. The **ameloblastoma** is characterized by slow growth and painless swelling that may reach huge proportions if untreated. The majority occur in the mandibular molar region, with some 60% extending into the ramus. The tumor is usually multilocular with bilocular, soap-bubble, and honeycomb variants; smaller lesions may be unilocular. Buccal and lingual expansion of the cortex occurs with larger lesions, and perforation of the cortical plate is possible. An impacted or displaced unerupted tooth is seen in about 40% of patients. Knife-edged resorption of adjacent teeth is characteristic. Ameloblastoma may metastasize; in this case, it is referred to as **malignant ameloblastoma**.

Odontogenic Myxoma (Fig. 40.5) is a benign but locally aggressive tumor that arises from odontogenic epithelial and mesenchymal (loose odontogenic pulp tissue) cells. Most occur in young adults less than 35 years, equally in men and women, and as a painless swelling associated with tooth displacement and cortical expansion of the posterior mandible. Maxillary lesions can involve the sinus and produce exophthalmos and nasal obstruction. Rare cases develop in the upper ramus and base of the condyle. Early lesions are unilocular. Advanced lesions are multilocular radiolucencies that have a soap-bubble appearance with internal septa that intersect at right angles, forming geometric shapes. Perforation of the outer cortex and invasion of local soft tissue can produce a honeycomb appearance. About 30% recur after surgical excision.

Central Hemangioma (Fig. 40.6) is a benign but destructive vascular tumor within bone that contains small capillaries (**capillary hemangioma**) or large blood-filled sinusoid spaces (**cavernous hemangioma**). Lesions often develop early in life. Jaw lesions can produce swelling, tooth mobility, blood oozing around an erupting tooth, warmer tissue temperature, and red, blue, or purple color to the overlying skin or mucosa. Pain, paresthesia, a pulsatile sensation, and bleeding in the local area are additional features. Most occur in the mandible and produce a variable radiographic appearance: an ill-defined or multilocular radiolucency that resorbs adjacent roots and the lamina dura and causes tooth displacement in the occlusal direction. Within the radiolucency, tubelike vascular channels can be seen, as well as a honeycomb pattern, a soap-bubble appearance, or a cystlike radiolucency. Surgery, sclerosing agents, and embolization have been used as treatment.

Glandular Odontogenic Cyst (Sialo-Odontogenic Cyst) (Fig. 40.7) is an aggressive and rare mucus-producing odontogenic cyst. These lesions arise in tooth-bearing areas. Most **glandular odontogenic cysts** appear in men after age 40 as unilocular intrabony radiolucencies that cross the midline of the mandible and extend posteriorly to the premolars bilaterally. Unilocular lesions often slowly expand and can become multilocular radiolucencies. Mature lesions are associated with epithelial-lined multicystic spaces, a painful or painless swelling (up to 6 cm in size), scalloping borders, and buccal expansion. They are well demarcated with a thin sclerotic rim along portions of the border and reactive denser bone along the remainder of the border. Treatment is enucleation with curettage; recurrence is rather common if there is incomplete removal of the epithelial lining.

Cherubism (Fig. 40.8) is an autosomal dominant condition transmitted by a mutation in a gene on chromosome 4. Affected children appear normal at birth, but between 1½ and 8 years, there is classical development of bilateral, multilocular, multicystic-appearing expansile lesions of the jaws. The fibro-osseous lesions proliferate through puberty but regress and fill with bone and remodel until age 30 years; at that point, lesions become rather nondetectable. Maxillary involvement can displace the eyes and produce a "cherub" facial appearance. Radiographically, cherubism produces soap-bubble or rounded multilocular radiolucencies with cortical expansion and cortical thinning, tooth displacement, delayed tooth eruption, and bilateral appearance. The full mandible can be involved, but the condyle is never involved. Because the condition is self-limiting, treatment is generally not necessary. Cosmetic recontouring is sometimes provided for esthetic reasons.

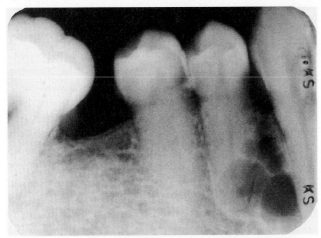

Fig. 40.1. Botryoid lateral periodontal cyst: often multilocular.

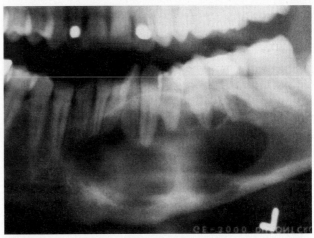

Fig. 40.2. Central giant cell granuloma: peripheral crenations.

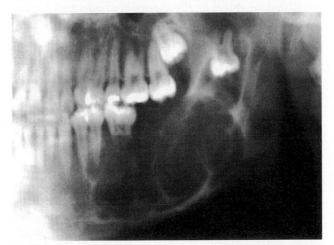

Fig. 40.3. Ameloblastoma: expansile, soap-bubble locules.

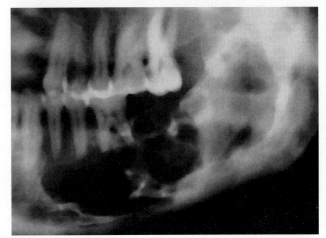

Fig. 40.4. Ameloblastoma: large and expansile, posterior mandible.

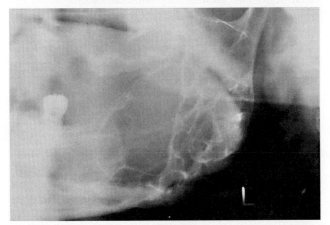

Fig. 40.5. Myxoma: septa shaped like letters X, Y, and V.

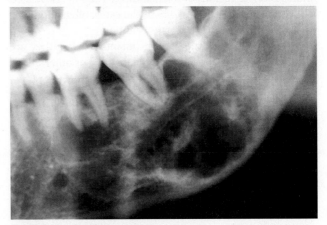

Fig. 40.6. Central hemangioma.

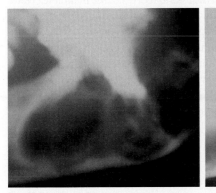

Fig. 40.7. Glandular odontogenic cyst.

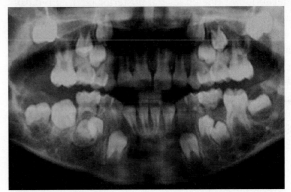

Fig. 40.8. Cherubism: multiple quadrants affected.

6

MIXED RADIOLUCENT-RADIOPAQUE LESIONS

Odontoma (Figs. 41.1 and 41.2), although usually classified as an odontogenic tumor, is not a true neoplasm. It is considered a developmental anomaly (hamartoma) of enamel and dentin that exhibits defective architecture. Two forms exist: **compound odontomas**, the components of which are assembled in an organized manner resembling teeth, and **complex odontomas**, amorphous *disorganized* radiopaque masses that do not resemble teeth. Most are identified in teenagers and young adults on routine radiographs or when a permanent tooth fails to erupt. They are usually asymptomatic and single, but multiple odontomas are possible. All are surrounded by a thin radiolucent zone corresponding to the follicular space and by an outer, thin corticated line. About two thirds occur in the anterior jaws.

Compound Odontoma (Fig. 41.1) is an organized mass resembling a conglomeration of rudimentary little teeth. They are twice as common in the maxilla as the mandible. They occur in the anterior maxilla and with an unerupted tooth in 65% of cases. The odontoma is most often located next to an impacted tooth. Less commonly, the odontoma arises adjacent to or between tooth roots. In about half of cases, the crown or root of an adjacent tooth is impinged on by the odontoma, which can delay or alter its eruption (Fig. 41.1B).

Complex Odontoma (Figs. 41.2 and 41.3) is a lesion containing gnarled densities of enamel, dentin, and pulp that appear as solid radiopaque masses within bone. Unlike compound odontomas, the majority of complex odontomas are found in the posterior regions of the mandible. They are associated with an impacted tooth in 70% of the cases, often above the impacted tooth, thus affecting its eruption.

Odontomas have little growth potential unless they are associated with a dentigerous cyst (Fig. 41.3) or other odontogenic lesions. Removal is curative and recurrence is rare.

Ameloblastic Fibro-Odontoma (Figs. 41.4 and 41.5) is a mixed odontogenic tumor composed of (1) neoplastic "ameloblastoma-like" epithelium, (2) mesenchyme, and (3) an odontoma. It is histologically similar to the ameloblastic fibroma; however, the ameloblastic fibroma lacks one or more odontomas. The **ameloblastic fibro-odontoma** occurs almost exclusively in tooth development years (i.e., younger than 20 years) and more often in the posterior jaw. Males are affected slightly more often. The most frequent symptom is noneruption of one or several posterior teeth. It typically appears as a well-circumscribed pericoronal radiolucency with internal radiopacities above a crown of an inferiorly displaced molar. The margin is hyperostotic and often surrounds an unerupted tooth. The internal opacities contain variable amounts of calcified material (enamel and dentin) that are histologically either a compound (toothlike) or complex odontoma. Expansion occurs with larger lesions. There is little tendency to recur after excision.

Adenomatoid Odontogenic Tumor (Fig. 41.6) is a slow-growing, mixed odontogenic neoplasm, derived from epithelial remnants of the enamel organ, that produces sheets of polyhedral pale or clear epithelial cells and prominent duct-like structures. Most occur in young females (12 to 16 years). It has a striking tendency to produce a radiolucent lesion in the anterior jaw, often involving an unerupted canine tooth (75% of cases), and two thirds occur in the maxilla—features which aid in the diagnosis. Lesions of longer duration can cause symptoms, swelling or perforation of the cortex. In about 65% of cases, radiopaque (enamel) flecks or patchy areas of calcification occur within the central part of the lesion. The margin of the tumor is radiopaque and may be thick, thin, or absent focally as a result of infection. Tumors contain a thick myxoid or fibrous capsule; thus, they are easily enucleated and tend not to recur.

Cemento-Ossifying Fibroma (see Fig. 39.7) is a fibro-osseous lesion common to the mandible at a location inferior to the premolars and molars. It produces a well-demarcated radiolucency that slowly expands and deposits mineralized matrix (osteoid, trabecular bone, and cementum), making mature lesions appear as unilocular radiolucency with radiopaque foci.

Calcifying Odontogenic (Gorlin) Cyst (Fig. 41.7) is a non-aggressive but enlarging lesion that displays variable behavior—some being like cysts, others like tumors, and sometimes associating with odontomas. Most **calcifying odontogenic cysts** occur in the jaws during the second and third decade of life. Radiographically, they usually appear as a well-demarcated unilocular radiolucency with radiopaque structures within the lesion. Some are multilocular, about a third are associated with an impacted tooth, and both the maxilla and mandible can be affected. The most characteristic microscopic feature is a variable number of ghost cells within the epithelial portion of the lesion. Treatment is surgical enucleation.

Calcifying Epithelial Odontogenic (Pindborg) Tumor (Fig. 41.8) is a painless, slow-growing swelling composed of sheets of large polyhedral neoplastic epithelial cells and pink amyloid deposits that tend to calcify. The cause of the tumor is unknown. It occurs predominantly as an intraosseous (central) neoplasm between 30 and 50 years of age. Males and females are affected equally, and, in two thirds of cases, the tumor arises in the mandibular molar area. Most are associated with an unerupted tooth and tumor-induced migration of an unerupted molar into the inferior cortex of the mandible creates a unique "bulge" in this area. Variable amounts of calcific foci are seen, with the radiopaque flecks appearing as small rounded structures within the mixed radiolucent-radiopaque mass. The flecks often cluster at the occlusal aspect of the tumor and form a linear "trail of driven snow" pattern. The **calcifying epithelial odontogenic tumor** is locally aggressive and can penetrate the cortex. After excision, recurrence occurs in about 15% of patients.

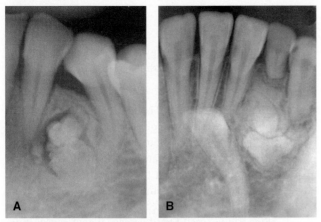

Fig. 41.1. Compound odontoma: affecting adjacent teeth.

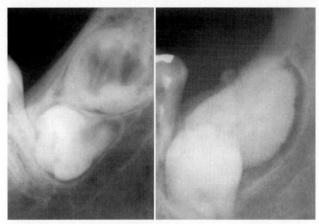

Fig. 41.2. Complex odontoma: related to impacted teeth.

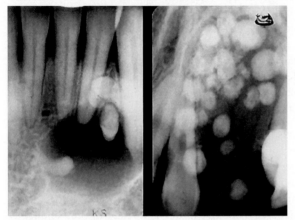

Fig. 41.3. Cystic odontoma: multiple odontomas.

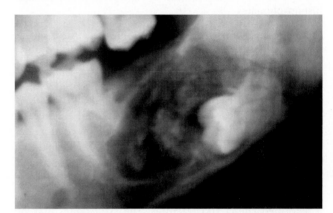

Fig. 41.4. Ameloblastic fibro-odontoma with nonerupted molar.

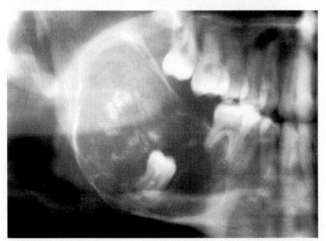

Fig. 41.5. Ameloblastic fibro-odontoma with nonerupted molar.

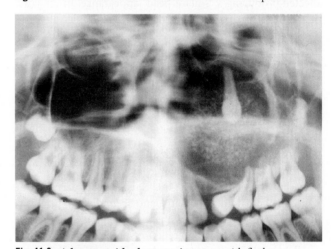

Fig. 41.6. Adenomatoid odontogenic tumor with flecks.

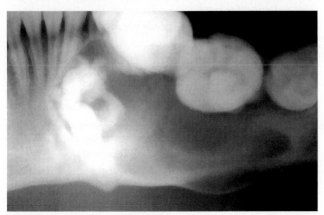

Fig. 41.7. Calcifying odontogenic cyst.

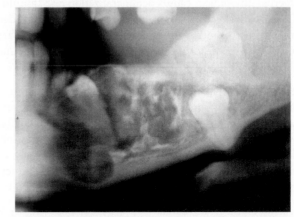

Fig. 41.8. Calcifying epithelial odontogenic (Pindborg) tumor.

6

GENERALIZED RAREFACTIONS

Osteoporosis (Fig. 42.1) is a condition associated with aging caused by a deficiency of organic bone matrix. It causes bones to become weak and brittle and is one of the most common disorders affecting postmenopausal women. Osteoporosis is associated with loss of height, stooped posture, and bone fracture(s). A bone density scan or dual x-ray absorptiometry (DXA) is used to measure bone loss. A DXA T-score below -2.5 indicates you likely have osteoporosis. In the jaws, osteoporosis causes thinning of the mandibular cortex and lamina dura, resorption of edentulous areas, and enlarged radiolucent medullary spaces. Treatment is directed toward increasing bone mass through exercise, calcium and vitamin D supplements, and antiresorptive drugs such as bisphosphonates.

Rickets (Fig. 42.2) is a disorder of defective mineralization that occurs in children before epiphyseal closure. It is caused by a deficiency or impaired metabolism of vitamin D, phosphorous, or calcium. Vitamin D deficiency from malnutrition is the most common cause; however, malabsorption or renal disease, which leads to excessive calcium excretion and other factors, can be causative. If the condition occurs after epiphyseal closure (i.e., in adults), it is called osteomalacia. In rickets, the mineralization of bone, cartilage, and dentin becomes disorganized. This leads to bony deformities (widening of the long ends of bones, bowing of the femurs, a deformed chest) and fractures. The skull bones may be affected producing a "square-head" appearance. In the jaws, the trabeculae become reduced in number, density, and thickness. The cortical bone appears thinned or absent, and the cortical outline of the mandibular canal may be lost. If the disease occurs during tooth formation, then enamel hypoplasia, dentin fissures, and enlarged pulp chambers lined by hyperdense dentin and long pulp horns are common. Bacterial invasion of these defects can lead to death of the pulp.

Hyperparathyroidism (Fig. 42.3) is the overproduction of parathormone by the parathyroid glands. Two forms exist: primary hyperparathyroidism, caused by hyperplasia or tumor of the parathyroid gland, and secondary hyperparathyroidism, which occurs often with kidney failure. The disease causes excessive secretion of parathyroid hormone, which in turn mobilizes calcium from bone. On radiographs, hyperparathyroidism causes demineralization and thinning of the jaw cortical boundaries (i.e., loss of inferior border, lamina dura, mandibular canal, and outline of maxillary sinuses). The trabecular patterns are thinned, granular, and grayish in appearance (also see Figs. 54.7 and 54.8).

Osteomyelitis (Figs. 42.4 and 43.4) is a rare inflammatory condition of bone that causes destruction of bone and marrow, and pus formation. Jaw osteomyelitis often follows trauma or untreated periapical/periodontal infection. Most patients have an underlying disease and reduced host defense. The mandible is most often affected; pain, tenderness, and swelling are common. The radiographic jaw bone changes include a grayish foggy lytic region with internal radiolucent tracts and dense radiopacities representing bone infarcts.

Sickle Cell Anemia (Fig. 42.5) is an inherited condition that affects the function and shape of red blood cells resulting in hemolytic anemia. It occurs almost exclusively in blacks and persons from the Mediterranean region and is the result of a single amino acid change in the β chain of hemoglobin. Affected red blood cells become sickle-shaped and sticky when poor oxygenation or infection occurs. The sticky red blood cells occlude small blood vessels, which causes pain, jaundice, shortness of breath, leg ulcers, and bony deformities. If the anemia is chronic, bone marrow can respond by becoming hyperplastic. This leads to rearrangement of the bone marrow spaces, widening and decreased number of trabeculae, and generalized osteoporosis of the jaws. Classically, two features are seen: stepladder configuration of the jaw trabeculae between the roots of teeth and "hair-on-end" hyperplasia of the outer cortex of the skull.

Thalassemia (Fig. 42.6) is a group of inherited disorders caused by a deletion or mutation in either the α or β globin gene of hemoglobin. This alteration results in a defect in globin synthesis. It occurs in many forms. Thalassemia major is due to inheritance of a faulty gene from both parents, and thalassemia minor is a result of only one faulty gene. The disease is most common in persons who originate from Africa, the Mediterranean, or Southeast Asia—sites where malaria is endemic. The minor type is not known to produce signs or symptoms. In contrast, thalassemia major produces jaw and skull bone changes similar to sickle cell anemia, that is, "hair-on-end appearance," and also produces bulbous enlargement of the maxillary bones.

Leukemia (Fig. 42.7) is discussed under Leukemic Gingivitis (Figs. 48.1 and 48.2). The radiographic jaw bone changes include diffuse osteopenia (fewer trabeculae and loss of lamina dura), destruction of tooth crypts, tooth displacement, and irregular radiolucent areas of alveolar bone that resemble periodontal disease.

Osteoradionecrosis (Fig. 42.8) is a disorder of nonhealing dead bone caused by high-dose radiation (greater than 65 Gy) to the jaws. It occurs in about 2% of patients who have received high-dose radiation for head and neck cancer. The affected bone is hypovascular and characteristically breaks down and is unable to heal after minor or major trauma or infection. Soft tissue necrosis leads to exposed necrotic bone, which can become secondarily infected. Risk is higher among those who are dentate, smoke, are malnourished, and have poor oral hygiene, after an extraction, or following the use of vasoconstrictors or dental trauma. The condition produces pain and an irregular radiolucency, usually in the mandible, with an indistinct border. Long-standing cases produce a moth-eaten lesion with ragged borders and bone sequestration or pathologic fracture. Treatment involves antibiotic therapy and hyperbaric oxygen.

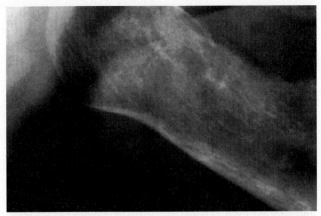

Fig. 42.1. Osteoporosis: posterior mandible.

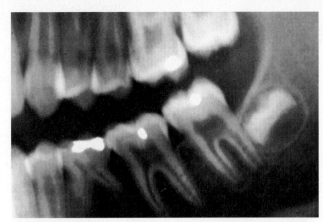

Fig. 42.2. Rickets/osteomalacia: large pulp chambers.

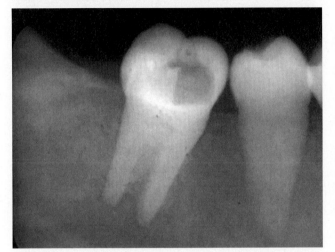

Fig. 42.3. Hyperparathyroidism: loss of trabeculations and lamina dura.

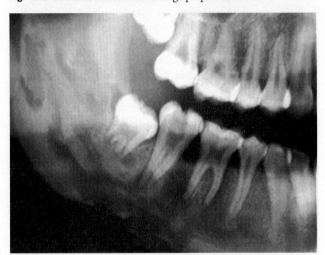

Fig. 42.4. Chronic osteomyelitis with radiolucent tracts.

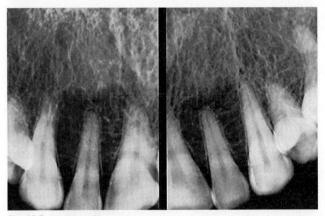

Fig. 42.5. Sickle cell anemia.

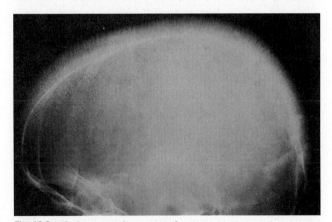

Fig. 42.6. Thalassemia: hair-on-end appearance.

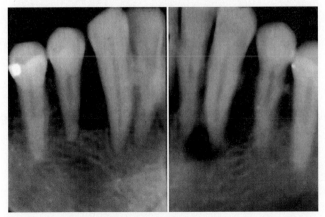

Fig. 42.7. Leukemia: bilateral bone loss.

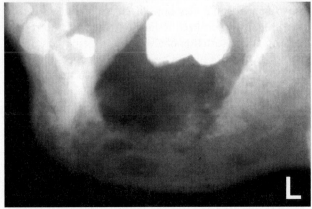

Fig. 42.8. Osteoradionecrosis: moth-eaten appearance.

Several conditions can cause "**floating teeth**" and each should be considered when dealing with this situation. In children, the clinician should also consider **hypophosphatasia**—a metabolic disorder that can affect bone mineralization and can result in premature loss of teeth.

Chronic Periodontitis (Fig. 43.1), defined as long-standing inflammation of the periodontium that extends into and destroys the attachment apparatus, can cause sufficient destruction of the supporting alveolar bone to produce the appearance of a "*floating tooth*." In this instance, increased tooth mobility, periodontal probing depths exceeding 8 mm, and gingival bleeding upon probing are present. Affected teeth may be tilted or supraerupted, have clinically exposed root surfaces, and display subgingival calculus. Radiographically, there is evidence of bone loss surrounding the entire root surface and involving the furcation region. The destruction produces a distinct scooped-out radiolucency with a curvilinear or wavy border. The apical portion of the lesion is often wider than the coronal aspect of the lucency and minor root resorption is common. The border of the radiolucency may show a reactive osteosclerosis and/or nutrient canals feeding the area. Diabetes mellitus, neutrophil disorders, and **Papillon-Lefevre syndrome** are conditions associated with advanced periodontal destruction and floating teeth.

Langerhans Cell Disease (Figs. 43.2 and 43.3) is a disease of dendritic cells, also known as Langerhans cells, that occurs in about 1 in 100,000 persons. Historically, the disease was known as **histiocytosis X** because the condition is characterized by proliferation of nonlipid histiocytes that later were identified to be mononuclear antigen-presenting (Langerhans) cells. There are three forms of this disorder: (1) **eosinophilic granuloma**, the mildest form of the disease, which occurs most commonly in older children and young adults and primarily involves lytic bone lesions, though about 20% have lung infiltration as well; (2) **chronic disseminated histiocytosis**, which usually begins in childhood but can appear in late middle age and classically produces a triad consisting of bone defects, exophthalmos, and diabetes insipidus; and (3) **acute disseminated histiocytosis**, previously known as Letterer-Siwe disease. The latter occurs in young children (less than 3 years) and produces infections, rashes, anemia, and fever. The rapid dissemination of the disease to skin, lymph nodes, bone, liver, and spleen indicates a poor prognosis. Localized lesions of the jaw often produce dull pain and destruction of alveolar bone, especially affecting the furcation of molars, resulting in scooped-out radiolucencies and "*floating teeth*." Bone lesions in the skull may cause vision or hearing loss. Localized bone lesions are often treated with corticosteroids and/or curettage. Chemotherapy is given for disseminated disease.

Osteomyelitis (Fig. 43.4) is inflammation accompanied by infection of the bone. There are two types: **acute** and **chronic osteomyelitis**. Both types are more common in the posterior mandible of men and are often associated with a nonvital tooth, a mobile tooth, blunt trauma, or jaw fracture. Less commonly, bacteremia can be causative. Pain, swelling, fever, and regional lymphadenopathy accompany the condition. Acute disease produces an irregular radiolucency and occasional periosteal reaction or new bone formation. However, as the infection spreads through the bone and the condition becomes chronic, a "moth-eaten" pattern is seen with localized sites of nonviable or sequestrating dense infarcted bone. Long-standing cases are associated with conditions that produce poor vascularity (which contributes to the bone infarcts), including high-dose jaw irradiation, Paget disease, or sickle cell disease. Chronic osteomyelitis is painful, can cause swelling and tenderness and "floating teeth," and is associated with an irregular, diffuse, wavy, or geographic radiolucent border. Treatment involves debridement and a long course of systemic antibiotics.

Malignancy (Figs. 43.5 and 43.6) can produce destruction of alveolar bone and "*floating teeth*." Malignant tumors that destroy alveolar bone can result (1) from a local tumor that invades from the soft tissue into bone, (2) from a tumor that arises within the jaw bone, or (3) as a metastatic tumor that travels from a distant site. If the malignancy produces bone-resorbing peptides like interleukin-1 beta (IL-1β), receptor activator of nuclear factor kappa B ligand (RANKL), and/or macrophage inhibitory protein 1 alpha (MIP-1α) that stimulate and activate osteoclasts, then the result is bone destruction. Local tumors such as **gingival carcinoma** that arise from within the gingiva can invade downward and destroy bone. This form of carcinoma produces a localized radiolucency within which flecks of resorbed bone may be seen and lacks a margin of reactive sclerotic bone. In fact, all three categories of malignancies mentioned above typically produce an irregular and infiltrating radiolucency, trabecular remnants (bone flecks) within the lucency, and cortical bone destruction that can result in a tooth floating in bone (also see Malignant Disease Figs. 53.7 and 53.8 under Radiographic Alteration of Periodontal Ligament and Lamina Dura). Treatment of malignancies often involves chemotherapy and/or radiation therapy.

Multiple Myeloma (Figs. 43.7 and 43.8) is a neoplastic proliferation of plasma cells. The abnormal neoplastic plasma cells tend to proliferate in bone and make monoclonal immunoglobulin. These immunoglobulins appear in blood and as fragments in urine (Bence Jones protein). Men over age 50 are more commonly affected. Multiple myeloma produces plasma cell tumors that invade and destroy bone producing sharply punched-out lytic radiolucencies. The skull bones are commonly affected, and the mandible is involved in about 20% to 33% of patients. Lesions are painful, multiple, noncorticated radiolucencies of varying size, which can produce a moth-eaten appearance as well as "*floating teeth*." Affected teeth can show root resorption. Treatment involves chemotherapy and immune modulators, which have increased survival to beyond 5 years.

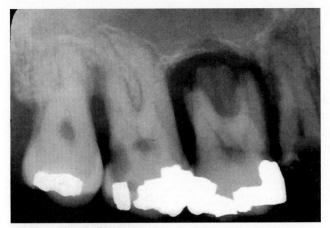

Fig. 43.1. **Advanced periodontitis:** floating tooth.

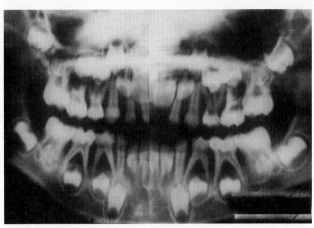

Fig. 43.2. **Langerhans cell disease:** chronic disseminated histiocytosis.

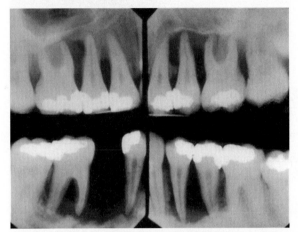

Fig. 43.3. **Langerhans cell disease:** eosinophilic granuloma.

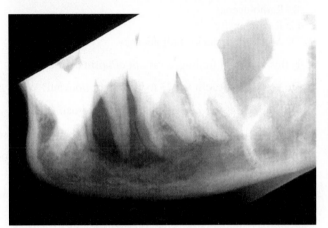

Fig. 43.4. **Chronic osteomyelitis** with premolar lacking support.

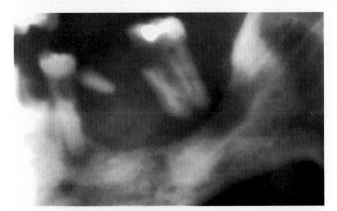

Fig. 43.5. **Gingival carcinoma.**

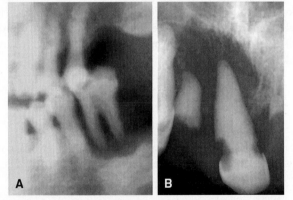

Fig. 43.6. **A: Gingival carcinoma. B: Metastatic adenocarcinoma.**

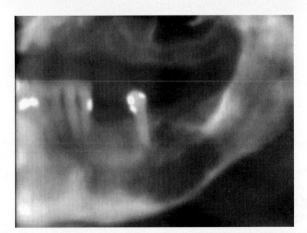

Fig. 43.7. **Multiple myeloma.**

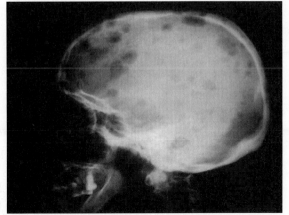

Fig. 43.8. **Multiple myeloma:** punched-out lesions.

CASE 26. (FIG. 43.9)

This 43-year-old African American woman came to the dental clinic because she wants her teeth cleaned and is interested in getting a crown on tooth no. 27. She had a root canal completed on tooth no. 27 (right mandibular canine) a few months ago by an endodontist in another city and just moved to your town. She is a good dental patient who goes to the dentist every 6 months for cleanings.

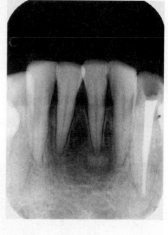

1. Describe the radiographic findings.

2. Which term best describes the lesion at the apex of no. 25?
   A. Radiopacity
   B. Radiolucency
   C. Radiodensity
   D. Mixed radiopacity-radiolucency

3. Is this a normal finding, a variant of normal, or disease?

4. Do you expect tooth no. 25 to be vital or nonvital? Why? And how can you determine the vitality of tooth no. 25?

5. Do you expect this condition to be symptomatic?

6. List conditions you should consider in the differential diagnosis, and note which condition is most likely the correct diagnosis.

7. What precautions should be taken when performing periodontal instrumentation? For example, is tooth no. 25 likely to be mobile?

8. Why do you think a root canal was performed on tooth no. 27?

CASE 27. (FIG. 43.10)

You take this radiograph of a 55-year-old man in your dental office. He had the bridge constructed at another dental office and has no dental symptoms. He is hypertensive and takes a diuretic.

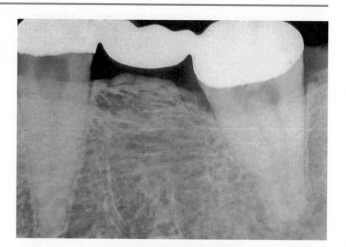

1. Describe the radiographic findings. Include normal and abnormal findings.

2. Do you expect this condition to be symptomatic? Why?

3. Is this a normal finding, a variant of normal, disorder, or disease?

4. Which of the following is the most likely diagnosis?
   A. Mandibular enostosis
   B. Reactive subpontine exostosis
   C. Irreversib le pulpitis
   D. Condensing osteitis

5. This condition is more common in:
   A. The maxilla of an older men
   B. The mandible of an older men
   C. The maxilla of a younger men
   D. The ramus of an older men

6. What periodontal findings are associated with this condition?

7. If the bridge is removed and reconstructed, would the lesion regress?

Additional cases to enhance your learning and understanding of this section are available Online through the book's Navigate 2 Advantage Access site.

Disorders of Gingiva and Periodontium

Objectives:

- Define the terms *plaque biofilm, aerobe, and anaerobe*, and know the constituents of plaque biofilm.
- Name the two major categories of periodontal disease.
- Define, compare, and contrast the terms *gingival disease, gingivitis, periodontal disease, periodontitis,* and other important clinical terms (i.e., *abscess, dehiscence,* and *fenestration*).
- Define and contrast the terms gingival disease, periodontal disease, and periodontitis.
- Recognize the causes and clinical and radiographic features of the different types of diseases that affect the periodontium.
- Use the diagnostic process to distinguish the different classifications of periodontal diseases.
- Recommend appropriate treatment options for the different types and classifications of gingivitis, periodontitis, and diseases of the periodontium.
- Identify conditions discussed in this section that (1) require the attention of the dentist and/or (2) affect the delivery of invasive and noninvasive dental procedures, including periodontal instrumentation.

In the figure legends, *†§ denotes the same patient.

PERIODONTAL DISEASE: DENTAL PLAQUE, CALCULUS, AND ROOT EXPOSURE

Periodontal disease is a broad term that refers to a bacterial infection of the periodontium. The two major diagnostic categories of periodontal disease are (1) gingivitis and (2) periodontitis. Specific types of diseases are identified within each of these major categories (see preceding page).

Plaque (Figs. 44.1 and 44.2) is a microbial biofilm that adheres tenaciously to tooth surfaces, restorations, and prosthetic appliances. The development of plaque biofilm is a well-characterized, stepwise process. The first step is the attachment of the **acquired pellicle**, a thin film of salivary proteins. Within a few days, gram-positive facultative cocci overlay and colonize the pellicle, then additional bacteria, such as *Veillonella* species (a gram-negative anaerobe), *Actinomyces* species (a gram-positive rod), and *Capnocytophaga* species (a gram-negative rod), enter the region and colonize plaque. *Prevotella intermedia* and filamentous *Fusobacterium* species colonize between the first and third weeks as a subgingival **anaerobic** environment becomes established. Undisturbed plaque is colonized with *Porphyromonas gingivalis*, motile rods, and *Treponema* species (spirochetes) during and after the 3rd week. The exact microbial composition varies according to site, available substrate, salivary components (adhesins and secretory immunoglobulin), duration, and the patient's oral hygiene practices.

Plaque biofilm is soft, translucent to white, and contains an extracellular, sticky matrix called **glucan**. Glucans are secreted by streptococci and promote adherence of bacteria to the pellicle. Clinically, plaque is classified by location as **supragingival plaque**, adhering to tooth structure above the gingiva, and **subgingival plaque**, found below the gingiva. Growth in supragingival plaque biofilm results from nutrients obtained from ingested simple carbohydrates (glucose) and lactic acid. In contrast, subgingival (plaque) bacteria preferentially use metabolized peptides and amino acids that are obtained from tissue breakdown products, the **gingival crevicular fluid**, and interbacterial feeding. Inflamed gingival tissues produce more gingival crevicular fluid, which favors the proliferation of subgingival bacterial replication. Subgingival bacteria prefer an anaerobic environment, whereas supragingival bacterial populations prefer a low-oxygen environment. The latter are called **facultative anaerobes**. Long-standing plaque is mostly composed of gram-negative anaerobes (e.g., *Fusobacterium nucleatum*, *Tannerella forsythia*, *Porphyromonas gingivalis*, *Prevotella intermedia*). Persistent microbial plaque biofilm can lead to stain, caries, gingivitis, calculus formation, gingival recession, and periodontitis. Poor esthetics, halitosis, and bacterial sepsis may be accompanying problems.

Calculus (Figs. 44.3 and 44.4) consists primarily of mineralized, dead bacteria with a small amount of mineralized salivary proteins. Its chemical components are mostly calcium phosphate, calcium carbonate, and magnesium phosphate. Calculus is hard, mineralized, and firmly adheres to the tooth. Above the gingival margin, calculus is called **supragingival calculus**. It appears yellow or tan and is usually located near

large salivary sources in patients who do not mechanically remove plaque regularly. Supragingival calculus accumulates preferentially along the lingual of the mandibular incisors adjacent to the duct for the sublingual and submandibular glands and along the buccal of maxillary molars adjacent to Stensen duct of the parotid gland. Radiographically, it appears as a pointy radiopaque spicule adherent to tooth near the CEJ. With age, it darkens and increases in size. A **calculus bridge** is an extensive matrix of calculus that extends across several teeth. It is often associated with gingival recession and periodontal disease. Removal of a calculus bridge may reveal several mobile teeth. Patients should be advised of this possibility before debridement.

Subgingival calculus forms below the gingival margin. It is not usually visible unless gingival recession has occurred. Subgingival calculus is detected with an explorer, as a rough mass projecting from the cementum. It appears brown, black, or green because of its chronic exposure to gingival crevicular fluid, blood, and blood breakdown products. It is associated with the development of a **pyogenic granuloma** (Fig. 49.1), an epulislike lesion on the gingiva.

Gingival Recession (Recession of the Gingival Margin) (Figs. 44.5–44.7) In health, the gingival margin normally extends about 1 mm above the cementoenamel junction. **Gingival recession** is the migration of the free gingival margin to a position apical to the cementoenamel junction. Gingival recession is an indication of the apical migration of the junctional epithelium in the presence of disease and/or trauma. By definition, recession results in loss of attachment and exposure of the root (i.e., cementum). It usually occurs in persons older than age 30 on the facial aspect of teeth and less commonly on the lingual aspect. Recession may be localized or generalized and often progresses during periods of inflammation that may be combined with improper toothbrushing. Prominently located teeth with thin gingiva, inadequate bands of attached gingiva, high muscle or frenum attachments, bony fenestrations, and dehiscences are commonly affected. Excessive occlusal loading, temporary crowns, plaque biofilm, and calculus are also contributing factors. A variant form is **clefting**—a limited zone of narrow recession. Clefting can be caused by fingernail injuries, oral jewelry, or calculus. Surgical grafting is one treatment option that can provide root coverage for areas of clefting or recession.

Dehiscence and Fenestration (Fig. 44.8) A **dehiscence** is loss of alveolar bone on the facial—rarely lingual—aspect of a tooth that leaves a characteristic oval, root-exposed defect apical to the cementoenamel junction. The defect may be 1 or 2 mm long or extend the full length of the root. The three features of a dehiscence are gingival recession, alveolar bone loss, and root exposure.

A **fenestration** is a window of bone loss on the facial or lingual aspect of a tooth that places the exposed root surface directly in contact with gingiva or alveolar mucosa. It can be distinguished from dehiscence in that the fenestration is bordered by alveolar bone along its coronal aspect.

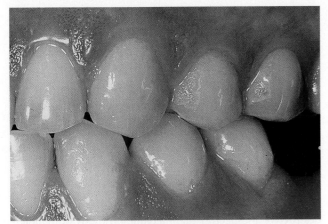

Fig. 44.1. Plaque: stained pink by disclosing solution.

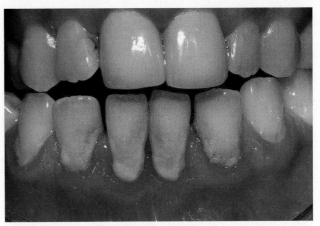

Fig. 44.2. Plaque: along gingival margins.

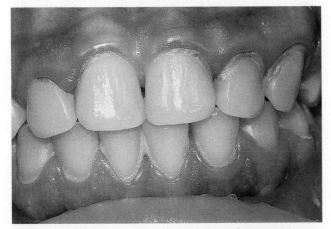

Fig. 44.3. Calculus: at interproximal and gingival margins.

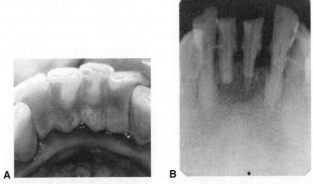

A   B

Fig. 44.4. A: Calculus bridge. B: Associated bone loss.

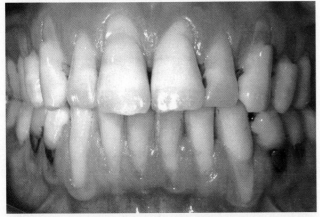

Fig. 44.5. Generalized gingival recession: 2 to 6 mm.

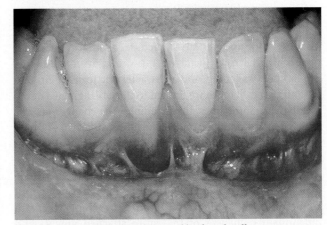

Fig. 44.6. Gingival recession: caused by frenal pull.

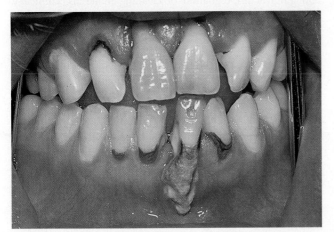

Fig. 44.7. Gingival clefting: beyond mucogingival junction.

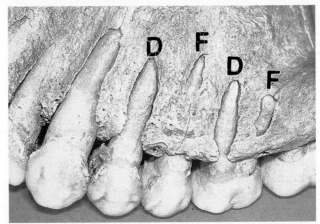

Fig. 44.8. Dehiscences (*D*) and fenestrations (*F*).

GINGIVAL DISEASES AND GINGIVITIS

Gingival diseases are classified by the American Academy of Periodontology into two major groups: **plaque induced** and **non–plaque induced**. These two conditions are exacerbated by over-contoured crowns, open contacts, overhanging margins, and tooth malposition. The term **gingivitis** is used in this text because it is the common clinical term used when describing many of these gingival diseases.

Plaque-Induced Gingival Diseases

Plaque-induced gingivitis (Figs. 45.1–45.4) is the most common form of gingivitis. It is a mixed bacterial infection that results in inflammation and reversible damage to the gingival tissues without loss of connective tissue attachment. It occurs at any age but most frequently arises during adolescence. It requires the presence and maturation of dental plaque. Gingivitis is diagnosed by bleeding and changes in the **color, contour,** and **consistency** of the gingiva. Features include red swollen marginal gingiva; loss of stippling; red-purple, bulbous interdental papillae; and increased fluid flow from the gingival crevice. Bleeding and pain are induced by toothbrushing and slight probing.

Plaque-induced gingivitis has no sex or racial predilection and is classified according to distribution, duration, cause, and severity. The distribution may be general, local, marginal, or papillary (involvement of interdental papillae). The duration may be acute or chronic. Treatment of plaque-induced gingivitis consists of frequent and regular removal of bacterial plaque and calculus. Untreated gingivitis can advance to periodontitis.

Mouth Breathing–Associated Gingivitis (Fig. 45.4)

Mouth Breathing–Associated Gingivitis (Fig. 45.4) is a plaque-induced condition characterized by nasal obstruction, a high narrow palatal vault, snoring, dry mouth, sore throat upon wakening, and a characteristic form of gingivitis. Soft tissue changes are limited to the labial gingiva of the maxilla and, sometimes, the mandible. The changes may be an incidental finding or noticed together with caries limited to the incisors. Plaque accumulation at the gingival margin and multiple anterior restorations also serve as a diagnostic clue. Early changes consist of diffuse redness of the labial, marginal, and interdental gingiva. The interproximal papillae become red, swollen, and bleed. Progression results in inflammatory changes of the entire attached gingiva and bleeding on probing. Improved oral hygiene reduces these signs but does not resolve the condition. Protective dressings (i.e., emollients) placed on the affected gingiva promote healing. However, definitive treatment should address re-establishment of a patent (unobstructed) nasal airway.

Focal Eruption Gingivitis (Localized Juvenile Spongiotic Gingival Hyperplasia) (Fig. 45.5)

Focal Eruption Gingivitis (Localized Juvenile Spongiotic Gingival Hyperplasia) (Fig. 45.5) is a specific type of plaque-induced gingivitis seen around erupting teeth, usually canines or premolars. It occurs as a hyperplastic reaction to microbial biofilm around teeth that do not have adequate marginal and attached gingiva. It occurs most often in adolescents, whose dental arch lacks space for a late erupting tooth. Because the canines and premolars erupt late within the confined space, their eruption tends to be superior and facial. At this location, the collar of the tooth is surrounded by alveolar mucosa, which lacks the tensile and compressive properties of attached gingiva. The accumulation of plaque biofilm causes the tissue to become inflamed, fiery red, and friable. Inspection reveals minute red papules and a band-like appearance around the collar of the tooth. The condition improves with meticulous oral hygiene and eruption into the normal position. Orthodontics may be required to position the tooth properly to allow attached gingiva to form.

Necrotizing Ulcerative Gingivitis (Fig. 45.6) (NUG)

Necrotizing Ulcerative Gingivitis (Fig. 45.6) (NUG) is a destructive and necrotizing infection, primarily of the interdental and marginal gingiva, characterized by partial loss of the interdental papillae, gingival bleeding, and pain. The condition is also known as **Vincent infection, pyorrhea,** or **trench mouth,** owing to its occurrence in men in battlefield trenches during World War I. This multifactorial disease has a bacterial population high in fusiform bacilli, *Prevotella intermedia,* and spirochetes. The condition is characterized by fever, lymphadenopathy, malaise, fiery red gingiva, extreme oral pain, hypersalivation, and an unmistakable fetor oris. The interdental papillae are punched out, ulcerated, and covered with a grayish pseudomembrane. The condition is common in persons between the ages of 15 and 25 years, particularly students and military recruits enduring times of increased stress and reduced host resistance, and in HIV-infected patients. Smoking, poor nutrition, lack of sleep, and poor oral hygiene are contributory. In rare instances (such as malnutrition, malignancy, or immunodeficiency), the infection can extend to other oral mucosal surfaces, where it is known as **necrotizing ulcerative mucositis (NOMA).** It can also recur if mismanaged. Treatment of NUG requires irrigation, gentle debridement, antibiotics (if constitutional symptoms are present), stress reduction, and rest. Partial loss of the interdental papillae can be expected despite normal healing.

Non–Plaque-Induced Gingival Disease

Prophy Paste (Foreign Body) Gingivitis (Fig. 45.7) is a rare form of gingivitis that occurs shortly after dental prophylaxis. It is caused by penetration of prophylaxis paste into the gingival tissue and the resulting inflammatory response to the foreign material. It may occur more often after air-powder abrasive system treatments, as these treatments can cause erosive changes and gingival impregnation of cleaning materials. Clinically, the affected tissue is focal or multifocal and appears red and friable. The well-demarcated red areas often are sore or burn. Treatment includes a tissue biopsy to confirm the diagnosis, topical steroids, careful debridement, and improved home care. If unresponsive, excision and a free gingival graft can be provided.

Actinomycotic Gingivitis (Fig. 45.8) is a rare form of gingivitis that presents with redness, intense burning pain, and lack of a response to normal therapeutic regimens. Biopsy of tissue reveals the non–acid-fast, gram-positive, anaerobic bacteria (*Actinomyces*) forming filamentous colonies. Gingivectomy or long-term antimicrobial therapy provides effective treatment.

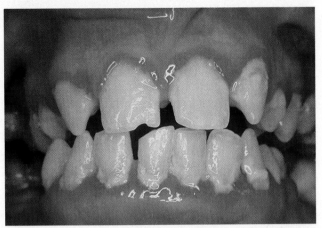

Fig. 45.1. Plaque-induced gingivitis: marginal gingiva bright red and swollen.

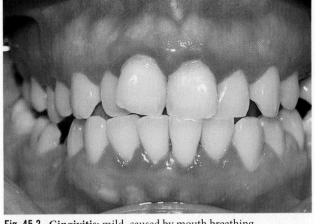

Fig. 45.2. Gingivitis: mild, caused by mouth breathing.

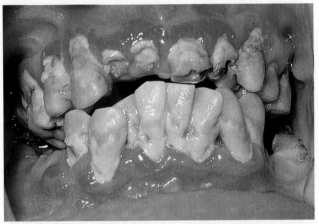

Fig. 45.3. Chronic gingivitis: severe and plaque induced.

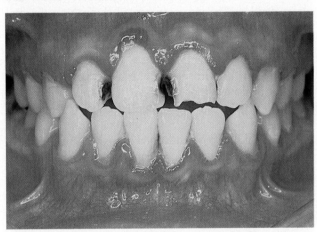

Fig. 45.4. Gingivitis: severe, caused by mouth breathing.

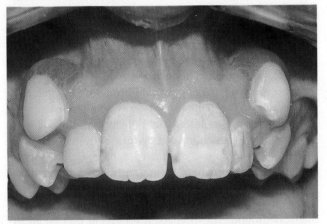

Fig. 45.5. Focal eruption gingivitis: fiery red above canines.

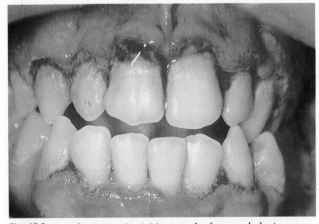

Fig. 45.6. Prophy paste gingivitis: 1 week after prophylaxis.

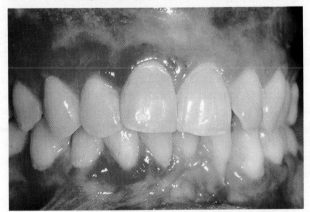

Fig. 45.7. Acute necrotizing ulcerative gingivitis: with fetid mouth odor

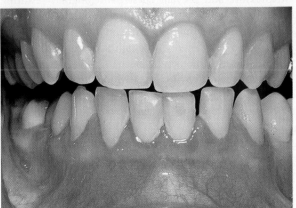

Fig. 45.8. Actinomycotic gingivitis: affecting marginal gingiva.

7

GINGIVAL DISEASES: GENERALIZED GINGIVAL ENLARGEMENTS

Primary Herpetic Gingivostomatitis (Fig. 46.1) **Herpes simplex virus** is a large DNA virus that infects human epithelium. Transmission is by contact with infected secretions such as saliva. The initial infection is usually subclinical (not readily visible) but can be prominent depending on the initial dose, location, integrity of the epithelium, and host response. **Herpetic gingivostomatitis** is a prominent manifestation of the primary oral infection. It is classified as a non–plaque-induced (viral infection) gingival disease. Replication of the virus in gingival epithelium causes generalized swelling, redness, and pain of the marginal gingiva. The interdental papillae become bulbous and bleed easily about 4 days after infection, and several oral vesicles and ulcers develop. The virus can spread throughout the oral mucosa and invade peripheral nerve endings. Once inside the infected nerve endings, the virus travels intra-axonally to the trigeminal ganglion, where it enters into a latent state. Systemic antiviral agents such as acyclovir (Zovirax), famciclovir (Famvir), or valacyclovir (Valtrex) are recommended early during the herpetic infection. Antimicrobial mouth rinses with chlorhexidine gluconate 0.12% (Peridex, PerioGard) also help to reduce oral sepsis. Systemic antibiotics are occasionally needed when patients become septic and their temperature is persistently elevated. Healing normally takes about 14 to 21 days. Thereafter, 30% to 40% of latently infected patients develop **recurrent herpes simplex virus infections** that reappear at sites previously infected (see Figs. 83.4–83.6 for more information).

Drug-Induced Gingival Overgrowth (Figs. 46.2–46.6) is a plaque-induced disease associated with use of specific prescription medications. Three drug categories have been implicated: anticonvulsants, immunosuppressants, and calcium channel blockers. The condition occurs in 25% to 50% of patients taking phenytoin (Dilantin) and cyclosporine (Sandimmune). Phenytoin is an antiseizure medication. Cyclosporine is taken by organ transplant patients to inhibit T-cell proliferation and prevent transplant rejection.

Gingival overgrowth also occurs in 1% to 10% of patients who take calcium channel blocker drugs (such as nifedipine [Procardia], diltiazem [Cardizem], verapamil [Calan], felodipine [Plendil], and amlodipine [Norvasc]). These drugs relax and dilate artery muscles and are used to lower blood pressure and prevent chest pain (angina) resulting from coronary artery spasm. Valproate sodium (Depakene), an antiseizure medication, and estrogen in birth control pills have also been associated with gingival overgrowth, generally at high doses. Although the mechanism of drug-induced gingival overgrowth remains unknown, many of these drugs affect calcium ion flux in gingival fibroblasts and appear to alter collagen metabolism, collagenase activity, and the local immune response. Estrogen may work separately by increasing the blood supply and inflammatory mediators to the gingiva. *Note:* Modern low-dose birth control pills rarely cause gingival overgrowth.

Drug-induced gingival overgrowth occurs at any age and in either sex. Although the overgrowth results from a hyperplastic response, an inflammatory component induced by dental bacterial plaque often coexists and tends to exacerbate the condition. The gingival overgrowth is usually generalized and begins at the interdental papillae. It appears most exaggerated on the labial aspects of the anterior teeth. The overgrowths form soft, red, lumpy nodules that bleed easily. Progressive growth results in fibrotic changes: the interdental tissue becomes enlarged, pink, and firm. With time, the condition can completely engulf the crowns of the teeth, which restricts home care, limits mastication, and compromises esthetics.

The condition can be minimized by instituting excellent patient oral hygiene care upon initiation of drug therapy. Once overgrowth develops, treatment may involve changing drug therapy and the provision of meticulous and frequent plaque control measures. The gingival swelling may completely regress by discontinuing drug use. However, excess fibrotic tissue unresponsive to changes in drug therapy should be surgically removed.

Gingival Fibromatosis (Figs. 46.7 and 46.8) is a rare, slowly progressive, fibrous enlargement of the gingiva classified as a non–plaque-induced gingival disease. It occurs more commonly as **hereditary gingival fibromatosis** but can be **idiopathic**. The gingival tissues contain fibroblasts that have low growth activity, dense collagen, and minimal inflammation. The condition begins with tooth eruption and becomes more prominent with age. The enlargement is usually generalized and noninflammatory, affecting the buccal and lingual surfaces of one or both jaws. The free, interproximal, and marginal gingiva are enlarged, uniformly pink, firm, nonhemorrhagic, and often nodular.

There are two types of **gingival fibromatosis**: generalized and localized. The generalized type is nodular and diffuse, exhibiting several coalesced areas of globular gingival overgrowths that encroach on and eventually cover the crowns of the teeth. In the less common localized variety, solitary overgrowths are limited to the palatal vault of the maxillary tuberosity or the lingual gingiva of the mandibular arch. These gingival overgrowths appear smooth, firm, and symmetrically round. The localized involvement may be unilateral or bilateral.

Gingival fibromatosis may interfere with tooth eruption, mastication, and oral hygiene. In severe cases, noneruption of the primary or permanent teeth may be the chief symptom. Regression in dentate patients is not a feature of this disease, even with effective oral hygiene measures. However, in areas of tooth loss, gingival size tends to decrease. Gingivectomy, with either a blade or a carbon dioxide laser, is the usual treatment. Continued growth may require several operations. The condition may be accompanied by acromegalic facial features, hypertrichosis, mental deficits, deafness, and seizures or associated with other syndromes.

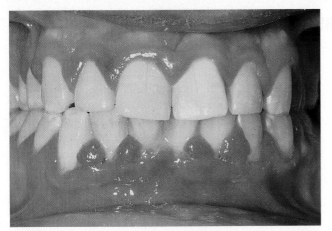

Fig. 46.1. Primary herpetic gingivostomatitis: painful.

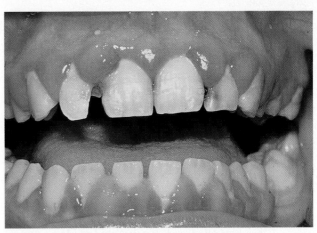

Fig. 46.2. Dilantin-induced gingival overgrowth.

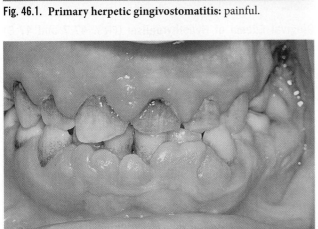

Fig. 46.3. Dilantin-induced gingival overgrowth.

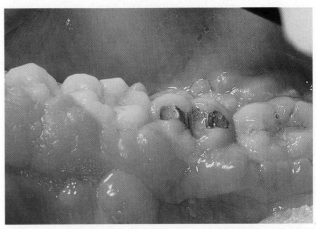

Fig. 46.4. Cyclosporine-induced gingival overgrowth.

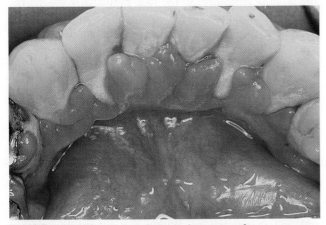

Fig. 46.5. Nifedipine-induced gingival overgrowth.

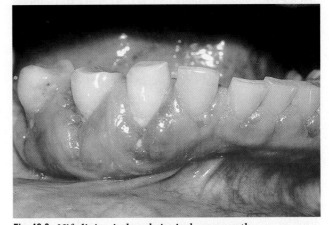

Fig. 46.6. Nifedipine-induced gingival overgrowth.

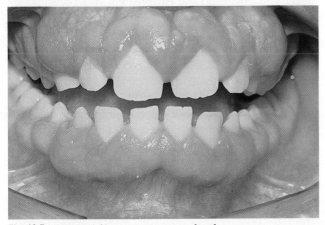

Fig. 46.7. Gingival fibromatosis: generalized.

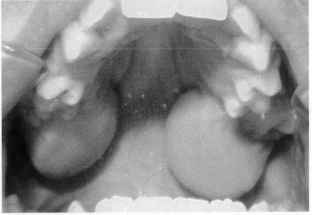

Fig. 46.8. Gingival fibromatosis: localized variant.

105

Pregnancy-Associated Gingivitis (Figs. 47.1–47.3) is a hyperplastic reaction to microbial plaque and hormone levels that affects women during pregnancy and, to a lesser extent, women during puberty and menopause. Elevated estrogen or progesterone levels resulting from hormonal shifts and use of (previously marketed versions of) birth control pills have been implicated. These hormones enhance tissue vascularity, which permits an exaggerated inflammatory reaction to plaque.

Pregnancy-associated gingivitis begins at the marginal and interdental gingiva, usually in the 2nd month of pregnancy. It produces fiery red, swollen, and tender marginal gingiva and compressible and swollen interdental papillae. The tissue is tender to palpation and bleeds easily on probing. The severity is related to plaque accumulation and poor oral hygiene. This is often the case during pregnancy when toothbrushing may be less frequent because it precipitates nausea.

Hormonal/pregnancy gingivitis is usually transitory and responds to meticulous home care, oral prophylaxis, and a decrease in hormone levels—which occurs after parturition or with a change of hormone medication. Persistence can result in fibrosis and pinker, firmer, and lumpy tissues. In a small percentage of pregnant women, the hyperplastic response may exacerbate in a localized area resulting in a **pyogenic granuloma** (pregnancy tumor) (Fig. 49.2). Gingivectomy is used to reduce fibrotic gingivae and excise tumorous growths.

Diabetes-Associated Gingivitis (Figs. 47.4–47.6) **Diabetes mellitus** is a common metabolic disease, affecting approximately 9% of the U.S. population and a high percentage of Hispanic Americans, African Americans, and Pacific Islanders. It is characterized by diminished insulin production (type 1) or diminished insulin use (type 2) that results in poor control of blood glucose levels. Before diagnosis, patients may present with hyperglycemia, glucosuria, polyuria, polydipsia, pruritus, weight gain or loss, loss of strength, visual problems, and loss of peripheral nerve sensation (neuropathy). It can also be a feature of **metabolic syndrome**—a cluster of disorders including insulin resistance, obesity, hypertension, cholesterol abnormalities, and increased risk for clotting. Because diabetes is a progressive disorder affecting large and small blood vessels, complications include many vascular-related problems, such as heart disease and stroke, blindness, high blood pressure, kidney failure, risk for infection, dry mouth, burning tongue, and persistent gingivitis.

The severity of **diabetic gingivitis** is dependent on the level of glycemic (blood glucose) control. In the patient with uncontrolled or poorly controlled diabetes, peculiar proliferations of swollen tissue arise from the marginal and attached gingiva. The well-demarcated swellings are soft, red, irregular, and sometimes hemorrhagic. The surface of the hyperplastic tissue is bulbous or lobular. The base of the tissue may be sessile or stalk-like. The condition is often accompanied by dry mouth, breath odor changes, and alveolar bone loss because of periodontitis. The gingivitis is difficult to manage when blood glucose levels remain elevated as the inflammatory response in the periodontal tissues is altered. Successful treatment requires meticulous patient self-care and control of the blood glucose level with diet, hypoglycemic agents, or insulin. *Note:* A well-controlled diabetic patient will have a fasting blood glucose level below 126 mg/dL and a glycosylated hemoglobin (HbA_{1c}) below 7%. Oral surgical procedures should be limited to when the blood glucose level is below 200 mg/dL and the patient's condition is considered stable.

Gingival Edema of Hypothyroidism (Figs. 47.7 and 47.8) **Hypothyroidism** is a relatively common disorder that is characterized by low levels of thyroid hormone. The clinical manifestations depend on the age at onset, duration, and severity of thyroid insufficiency. When thyroid hormone (triiodothyronine [T3] or thyroxine [T4]) deficiency occurs during infancy, **cretinism** results. This disease is characterized by short stature, mental retardation, disproportionate head-to-body size, delayed tooth eruption, mandibular micrognathism, and swollen face, lips, and tongue. Regardless of the age at onset, hypothyroid patients are intolerant to cold and have coarse, yellowish skin that feels cool and dry to the touch, coarse hair, and lethargy. Adult-onset hypothyroidism is also characterized by dull expression, loss of eyebrow hair, slow physical and mental activity, and elevated cholesterol. Soft tissue swelling is the classic feature and is most prominent in the face, particularly around the eyes. It is caused by accumulation of subcutaneous fluid.

Hypothyroidism can be primary or secondary. In primary, the thyroid gland is abnormal or forms incorrectly. Secondary hypothyroidism is due to lack of production of thyroid-stimulating hormone (TSH) by the pituitary gland. Hypothyroidism in children is most commonly caused by primary disease—hypoplasia or agenesis of the thyroid gland. Hypothyroidism in adults is commonly caused by medical therapy that is used to eliminate an overactive thyroid gland (hyperthyroidism), as well as by autoimmune lymphocytic infiltration (**Hashimoto thyroiditis**), in which the thyroid glandular cells are replaced by lymphocytes.

Hypothyroidism can produce an enlarged thyroid gland and oral manifestations. Within the mouth, an enlarged tongue (macroglossia) and enlarged lips (macrocheilia) are common and may cause an altered speech pattern. The gingiva appears uniformly enlarged, pale pink, and compressible. Swelling occurs in all directions on both the facial and lingual sides of the dental arches. When secondary inflammation is present, the tissues become red and boggy and have a tendency to bleed easily. Treatment for the gingival condition depends on the degree of thyroid deficiency. Patients with marginal deficiency require only strict oral hygiene measures, whereas frank cases require supplemental replacement thyroid therapy (thyroxine or levothyroxine) to achieve resolution of the systemic and oral condition.

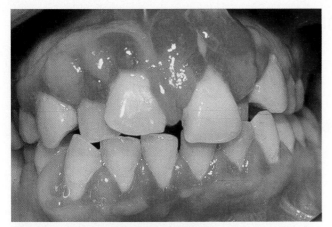

Fig. 47.1. Pregnancy-associated gingivitis.

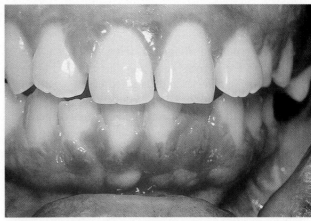

Fig. 47.2. Pregnancy-associated gingivitis: 3 weeks postpartum.

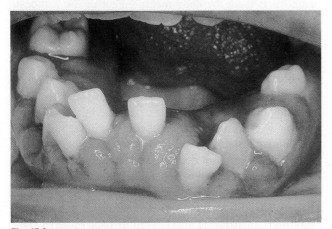

Fig. 47.3. Oral contraceptive–associated gingivitis.

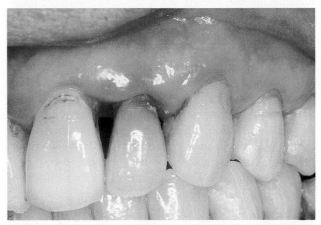

Fig. 47.4. Diabetes-associated gingivitis: advanced periodontitis.

7

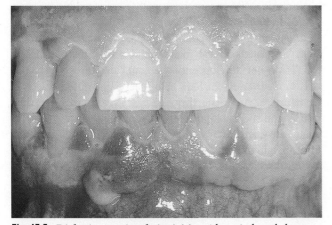

Fig. 47.5. Diabetic-associated gingivitis: with periodontal abscess.

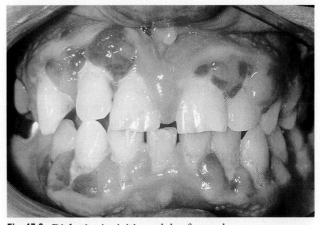

Fig. 47.6. Diabetic gingivitis: nodular, fiery red.

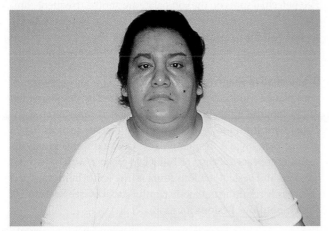

Fig. 47.7. Hypothyroidism: edema, thick skin.*

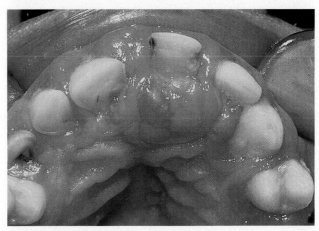

Fig. 47.8. Hypothyroidism: gingival edema.*

Leukemia-Associated Gingivitis (Figs. 48.1 and 48.2)

Leukemia is a malignant condition characterized by overproduction of leukocytes and classified by the white blood cell type involved and the clinical course (acute or chronic). Oral manifestations are more frequently encountered in acute leukemia of the monocytic and myelogenous subtypes. Oral features occur early in the course of the disease because of neoplastic proliferation of the white blood cells that deposit in oral tissue. Systemic symptoms develop as the neoplastic cells overwhelm the normal production of the other hematopoietic cells.

Consistent signs of acute leukemia are cervical lymphadenopathy, malaise, anemic pallor, leukopenia-induced ulcerations, recurrent infections, and gingival changes. Multiple adjacent gingival sites are affected and appear red, tender, and spongy. With progression of the disease, the swollen gingiva becomes shiny purple and tends to lift away from the teeth. Stippling of the tissue is lost, and spontaneous bleeding from the gingival sulcus eventually occurs. The edematous tissue is most prominent interdentally and results from leukemic infiltration of malignant cells. In certain patients, the neoplastic cells may invade pulpal and osseous tissue, inducing vague symptoms of pain without corresponding radiographic evidence of pathosis. Purpuric features, such as petechial lesions and ecchymoses on pale mucosal membranes, together with gingival hemorrhage, occur frequently. Systemic control of leukemia often involves intensive radiotherapy, chemotherapy, blood transfusions, and bone marrow transplantation. Difficulty may be encountered in maintaining optimal oral health because of chemotherapy-induced oral ulcerations. Meticulous oral hygiene combined with antimicrobial rinses is recommended to reduce oral inflammation and ulcerations caused by chemotherapy.

Agranulocytosis (Neutropenia) is a disease characterized by a marked decrease in the number of circulating granulocytes (less than 500 cells/mm^3), most commonly neutrophils—cells that defend against infection. Most often, the condition is recognized by clinical symptoms, which consist of chronic infections and an almost complete absence of neutrophils in lab blood tests. Cytotoxic drugs and disorders that decrease bone marrow production or destroy neutrophils are causative agents in the majority of cases. Rarely, the condition may be congenital. Uncontrollable infection in the neutropenic patient can result in bacterial pneumonia, sepsis, and death.

Cyclic Neutropenia (Figs. 48.3 and 48.4)

A distinct form of agranulocytosis is **cyclic neutropenia**, an inherited disorder characterized by a periodic decrease in circulating neutrophils that occurs about every 3 weeks and lasts for about 5 days. The condition is caused by an inherited (autosomal dominant) mutation in the *ELANE* gene that encodes for neutrophil elastase. Cyclic neutropenia appears in childhood and is often accompanied by pharyngitis, fever, headache, lymphadenopathy, and arthritis. A history of repeated infections of the skin, ear, and upper respiratory tract is common. Oral manifestations include recurrent episodes of inflammatory gingival changes and mucosal ulcerations. The ulcerations are usually large, oval, and persistent. They vary in size and location. Sometimes, they are found on the attached gingiva and other times on the tongue and buccal mucosa. At stages that correspond to elevated levels of circulating neutrophils, minimal inflammation is evident. In contrast, when the neutrophil count decreases precipitously, generalized inflammatory hyperplasia and erythema occur. If left untreated, the condition is exacerbated by the presence of local factors, such as plaque and calculus, which result in alveolar bone loss, tooth mobility, and early exfoliation of teeth.

Recurrent episodes and spontaneous regression of signs and symptoms are characteristic of cyclic neutropenia. The diagnosis is made by daily measurement of the leukocyte count. Treatment involves use of the blood growth factor known as *granulocyte colony–stimulating factor*, along with antimicrobial agents and a strict oral hygiene program.

Thrombocytopathic and Thrombocytopenic Purpura (Figs. 48.5–48.8)

Platelets help maintain hemostasis by providing the primary hemostatic plug and by activating the intrinsic system of coagulation. A decrease in the number of circulating platelets (**thrombocytopenia**) may be idiopathic or may be the result of decreased platelet production in the bone marrow, increased peripheral destruction, or increased splenic sequestration. Decreased function of circulating platelets (**thrombocytopathia**) is often related to hereditary syndromes or acquired states, such as drug-induced bone marrow suppression, liver disease, or dysproteinemic states like uremia. Mild thrombocytopathia is caused by daily use of aspirin or clopidogrel (Plavix).

The normal platelet count is 150,000 to 400,000 cells/mm^3. Vascular-related clinical manifestations of platelet disorders usually do not develop until the count decreases to <75,000 cells/mm^3. Features include petechiae, ecchymoses, epistaxis, hematuria, hypermenorrhea, and gastrointestinal bleeding resulting in melena. **Spontaneous gingival bleeding** is a frequent, early, and dramatic occurrence. Blood oozes profusely from the gingival sulcus, either spontaneously or after minor trauma, such as toothbrushing. The fluid then turns into purplish black globs of clotted blood that adhere to the oral structures. Clotted blood is sometimes swallowed, which can cause nausea. Mild traumas, particularly at the occlusal line of the buccal mucosa and tongue, are sites of extensive hemorrhage. Red petechial spots on the soft palate are another frequent clinical sign. Measurement of the platelet count and platelet function should be done to assess platelet disorders. Platelet transfusions may be necessary if local measures do not control oral bleeding.

Desquamative Gingivitis (Figs. 87.5–87.7)

is another form of non–plaque-induced gingivitis characterized by desquamation of the gingival epithelium. The condition is most often associated with immunologically mediated disease such as lichen planus, pemphigoid, or pemphigus. **Desquamative gingivitis** typically appears as bright red attached gingiva, with or without erosions and vesiculobullous lesions. The epithelium may peel away easily resulting in bloody painful surfaces (see **Section 10, Vesiculobullous Lesions** for more details).

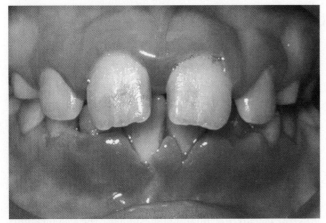

Fig. 48.1. Leukemia-associated gingivitis: acute myelogenous leukemia.

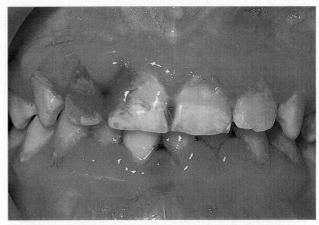

Fig. 48.2. Leukemia-associated gingivitis: acute lymphocytic leukemia.

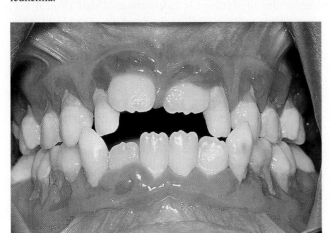

Fig. 48.3. Cyclic neutropenia: gingival erythema.*

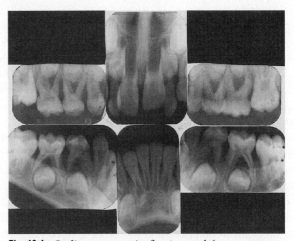

Fig. 48.4. Cyclic neutropenia: floating teeth.*

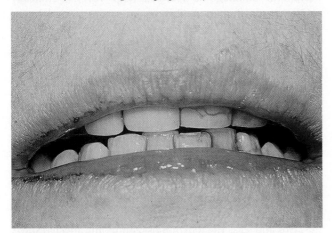

Fig. 48.5. Thrombocytopathia and cirrhosis.‡

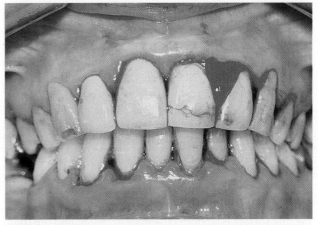

Fig. 48.6. Thrombocytopathia: spontaneous bleeding.‡

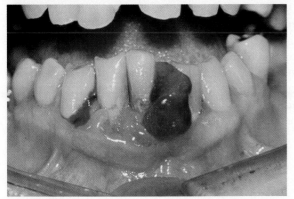

Fig. 48.7. Thrombocytopenia: 26,000 platelets/mm³.§

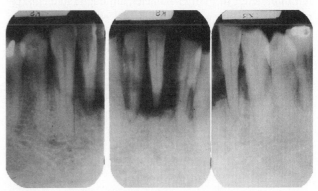

Fig. 48.8. Thrombocytopenia evidence of chronic irritants.§

Pyogenic Granuloma (Figs. 49.1 and 49.2) is a common, benign mass of inflamed tissue that bleeds easily because of an abnormally high concentration of blood vessels. The name *pyogenic granuloma* is a misnomer because the condition is neither a granuloma nor pus filled. The growth is an exaggerated response to a chronic irritant, such as overhanging restorations or calculus. Often, they develop rapidly and in patients who have poor oral hygiene. Women are more susceptible to the condition because of hormonal imbalances that occur during puberty, pregnancy, or menopause. In such cases, the granulomas are called **hormonal** or **pregnancy tumors**. About 1% of pregnant women develop this lesion. A limited number of cases have occurred in patients who take cyclosporine.

Pyogenic granulomas appear as bright red to purple, fleshy-soft nodules. The surface is glossy, ulcerated, and often lobulated. The base is polypoid or pedunculated. Although usually asymptomatic, the condition bleeds easily after minor manipulation because of the thinned epithelium and highly vascular tissue. Mature lesions become fibrotic, less vascular, and less red in color.

Pyogenic granulomas most frequently arise from the interdental papilla anterior to molar sites and can enlarge from the labial and lingual aspects to several centimeters. Other sites of development include the tongue, lips, buccal mucosa, and edentulous ridge. Treatment is surgical excision with removal of local irritants to prevent recurrence. In the pregnant woman, excision should be delayed until after childbirth.

Peripheral Giant Cell Granuloma (Figs. 49.3 and 49.4) is a reactive lesion that develops exclusively on the gingiva. It is generally associated with a history of trauma or irritation and is thought to originate from the mucoperiosteum or periodontal ligament. Therefore, the **peripheral giant cell granuloma** demonstrates a restricted area of development—the dentulous or edentulous ridge. The mandibular gingiva anterior to the molars is particularly affected, especially in women between the ages of 40 and 60. Histologic examination shows sheets of multinucleated giant cells and numerous fibroblasts.

The peripheral giant cell granuloma is a well-defined, firm, epulislike growth that seldom ulcerates. The base is sessile, the surface is smooth or slightly granular, and the color is pink to dark red-bluish purple. The nodule is usually a few millimeters to 1 cm in diameter, although rapid enlargement may produce a large growth that encroaches on adjacent teeth. The lesion is generally asymptomatic. However, because of its aggressive nature, the underlying bone is often involved, producing a characteristic superficial "cupping" resorptive radiolucency of the alveolar bone. Treatment is excision that includes the base of the lesion and curettage of the underlying bone. Incomplete removal may result in recurrence. On histologic examination, this lesion cannot be distinguished from the **central giant cell granuloma** and the **brown tumor of hyperparathyroidism**.

Peripheral Ossifying Fibroma (Figs. 49.5 and 49.6) is a reactive growth, unrelated to the central ossifying fibroma, that is especially prone to occur in the anterior region of the maxilla of females in the second decade of life. The cause of the peripheral ossifying fibroma is uncertain, but inflammatory hyperplasia of superficial periodontal ligament origin has been suggested. The condition arises exclusively from the gingiva, usually the interdental papillae. The calcifications seen within the fibrous lesion may consist of woven bone, cementum, or dystrophic calcification. Usual clinical features of this solitary swelling are firmness, pink to red color, possible ulceration, and sessile attachment. An important diagnostic clue is the marked tendency of the condition to cause displacement of adjacent teeth. The chief sign is often an asymptomatic, slow-growing round or nodular swelling. Immature lesions are soft and bleed easily, whereas older lesions become firm and fibrotic. Radiographs may reveal central radiopaque foci, mild resorption of the crestal bone (peripheral cuff of bone), and wispy trabeculae. Treatment is excision. The recurrence rate is about 15%.

Irritation Fibroma is a common benign oral lesion that occasionally develops on gingival tissues. It is more typically seen on moveable mucosa and is discussed in Section 10 (Fig. 81.1).

Peripheral Odontogenic Fibroma (Fig. 49.7) is clinically similar to the irritation fibroma but characterized by its unique location and tissue of origin. In most cases, it presents as a firm, dome-shaped swelling on the facial aspect of the interdental papilla, generally located anterior to the molar teeth. A cuplike erosion of the underlying alveolar bone may be seen radiographically. The lesion probably arises from cellular components of the periodontal ligament. Microscopically, it shows strands of odontogenic epithelium among dense collagenous tissue and occasional mineralized products.

Desmoplastic Fibroma (Fig. 49.8) is a rare tumor composed of dense fibroblasts and abundant collagen that most frequently affects the metaphyseal regions of the long bones of the arms and legs. The fourth most commonly affected site is the mandible. Most cases occur in adults younger than age 30. The posterior jaw is the most common intraoral location. The tumors begin as painless firm swellings within bone that expand and produce unilocular radiolucencies. Erosion of the cortical bone results in root resorption and a pink, firm soft tissue mass of the alveolar ridge or gingiva. The tumor is locally aggressive and recurs in about 5% of patients after surgical excision. Thus, resection with clear margins is recommended to minimize recurrences.

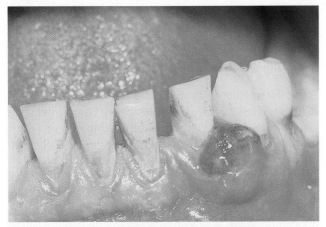

Fig. 49.1. **Pyogenic granuloma** at interdental papilla.

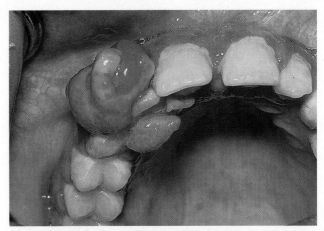

Fig. 49.2. **Pregnancy tumor:** 3 days after parturition.

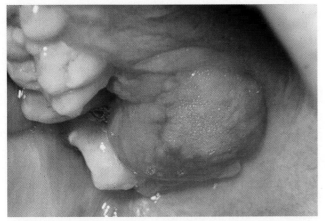

Fig. 49.3. **Peripheral giant cell granuloma** on gingival margin.

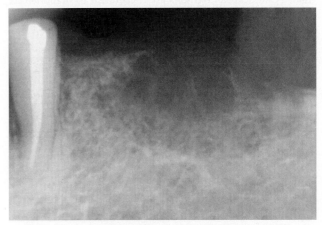

Fig. 49.4. **Peripheral giant cell granuloma:** "cuffing of bone."

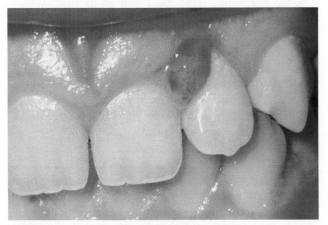

Fig. 49.5. **Peripheral ossifying fibroma:** typical location.

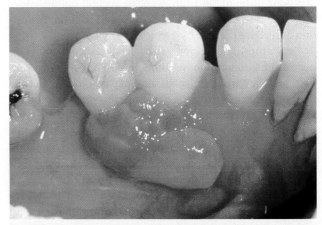

Fig. 49.6. **Peripheral ossifying fibroma:** pink and firm.

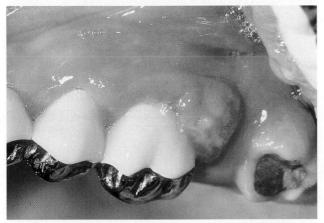

Fig. 49.7. **Peripheral odontogenic fibroma:** arising from PDL.

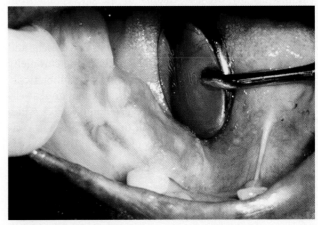

Fig. 49.8. **Desmoplastic fibroma:** aggressive, firm lesion.

LOCALIZED GINGIVAL LESIONS

Parulis (Figs. 50.1 and 50.2) or **Gumboil**—the latter term being reserved for children (Fig. 15.8)—is a localized area of inflamed granulation tissue that occurs at the end point of a sinus tract that is draining from a nonvital tooth. It appears as a soft, solitary reddish papule, located apical and facial to a chronically abscessed tooth, usually on or near the labial mucogingival junction. The parulis can be slightly yellow in the center and emit a purulent yellowish exudate on palpation. Acute swelling and pain may accompany the condition if the sinus tract is obstructed.

To locate the nonvital tooth from which the parulis arises, a sterile gutta-percha point may be inserted into the sinus tract. Periapical radiographs are then taken to demonstrate the proximity of the gutta-percha point to the apex of the offending tooth. After the nonvital tooth is diagnosed, the treatment of choice is root canal therapy or extraction. Treatment results in healing of the parulis. If the problematic tooth is left untreated, the parulis may persist for years. A persistent lesion may mature into a pink-colored fibroma.

Pericoronitis (Operculitis) (Figs. 50.3 and 50.4) is inflammation of the soft tissue surrounding the crown of a partially erupted or impacted tooth. Pericoronitis may develop at any age but most frequently occurs in children and young adults whose teeth are erupting. Generally, it is associated with an erupting mandibular third molar that is in good alignment but is limited in its eruption by insufficient space. Radiographs reveal a flame-shaped radiolucency in the alveolar bone distal to the tooth, with the cortical outline either absent or distinctly thickened because of infection, deposition of reactive bone, or cyst formation.

Pericoronitis develops from bacterial contamination beneath the **operculum**, resulting in gingival swelling, redness, and halitosis. Pain varies and may be extreme, but the discomfort usually resembles that of gingivitis, a periodontal abscess, or tonsillitis. Regional lymphadenopathy, malaise, and low-grade fever are common. If edema or cellulitis extends to involve the masseter muscle, trismus accompanies the condition. Pericoronitis is frequently complicated by dysphagia (difficulty swallowing) and pain induced by trauma from the opposing tooth during closure.

Pericoronitis is best managed by flushing the purulent material from the gingival sulcus with saline solution and eliminating any occlusal trauma to the operculum from the opposing third molar. Definitive treatment is usually extraction of the involved tooth. Antibiotic coverage is recommended when constitutional symptoms are present and the spread of infection is likely. Recurrences and chronicity are likely if the condition is managed only with antibiotics.

Periodontal Abscess produces a localized gingival swelling. The American Academy of Periodontology classifies abscesses as gingival, periodontal, or pericoronal. In contrast, the American Association of Endodontists classifies them as either acute or chronic apical abscess. For more information, see Figure 51.7.

Epulis Fissuratum (Figs. 50.5 and 50.6) is an overgrowth of fibrous connective tissue resulting from chronic irritation usually from the flange of an ill-fitting complete or partial denture. The overextended denture margin initially produces an ulcer that is repeatedly traumatized. Hyperplastic healing results in a pink-red, fleshy exuberance of mature granulation tissue. The hyperplastic lesion, located where the denture flange rests, is found mostly in older women. It is nonpainful, grows slowly on either side of the denture flange, and causes the patient little concern.

The epulis fissuratum in the early stages consists of a single fold of smooth soft tissue. As the swelling grows, a central cleft or several clefts become apparent, the boundaries of which may drape over the denture flange. The mucolabial fold of the anterior maxilla is the most common location, followed by the mandibular alveolar ridge and the mandibular lingual sulcus. Adjustment of the denture, a reline, or construction of a new denture may reduce the trauma and inflammation but will not cause the underlying fibrous tissue to regress. Likewise, surgical excision without alteration of the dentures promotes recurrence. Successful treatment usually requires surgical removal of the redundant tissue, microscopic examination of the excised tissue, and correction or reconstruction of the denture.

Gingival Carcinoma (Figs. 50.7 and 50.8) The gingiva is the site of about 5% to 10% of all cases of oral squamous cell carcinoma. Generally, at the time of diagnosis, the disease is advanced because of its asymptomatic nature, posterior location, and delay in examination.

Gingival carcinoma varies in appearance. It usually appears as a reddish proliferative mass with focal white areas arising from the gingiva that can mimic benign inflammatory and reactive gingival conditions, such as a pyogenic granuloma, erythroplakia, leukoplakia, or a simple ulceration. Carcinoma should be suspected when close examination reveals a pebbly surface, many small blood vessels in the overlying epithelium, and surface ulceration. Etiologic factors include tobacco use, alcoholism, and poor oral hygiene. Elderly men are especially susceptible, and the condition has a slight predilection for the alveolar ridge of the posterior mandible. Completely dentate persons rarely have this disease.

Gingival carcinoma may extend onto the floor of the mouth or mucobuccal fold or invade the underlying bone. Radiographs may reveal a cupping out of the alveolar crest. Metastasis to regional lymph nodes occurs frequently. Metastatic lymph nodes are firm, rubbery, matted, nonmovable, and nonpainful. Treatment consists of surgery and radiotherapy.

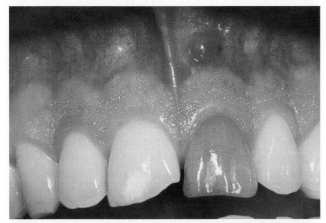

Fig. 50.1. Parulis: reddish papule above nonvital central.

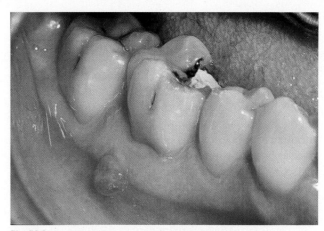

Fig. 50.2. Parulis: adjacent to nonvital first molar.

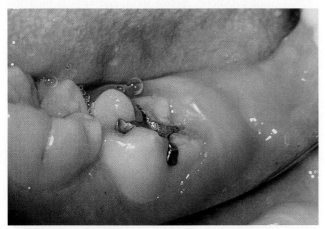

Fig. 50.3. Pericoronitis: distal to partially erupted molar.

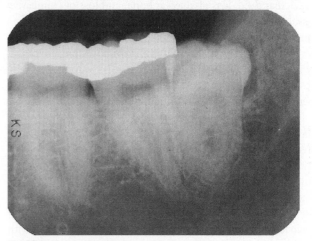

Fig. 50.4. Pericoronitis: flame-shaped radiolucency.

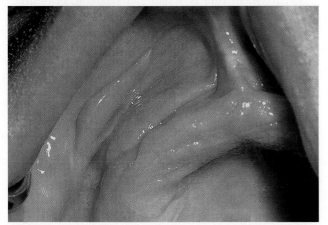

Fig. 50.5. Epulis fissuratum in maxillary labial fornix.

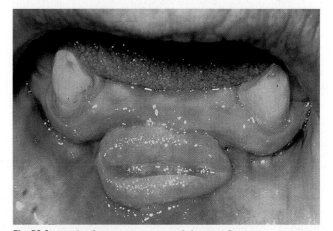

Fig. 50.6. Epulis fissuratum at partial denture flange.

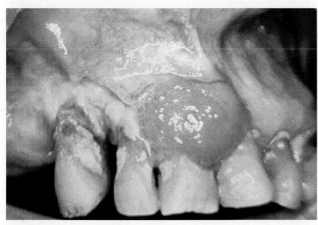

Fig. 50.7. Gingival carcinoma: poor oral hygiene.

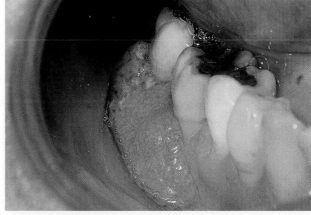

Fig. 50.8. Gingival carcinoma: squamous cell type.

PERIODONTITIS

Periodontitis (Figs. 51.1–51.8) is an inflammatory disease of the supporting structures of the periodontium including the gingiva, periodontal ligament, bone, and cementum. It results in irreversible destruction to the tissues of the periodontium. It is characterized by progressive loss of epithelial attachment and destruction of the periodontal ligament and alveolar bone. It is preceded by gingivitis and dental plaque that contains many anaerobic species. The most common form, **chronic periodontitis**, increases in prevalence with age and progresses episodically. During exacerbations, there is apical migration of the epithelial attachment, increased periodontal pocket depth (greater than 3 mm), increased gingival crevicular fluid, loss of alveolar bone, and loss of connective tissue attachment. Disease activity is assessed by monitoring these findings clinically, radiographically, and supplementally by analyzing the content of gingival crevicular fluid and saliva, which contain inflammatory mediators. Periodontitis usually results in mobility, shifting, and loss of teeth. Nonvitality and periodontal abscess are two less common outcomes.

Chronic periodontitis is divided into three types (mild, moderate, and advanced) based on severity and can be localized or generalized. The other categories of periodontitis include *aggressive periodontitis* (previously termed prepubertal, juvenile, or early-onset periodontitis), *periodontitis as a manifestation of systemic diseases, necrotizing periodontal diseases, abscesses of periodontium,* and *periodontitis associated with endodontic lesions.* The predominant species associated with chronic periodontitis are *Actinomyces naeslundii, Tannerella forsythia, Campylobacter rectus, Eikenella corrodens, Eubacterium* species, *Fusobacterium nucleatum, Peptostreptococcus micros, Prevotella intermedia, Porphyromonas gingivalis, Selenomonas sputigena, Streptococcus intermedius,* and *Treponema* species (*T. denticola*). Certain species such as *Aggregatibacter (Actinobacillus) actinomycetemcomitans* are detected more often with specific types of periodontitis (i.e., aggressive periodontitis). Risk factors for periodontal disease include smoking, aging, genetic factors, and certain systemic diseases (diabetes mellitus, white blood cell disorders, and Ehlers-Danlos syndrome). Treatment involves the removal of plaque, calculus, and diseased cementum by periodontal instrumentation. Antibiotics (tetracycline and metronidazole) are used with aggressive periodontitis. Periodontal surgery is recommended for unresponsive sites after periodontal instrumentation is complete and good patient self-care is in place.

Mild Periodontitis (Figs. 51.1 and 51.2) is characterized by mild breakdown of pocket epithelium, migration of neutrophils, increasing population of plasma cells, apical migration of junctional epithelium, minor destruction of the connective tissue attachment, and localized resorption of alveolar bone. This stage is defined by **1 to 2 mm of clinical attachment loss** (measured from the CEJ to the base of the pocket), periodontal probe pocket depths of 4 mm, class I furcation involvement, and alveolar crestal bone loss of 2 mm or less. The **class I furcation** is limited destruction of bone between the superior aspect of the roots and the tooth crown that is detectable by 1-mm entry of an explorer or probe. Alveolar

bone loss is determined clinically by periodontal probing and supplemented by the use of vertical periapical bitewing radiographs or subtraction radiography.

Moderate Periodontitis (Figs. 51.3–51.5) is the second stage of chronic periodontitis. Microscopic examination shows ulceration of the pocket epithelium, infiltrating populations of plasma cells and T cells, significant apical migration of junctional epithelium, and destruction of the connective tissue attachment and alveolar bone. The condition is defined by **3 to 4 mm of clinical attachment loss**, periodontal pocket depths of 5 to 6 mm, alveolar bone loss that is 3 to 4 mm, gingival exudate, and bleeding. Horizontal bone loss, vertical bone loss, osseous defects (moats, craters), mobile teeth, and class II furcation involvement are additional radiographic and clinical features of the disease. The **class II furcation** is a 2 to 4 mm defect of cortical and alveolar bone located superiorly between the roots.

Advanced Periodontitis (Fig. 51.6) is characterized microscopically by major destruction of the pocket epithelium, connective tissue attachment, and alveolar bone and large populations of plasma cells and T cells. Advanced periodontitis is defined by **at least 5 mm of clinical attachment loss**. Typically, periodontal pocket depths exceed 6 mm; alveolar bone loss is more than 4 mm; and gingival recession, significant tooth mobility, and **class III furcation** involvement (a through-and-through bony defect) are seen. See Figures 37.4, 43.1, and 52.8 for radiographic examples of advanced periodontitis.

Recurrent disease is a sign and symptom of destructive periodontitis that reappears after periodontal therapy because the disease was not adequately treated and/or the patient did not practice adequate self-care.

Refractory Periodontitis refers to periodontal disease that is nonresponsive to treatment, despite longitudinal properly executed monitoring and therapy.

Periodontal Abscess (Figs. 51.7 and 51.8) is a collection of pus resulting from pathogenic bacteria that are occluded (trapped) in the periodontal pocket of a pre-existing periodontal lesion. The condition produces a rapidly progressing, red-purple fluctuant swelling that distends the attached gingiva. The gingival surface is typically smooth, with loss of stippling of the free marginal groove. Occasionally, the surface is necrotic or has pus emanating. Affected teeth usually have a deep pocket, subgingival calculus, an occluded entrance into the periodontal pocket, and furcation involvement and are mobile. Patients often report well-localized, dull, and continuous pain, especially if the purulent exudate has no avenue for escape. The pain intensifies when pressure is applied to the tooth or the overlying soft tissue. Use of a periodontal probe may initially produce discomfort but is often therapeutic for a short time because it may drain the abscess. Fever, malaise, lymphadenopathy, and an unpleasant taste may accompany the condition. The pulp of the affected tooth usually tests vital although the periodontal infection may spread to the pulp via the apex of a lateral canal. Treatment involves removal of necrotic material, adequate drainage, localized periodontal therapy, and improved plaque control measures.

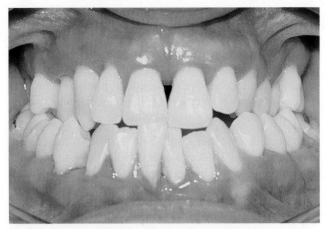

Fig. 51.1. **Mild periodontitis:** loss of attachment evident.

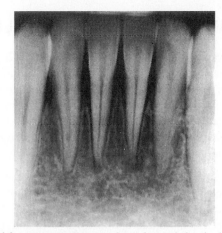

Fig. 51.2. **Mild periodontitis:** loss of crestal alveolar bone.

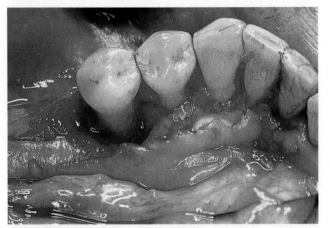

Fig. 51.3. **Moderate periodontitis:** 4-mm moat defect.

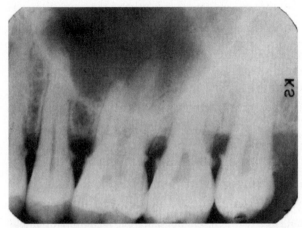

Fig. 51.4. **Horizontal bone loss** and calculus.

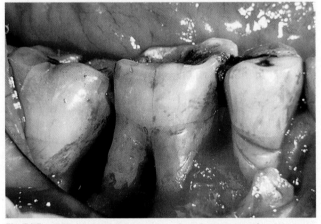

Fig. 51.5. **Class II furcation:** a sign of moderate periodontitis.

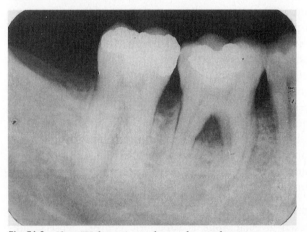

Fig. 51.6. **Class III furcation:** advanced periodontitis.

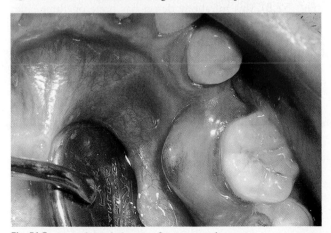

Fig. 51.7. **Periodontal abscess:** fluctuant and pointing.

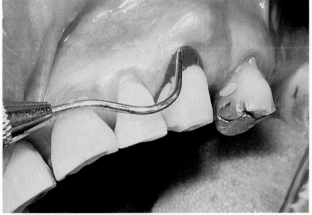

Fig. 51.8. **Periodontal abscess** with 12-mm pocket.

115

RADIOGRAPHIC FEATURES OF PERIODONTAL DISEASE

There are several radiographic features associated with periodontal disease, the most prominent being alveolar bone loss. This basic finding, although suggestive of periodontitis, is a nonspecific radiographic finding. It suggests that inflammatory and resorptive processes have been active. However, bone loss only provides historical reference. It is not indicative of whether the loss occurred years ago or recently.

Local Factors: Overhang (Fig. 52.1) Local factors can contribute indirectly to the development of periodontal disease. Examples include calculus (Fig. 51.4), crowding (Fig. 51.1), traumatic occlusion, supraeruption (Figs. 17.7 and 17.8), and restoration overhangs. An **overhang** is a specific portion of restoration that extends beyond the gingival preparation margin into the interproximal space. It is usually caused by inadequate banding and wedging of a prepared tooth before placement of the final restoration. Overhangs are seen with class II amalgams, as well as with composites and castings. Overhangs are **iatrogenic** because they are caused by a dental procedure. In Figure 52.1, a bone defect is associated with the mesial overhang of the maxillary second molar. There is also a small overhang on the mesial of the second premolar. However, it is associated only with a mild crestal irregularity. Overhangs should be removed and the margins smoothed either during periodontal procedures or as a new restoration.

Local Factors: Open Contact and Poor Restoration Contour (Fig. 52.2) Poor restoration contacts can contribute to food impaction, the accumulation of plaque, and the development of periodontitis. An **open contact** is an area between teeth where interproximal contact is absent. A poor restoration contact can be rough or have inappropriate width, length, height, or contour. Poor and open contacts can result from tooth mobility caused by malocclusion or periodontal disease, supraeruption, drifting of erupted teeth, and attrition and flattening of the interproximal contacts and iatrogenically (when a contact is improperly restored). In Figure 52.2, poor and open contacts are present between the first and second molars. Also, a bone defect is present, and the undercontoured restoration needs replacement.

Bone Loss: Localized (Figs. 51.2, 52.1, and 52.3) Healthy crestal alveolar bone is superiorly convex, densely radiopaque, continuous with the lamina dura on both sides, and located 1 to 1.5 mm apical to the cementoenamel junction. Localized bone loss occurs when inflammatory cytokines cause bone resorption. Radiographically, one sees crestal irregularities, triangulation (bone defect formation), loss of bone density, and interseptal bone changes. These changes may be localized or affect several areas. **Triangulation** is a wedge-shaped radiolucent defect that is a result of periodontal disease on the mesial or distal of the crestal interalveolar bone. Interseptal bone changes consistent with periodontal

disease are prominent **nutrient canals**, especially in the mandibular anterior region (Figs. 51.2 and 53.2). Nutrient canals appear as vertical radiolucent lines and indicate increased vascularity to the region and susceptibility to bone loss if treatment is not provided.

Bone Loss: Generalized (Figs. 51.4 and 52.4) Generalized bone loss indicates resorption of alveolar bone in multiple, often continuous sites. It occurs most frequently as **horizontal bone loss**. However, there may be areas of **vertical (or angular) bone loss**. In Figure 52.4, there are generalized horizontal bone loss; areas of vertical bone loss distal to the second premolar and mesial to the first molar; contact flattening caused by attrition, especially of the premolars; extrusion of the first molar with root caries; calculus; class III furcation involvement of the first molar; and furcation involvement of the second molar. The soft tissue outline of the gingiva seen along the cementoenamel junction indicates that deep periodontal pockets are present.

Bone (Infrabony) Defects Angular or vertical bone defects are classified by the number of walls remaining after destruction of alveolar bone by periodontal disease. Although radiographs are suggestive of an infrabony defect and its severity, defects are best delineated by careful probing or surgical exploration. A **crater** is simply a scooped-out area of alveolar bone anywhere along the circumference of a tooth and is not classified as a walled defect.

One-Wall Infrabony Defect (Figs. 52.3 and 52.5) This defect has only one wall of interseptal bone (hemiseptum) remaining. The wall may slope mesiodistally, as seen distal to the second premolar in Figure 52.3, or ramp buccal or lingually, as seen in Figure 52.5 between the molars. This defect is difficult to treat.

Two-Wall Infrabony Defect (Fig. 52.6) A two-wall bony defect has two walls of interseptal bone remaining. Radiographically, there is a combination of the ramping, as seen in Figure 52.6, and the vertical defect, as seen in Figure 52.3. The result is a combination of bony walls creating an osseous defect in the interseptal bone at the mesial or distal of a tooth. This defect makes up 35% of all defects and 62% of mandibular defects. In our example, the crater is mesial alongside the lower second molar.

Three-Wall Infrabony Defect (Fig. 52.7) and Moat Defect (Fig. 52.8) This infrabony defect has bone on three sides with the tooth root forming the fourth wall. The defect surrounds only a portion of the root. When it involves the buccal or lingual surface or completely surrounds the root, it is referred to as a **circumferential** or **moat** defect. In the case in which the defect involves the periapex, inflammation and vascular compromise can result in necrosis of the pulp. This coalescence of infections is known as a combined **periodontal-endodontic lesion**.

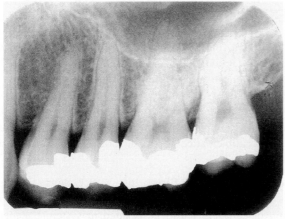

Fig. 52.1. Local factors: overhang and crestal defects.

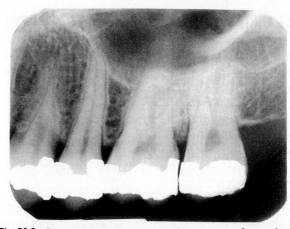

Fig. 52.2. Open contact, poor restoration contour: first molar.

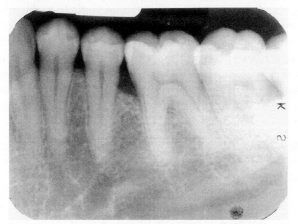

Fig. 52.3. Vertical one-wall defect: distal to premolar.

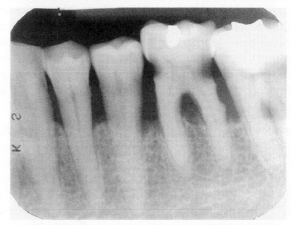

Fig. 52.4. Bone loss: generalized; extrusion and root caries.

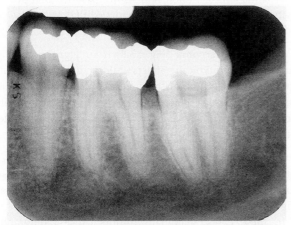

Fig. 52.5. One-wall bone defect: ramping between molars.

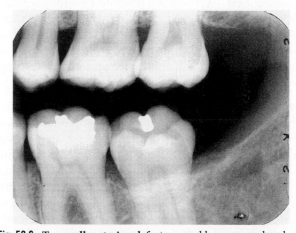

Fig. 52.6. Two-wall cratering defect: around lower second molar.

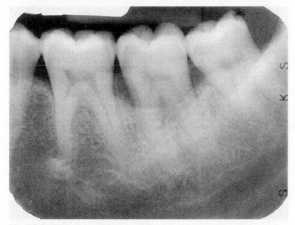

Fig. 52.7. Three-wall bone defect: second molar area.

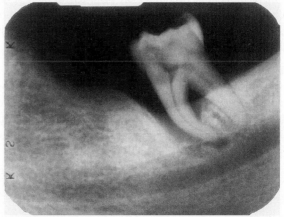

Fig. 52.8. Circumferential (moat) defect and nonvital tooth.

Periodontal Ligament and Lamina Dura The **periodontal ligament (PDL)** is composed of connective tissue fibers that attach the root to the alveolar bone. It appears as a 1-mm radiolucent space surrounding the root (see example in Fig. 5.5). The **lamina dura** is a thin dense radiopaque layer of cortical bone that lines the tooth socket. It is seen immediately outside the PDL space. Changes in the PDL space and lamina dura are caused by several diseases discussed below.

Acute Apical Periodontitis (Fig. 53.1) is the result of pulpal inflammation and early necrosis that is due to deep caries, trauma, or operative procedures that lead to death of the pulp. The first sign is a localized thickening of the PDL space. Then, osteoclasts resorb local bone, causing the lamina dura to become less distinct and ultimately fade. Subsequently, the apical PDL space widens, and resorption of apical alveolar bone occurs. Clinically, the tooth is tender to percussion. Without root canal treatment, a periapical abscess, cyst, or granuloma can be expected to develop.

Periodontitis (Figs. 53.2, 52.1–52.8) An early radiographic sign of **periodontitis** is the disappearance of the lamina dura along the interproximal aspects of the root beginning at the alveolar crest. Resorption of the lamina dura progresses apically. This initially produces a small triangular defect (**triangulation**) in the crestal bone with the apex of the triangle pointing apically. Another radiographic sign of periodontitis is the presence of prominent interdental **nutrient canals**. This feature is especially prominent in the mandibular anterior region. Nutrient canals are engorged blood vessels containing inflammatory elements that are prone to stimulate resorption and are risk factors for chronic active periodontitis.

Traumatic Occlusion (Figs. 53.3 and 53.4) is a condition where one or more teeth are placed under repeated, excessive biting force that results in inflammation and damage to the tooth and periodontium. It is often associated with extruded teeth, maligned teeth, bruxism, or clenching. Radiographically, the tooth with a premature or excessive contact has a prominent widened PDL space and a widened, more radiopaque lamina dura along one side of the involved tooth. Early involvement limits the findings to the cervical half of the tooth. As the trauma becomes more persistent or more severe, the whole side of the tooth or both sides of the tooth demonstrate widened PDL space. In this latter case, tooth mobility will be present, and pain upon biting may be a complaint.

Orthodontic Tooth Movement (Fig. 53.5) In an attempt to change the position of teeth, **orthodontic tooth movement** produces forces on the PDL and adjacent bone that alters blood flow and stimulates bone resorption. As a result, the PDL space changes shape and can be widened by orthodontic treatment (Fig. 17.2). The widening represents stretched PDL fibers. Radiographically, one sees widening of the PDL space and of the lamina dura on the tension side and thinning of the PDL space and resorption of the lamina dura on the pressure side. Teeth with widened PDL space often display some mobility. If too much force is applied to a tooth of a susceptible patient, external root resorption can result (Fig. 29.4).

Scleroderma (Fig. 53.6) is a disease that slowly produces loss of elasticity in the skin and sclerosis as a result of deposition of collagen. It can be isolated or systemic. Patients who have **scleroderma** develop difficulty in moving the fingers and in opening the mouth wide. In the jaws, the most prominent finding is a diffuse widening of the periodontal ligament space of multiple teeth in more than one quadrant. Bilateral resorption of the posterior border of the ramus, coronoid process, and condyle can occur as a result of chronic constrictive pressure arising from the sclerosing soft tissues of the face. When the condyles are resorbed, an anterior open bite will develop.

Malignant Disease (Figs. 53.7 and 53.8) can mimic radiographic aspects of periodontal disease and involve the periodontium. Notable examples are discussed below.

Chondrosarcoma affects a wide range of patients, with peak incidence around age 35 years. The tumor is slowly aggressive producing neoplastic cartilage that can appear radiopaque and/or radiolucent with ill-defined margins. In Figure 53.7, this tumor displays widened PDL with adjacent radiopaque cartilage deposition.

Osteogenic sarcoma (Fig. 53.8) is an aggressive malignant tumor that typically affects children and young adults and the jaws about 6% of cases. Lesions are destructive and commonly display a sclerotic and sunburst effect containing radiating tumor spicules. Adjacent to teeth, they can widen the PDL space and destroy adjacent alveolar bone.

Squamous cell carcinoma destroys alveolar bone by local extension (see Fig. 43.5), whereas **metastatic disease** arises from distant malignant sites—most commonly the breast (Fig. 43.6), lung, kidney, thyroid, or prostate.

In these cases, malignant tumors cause radiographic changes that classically appear as loss of the lamina dura and a thickened and irregular periodontal membrane space along the mesial or distal length of a tooth root. Sometimes, several adjacent teeth are affected as the tumor spreads. The tumor can also produce bone destruction that resembles a perio-endo lesion. Along with the radiographic features just mentioned, the clinical features of a malignant tumor are red or swollen gingiva, a palpable fungating mass or ulcer, loss of nerve sensation (paresthesia), and a range in pain from asymptomatic to deep, debilitating bone pain.

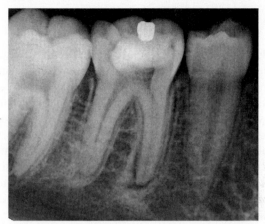

Fig. 53.1. Apical periodontitis: widened PDL, thickened lamina dura.

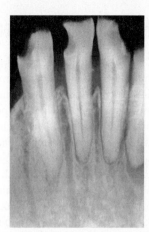

Fig. 53.2. Periodontitis: interradicular nutrient canals and funneling.

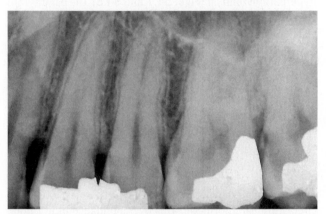

Fig. 53.3. Traumatic occlusion: widened PDL and lamina dura first premolar.

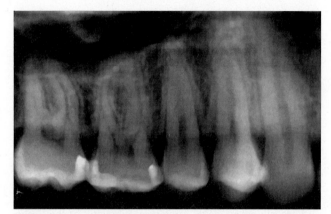

Fig. 53.4. Traumatic occlusion: thickened lamina dura second premolar.

7

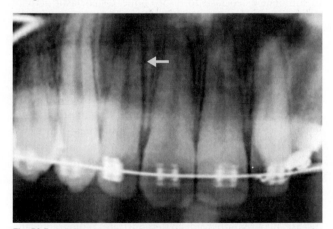

Fig. 53.5. Widened PDL: right lateral incisor, orthodontic associated.

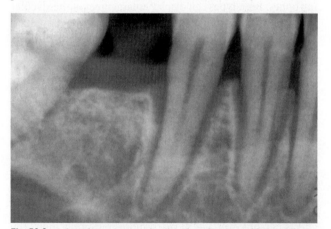

Fig. 53.6. Scleroderma: generalized widened PDL and lamina dura.

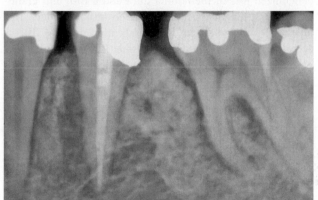

Fig. 53.7. Malignant disease: chondrosarcoma; wide PDL one side root.

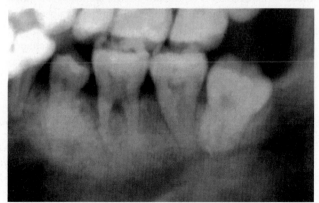

Fig. 53.8. Malignant disease: widened PDL associated with osteosarcoma.

Ankylosis (Figs. 54.1 and 54.2) is defined as fusion of the tooth root with the alveolar bone. The most common ankylosed tooth is the retained primary mandibular molar (Fig. 18.6). These teeth are most often affected when the permanent mandibular second premolar is absent. Also affected are impacted permanent teeth and transplanted teeth, particularly mandibular third molars that have been reimplanted into first molar positions. Ankylosis is characterized by an absence of the PDL space, absence of the lamina dura, along with fusion of the cementum to the adjacent alveolar bone. If a primary molar is affected, it is typically "submerged" below the normal plane of occlusion. Percussing an ankylosed tooth produces a characteristic dull sound.

Fibrous Dysplasia (Figs. 54.3 and 54.4) is classified as a benign fibro-osseous disease whereby bone is replaced with abnormal fibro-osseous connective tissue. Two types are described: **monostotic**, which affects a single bone, and **polyostotic**, which involves more than one bone. Both types develop in children and adolescents. The monostotic type often affects the mandible or maxilla producing a painless, bulging enlargement of the face in one or more quadrants. The polyostotic type affects the skull, clavicles, and long bones and produces **café au lait spots**, which are macules that have smooth regular borders said to resemble the coast of Maine. These patients can have varying severity of disease and are subject to visual impairment, bowing of the limbs, bone pain, and pathologic fractures in affected weight-bearing bones. Both types can display enlargement of the alveolar process and facial bones, which may create esthetic issues. The radiographic lesions can involve the jaws extensively with radiolucent, radiopaque, and mixed patterns. A diffuse radiopacity that (1) resembles ground glass, (2) blends with the adjacent normal bone, and (3) results in loss of the lamina dura is classically seen. These changes are limited to the bone(s) affected by fibrous dysplasia.

Paget Disease (Figs. 54.5 and 54.6) is a slowly progressive and chronic disease of irregular bone breakdown and formation that results in bone expansion, brittle bones that are prone to fracture, and bone pain. Other names for this condition are *osteitis deformans* and *leontiasis ossea*. The disease affects persons over age 50 years, more commonly men. The cause is not known. It affects any bones, including the jaws, facial bones, and skull. Affected bones symmetrically enlarge causing pain, headaches, dizziness, and possibly deafness. The symptoms are the result of the enlarged and misshapen bones impinging on the cranial nerves as they exit the foramen and foramina of the skull. The skin over the affected bone is warm to touch. Affected patients often develop diastemas and experience the need for a larger hat as their skull enlarges, and edentulous patients often complain that their dentures are too tight. The maxilla is more commonly affected than the mandible. Radiographically, there are three phases. The initial phase is characterized by lysis (loss of lamina dura and PDL space), thinned trabeculae, and the spaces between trabeculae narrowing often producing a granular (orange peel or ground-glass) appearance. The biphasic stage shows lytic and blastic elements: multiple rounded radiopaque masses that appear like "cotton rolls." The late stage shows dense sclerotic masses bilaterally within the jaws, with jaw enlargement, multiple radiopaque "cotton-wool" patches of bone, hypercementosis, and ankylosed teeth as a result of the deposition of abnormal bone around the roots of teeth. Patients with active disease have significantly elevated serum alkaline phosphatase levels, which helps in making the final diagnosis.

Hyperparathyroidism (Figs. 54.7 and 54.8) The parathyroid glands are located along the posterior poles of the thyroid gland and are responsible for regulating calcium levels in the blood through the production and release of parathormone. When there is abnormal increase in secretion of parathormone and circulating parathormone, the condition is known as hyperparathyroidism. Hyperparathyroidism is divided into two types: primary and secondary hyperparathyroidism. **Primary hyperparathyroidism** results from disease of the parathyroid glands themselves, as a result of hyperplasia, a noncancerous growth (adenoma), or a cancerous (malignant) tumor. It generally occurs after the age of 55 years. During primary hyperparathyroidism, there is too much circulating parathormone. This overabundance in hormone mobilizes calcium from the blood by the hormone's ability to stimulate osteoclasts to resorb bone. Osteoclastic activity in turn removes calcium from the bone and places into the bloodstream. In contrast, **secondary hyperparathyroidism** is a compensatory mechanism due to kidney disease or conditions associated with hypocalcium or vitamin D deficiencies, such as rickets, osteomalacia, calcium deprivation, or pregnancy. Hyperparathyroidism can cause bone pain or stiffness, kidney stones, nausea and gastrointestinal pain, lethargy, depression, and personality problems—hence, the description "bones, stones, abdominal groans, and psychic moans." In some cases, prolonged hypercalcemia can also result in calcification in the cornea of the eye.

The bony changes in hyperparathyroidism are identical whether the cause is primary or secondary. Like early Paget disease, hyperparathyroidism demonstrates radiographically generalized loss of the lamina dura and a thin and granular (ground-glass) appearance of the alveolar bone. This is a result of generalized demineralization of bone. This is accompanied by a thinned but visible PDL. As the disease progresses, the cancellous bone classically becomes "*ground glass*" in appearance, and brown tumors develop that contain hemosiderin from small hemorrhages. The brown tumors, which histologically resemble **central giant cell granulomas** and are more commonly seen in the mandible, can produce unilocular or multilocular radiolucencies and can resorb roots. Renal osteodystrophy produces similar radiographic findings.

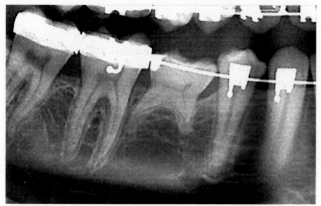

Fig. 54.1. **Ankylosis primary molar:** no lamina dura or PDL space.

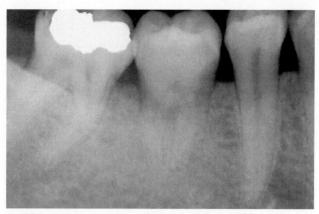

Fig. 54.2. **Ankylosis:** transplanted third molar, no lamina dura or PDL.

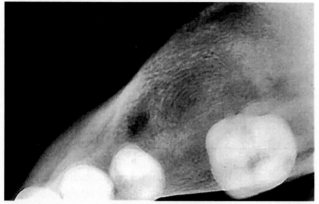

Fig. 54.3. **Fibrous dysplasia** with fingerprint pattern.

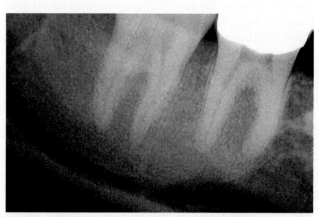

Fig. 54.4. **Fibrous dysplasia** and loss of lamina dura.

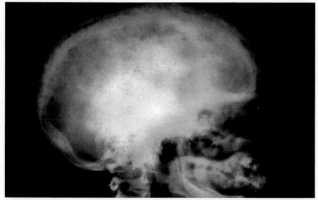

Fig. 54.5. **Paget disease:** cotton-wool appearance.

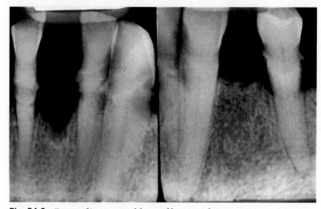

Fig. 54.6. **Paget disease** and loss of lamina dura.

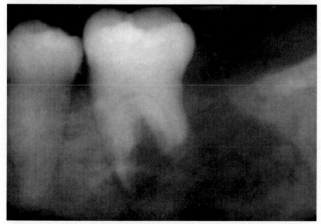

Fig. 54.7. **Hyperparathyroidism** and loss of lamina dura.

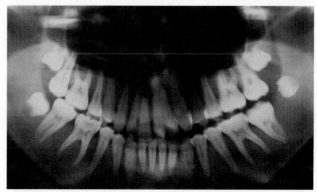

Fig. 54.8. **Hyperparathyroidism** and loss of lamina dura.

7

DENTAL IMPLANTS

Dental Implants (Figs. 55.1–55.5), also called **endosseous** or **endosteal implants**, are titanium structures inserted into alveolar bone that serve as roots for prosthetic reconstruction of missing teeth. Dental implants function as alternatives and adjuncts to fixed and removable partial dentures and are often used when a tooth is missing due to injury, periodontal disease, or other reason. In Figure 55.1, the second premolar has advanced periodontitis (a large moat defect and class II mobility). It was extracted and an endosteal implant was placed as illustrated in Figure 55.2. Some treatment plans include local bone grafting prior to implant placement.

Technically speaking, the **implant** is the metal component that is below the gum and interfaces with the alveolar bone. It is typically made of titanium because titanium fuses tightly with bone. The component that inserts into the top of the implant is called the **abutment,** and on top of the abutment is the **crown** (Fig. 55.3).

There are various types of endosteal implants including cylinders, screws, or blades. These are further categorized as long (greater than 10 mm) or short (less than 10 mm) and rough or smooth surface. Each relies on the biological process of osseous integration to succeed. **Osseointegration** generally takes several weeks and is evident by the deposition of woven bone adjacent to the entire length of the submerged dental implant (Fig. 55.4). Once osseointegration has been achieved, the prosthetic crown can be attached and loaded by teeth from the opposing arch. The convention is to follow the two-staged implant system, where stage 1 is placing the implant and stage 2 occurs after tissue healing and osseointegration when the abutment and crown can be placed.

Implants can succeed or fail. A successful endosseous implant is stable and serves to hold a prosthetic tooth in a manner that offers comfort and good esthetics and function to the patient (Fig. 55.5). Current data suggest that most dental implants succeed. That is, more than 90% of dental implants have life spans of greater than 10 years. Factors that contribute to success are good overall health, proper positioning and angulation of the implant, appropriate occlusal loading, healthy alveolar bone, and good oral hygiene. Implants that fail are more common in patients who are older (greater than 60 years), have systemic disease (diabetes), have inadequate or poor alveolar or cortical bone (e.g., due to osteoporosis or radiation therapy), take drugs that influence osseointegration (bisphosphonates, corticosteroids), smoke cigarettes, or have poor oral hygiene.

Clinically, a healthy implant should be stable, nonpainful, nonmobile, and in proper occlusion. Radiographically, dental implants lack a periodontal ligament and lamina dura but should demonstrate good alveolar bone in close apposition with the implant. Since implants lack a periodontal ligament, patients do not sense the amount of pressure they impart during biting. Thus, implants must be placed into optimal position and occlusion to prevent angular mechanical loading that can lead to traumatic occlusion. In addition, improperly placed implants or implants that are too long can contact or place pressure on the inferior alveolar nerve or maxillary sinus resulting in persistent pain.

Implant-Related Disease As stated, not all dental implants remain healthy. Like teeth, they require good home oral hygiene care and regular dental visits to keep them plaque-free. Implants that become diseased exhibit one of three conditions: (1) **peri-implant mucositis**, (2) **peri-implantitis**, or (3) a **failed implant**.

Peri-implant mucositis is plaque-induced inflammation of the soft tissue surrounding the dental implant. This condition exhibits bleeding on probing; however, the connective tissue attachment apparatus remains intact and there is no loss of supporting bone. Thus, the condition is reversible, if etiologic factors are removed and good oral hygiene measures are implemented.

Peri-implantitis (Figs. 55.6 and 55.7) is chronic inflammation affecting the soft and hard tissues surrounding a functioning osseointegrated dental implant, resulting in loss of supporting alveolar bone. The microbes present are similar with those detected with periodontitis; however, *Staphylococcus aureus* has also been detected more frequently around sites of peri-implantitis. The subgingival bacteria promote the inflammatory response; thus, clinically, one detects bleeding on probing and suppuration. Radiographically, there is decreased bone density around the implant and bone loss (50% or greater) that occurs along the surface of the implant, which jeopardizes osseointegration of the implant. Successful treatment relies on early diagnosis and the reduction or elimination of risk factors (smoking, traumatic occlusion, poorly controlled diabetes). Nonsurgical and surgical protocols have been reported. The former uses debridement with antiseptic oral rinses. The latter has involved the use of flap procedures, mechanical and chemical decontamination, lasers, guided bone regeneration, and antibiotics. In the absence of appropriate treatment, peri-implantitis can progress to becoming a failed implant.

Implant failure (Fig. 55.8) occurs when the progression of peri-implantitis is not halted and osseointegration fails. Implant failure is three times more common in the maxilla than the mandible. Causative factors include poor oral hygiene, defects of bone formation, insufficient bone density or volume, parafunctional activity, improper occlusal loading, incorrect implant positioning, sudden impact, or persistent microbial infection. Diabetics and smokers are at higher risk of implant failure. Features of a failed dental implant include deep probing depths, mobility, bleeding on probing, suppuration, pain in function, and radiographic bone loss of more than half the length of the implant. Clinically, one may see the metal implant exposed above the gingival margin. Most failed implants are removed, and the sites are surgically, mechanically, or chemically decontaminated. Bone augmentation is generally provided and once healed, another implant can be placed, if local or systemic factors are controlled.

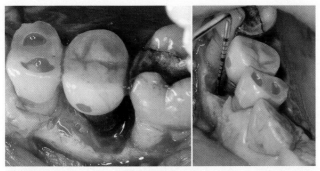

Fig. 55.1. Advanced periodontitis: an indication for implants.*

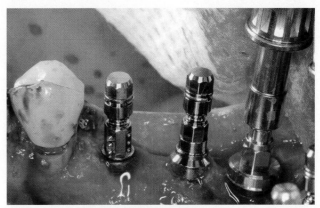

Fig. 55.2. Surgical placement of implants.*

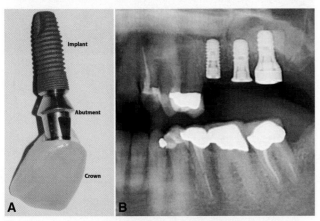

Fig. 55.3. A: Components. **B:** Maxillary implants healing stage.

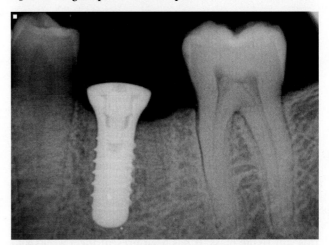

Fig. 55.4. Implant with healing abutment uncovered.

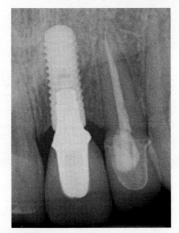

Fig. 55.5. Healthy incisor implant: restored with crown.

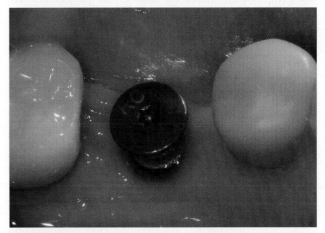

Fig. 55.6. Peri-implantitis: notice exposed threads.

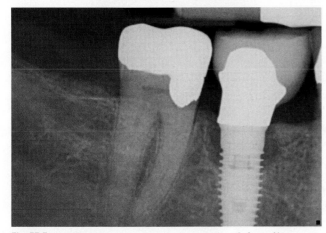

Fig. 55.7. Peri-implantitis: 5-mm saucerization defect of bone.

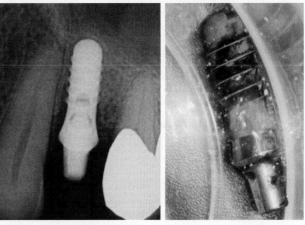

Fig. 55.8. Failed implant: radiolucency along entire length.

CASE STUDIES

CASE 31. (FIG. 55.9)

This is a 31-year-old patient. He has an intellectual disability and takes medication for seizures. His parents are deceased, and he has been institutionalized without proper oral care for several years.

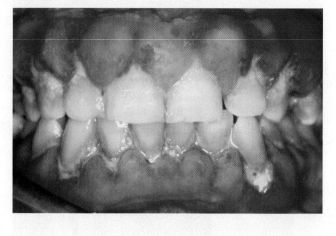

1. Describe the clinical findings.

2. Would these tissues bleed easily? What features provide a clue?

3. What features are suggestive that the condition has been present for some time?

4. What factors are contributing to the condition?

5. What medication is he likely taking?

6. What is abnormal about the teeth and suggestive of his medical condition?

7. What additional gingival abnormalities are present?

8. What should you communicate to his caregiver?

CASE 32. (FIG. 55.10)

A healthy 7-year-old boy appears at the dental clinic with this soft tissue mass. It has been present for 3 weeks and has progressively increased in size. The patient reports that "he spits out blood every time he brushes his teeth, so he stopped brushing his teeth." All the adjacent teeth are asymptomatic and test vital. Periapical radiographs of the area reveal no abnormalities.

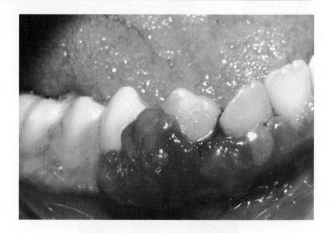

1. Describe the clinical findings.

2. Is this a normal finding, a variant of normal, or disease?

3. Do you expect this condition to be painful, and if so, why?

4. This lesion shows features of malignancy.
   A. True
   B. False

5. The most likely diagnosis for the condition is:
   A. Leukemic infiltrate
   B. Parulis
   C. Peripheral ossifying fibroma
   D. Pyogenic granuloma

6. List other intraoral sites where this can occur.

7. What are the treatment options for this tooth?

8. What clinical features are suggestive that this is a young patient?

9. What should you communicate to him and his parents

Additional cases to enhance your learning and understanding of this section are available Online through the book's Navigate 2 Advantage Access site.

Abnormalities by Location

Objectives:

- Define and use diagnostic terms that describe common disorders of the tongue, lip, floor of the mouth, palate, and face.
- Recognize the causes and clinical features of common lesions and swellings of the lip, tongue, floor of the mouth, palate, and face.
- In the clinical setting, document the characteristics of oral conditions or deviations from normal that affect the lip, tongue, floor of the mouth, palate, and face and provide the patient with information about the condition or deviation.
- Use the diagnostic process to distinguish similar-appearing lesions and swellings of the lip, tongue, floor of the mouth, palate, and face.
- Recommend appropriate treatment options for common lesions and swellings of the lip, tongue, floor of the mouth, palate, and face.
- Identify conditions discussed in this section that would (1) require the attention of the dentist, (2) affect the delivery of noninvasive and invasive dental procedures, or (3) need to be further evaluated by a specialist.

In the figure legends, *⁺ denotes the same patient.

CONDITIONS OF THE TONGUE

Scalloped Tongue (Crenated Tongue) (Figs. 56.1 and 56.2) is a common finding characterized by a series of indentations on the lateral border of the tongue. The condition is caused by abnormal pressure (e.g., suction) within the mouth of persons who clench or brux. It is usually bilateral but may be unilateral or isolated to a region where the tongue is held in close contact with the teeth. The abnormal pressure imprints a distinctive pattern: depressed ovals on the tongue that are sometimes circumscribed by a raised, white scalloped border. Causes of **scalloped tongue** include situations that produce abnormal tongue pressure, such as movement of the tongue against teeth, tongue thrusting, tongue sucking, clenching, bruxing, or an enlarged tongue (macroglossia). The pattern can be accentuated when pressure is applied in areas of **diastemata** (spacing between teeth). A scalloped tongue is seen in normal patients, as well as in association with temporomandibular joint disorders, and conditions that result in an enlarged tongue such as acromegaly, amyloidosis, and Down syndrome. The condition is harmless and asymptomatic. Treatment is aimed at habit elimination. A prominent linea alba on the buccal mucosa, a frequent coexisting finding, is caused by the same negative intraoral pressure associated with tongue sucking in persons who clench or brux their teeth.

Macroglossia (Figs. 56.3 and 56.4) involves an abnormally enlarged tongue. To assess tongue size, the tongue should be completely relaxed. The normal height of the dorsum of the tongue should be even with the occlusal plane of the mandibular teeth. The lateral borders of the tongue should contact, but not overlap, the lingual cusps of the mandibular teeth. A tongue that extends beyond these dimensions is enlarged.

Macroglossia is either congenital or acquired. Congenital macroglossia can be caused by idiopathic muscular hypertrophy, muscular hemihypertrophy, benign tumors, vascular malformations, hamartomas, allergic reactions, or cysts. Congenital macroglossia that develops at an early age is a component of Beckwith-Wiedemann syndrome and Down syndrome. Acquired macroglossia may be the result of passive enlargement of the tongue when mandibular teeth are lost. In this case, the enlargement may be localized or diffuse, depending on the size of the edentulous area. Systemic disease, such as acromegaly, amyloidosis, hypothyroidism, or neoplasms, which can occlude lymphatic drainage and produce a swollen tongue, can cause macroglossia. Indicators of an enlarged tongue are focal or diffuse enlargement of the tongue, speech difficulties, displaced teeth, malocclusion, or a scalloped tongue. If the enlarged tongue is hindering function, elimination of the primary cause or surgical correction may be necessary. An enlarged tongue can cause patients to have difficulty accommodating a removable prosthesis.

Hairy Tongue (Lingua Villosa, Coated Tongue) (Figs. 56.5 and 56.6) is an abnormal elongation of the filiform papillae that gives the dorsum of the tongue a hairlike appearance.

It is a hypertrophic response associated with increased keratin deposition or delayed shedding of the cornified layer. Patients who do not cleanse their tongues, which allows colonization and growth of chromogenic microbes, are most commonly affected. Cancer therapy, infection with *Candida albicans*, irradiation, poor oral hygiene, change in oral pH, smoking, and use of antibiotics, bismuth, or oxidizing mouthwashes are associated with this condition.

Hairy tongue may be white, yellow, green, brown, or black, hence the names white-coated tongue and yellow, brown, or black hairy tongue. The color of the lesion is a result of intrinsic factors (chromogenic organisms) combined with extrinsic factors (food, drink [coffee, tea], and tobacco stains). Hairy tongue occurs more frequently in men and primarily in persons older than age 30 years. It increases in frequency with age and consumption of hot drinks and a soft diet. The condition begins in the midline of the tongue near the foramen cecum and spreads laterally and anteriorly. The affected filiform papillae discolor, progressively elongate, and may reach a length of several millimeters. Generally, hairy tongue is only of cosmetic concern, and the tongue remains asymptomatic. Symptoms can include a tickling or gagging sensation or altered taste or halitosis. Brushing the tongue daily with abrasive pastes along with elimination of predisposing factors leads to resolution. In refractory cases, an underlying condition, such as a dry mouth or diabetes mellitus, should be investigated.

Hairy Leukoplakia (Figs 56.7 and 56.8) is a disorder characterized by raised, white, corrugated lesions on the lateral border of the tongue. It is caused by replication of Epstein-Barr virus within the affected epithelial cells. The lesion is a sign of immunosuppression and is most common in persons infected with human immunodeficiency virus (HIV) or who are immunosuppressed from drugs taken for organ transplantation, chemotherapy, or systemic disease. The white lesion is primarily located on the lateral borders of the tongue but may extend to cover the dorsal and ventral surfaces and has been documented on the palate and buccal mucosa. Hairy leukoplakia is so named because hairlike peeling of the parakeratotic surface layer is evident histologically. Biopsied lesions frequently show an association with the fungal organism *C. albicans* but have few Langerhans cells.

Early lesions have alternating faint white folds and adjacent normal pink troughs that produce a characteristic vertical white-banded washboard appearance. The bands eventually coalesce to form discrete white plaques or extensive thick white corrugated patches. Large lesions are usually asymptomatic, have poorly demarcated borders, and do not rub off. Bilateral occurrence is common, but unilateral lesions are possible. Antiviral agents that block or limit replication of Epstein-Barr virus are useful in reducing the size of or eliminating the lesions. Therapies that return immune health also lead to resolution.

126

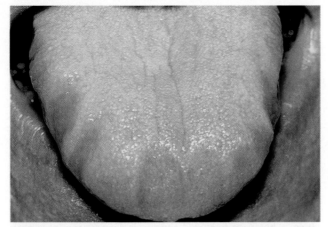

Fig. 56.1. Scalloped tongue: associated with clenching.

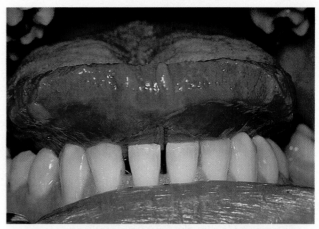

Fig. 56.2. Scalloped tongue: caused by tongue sucking.

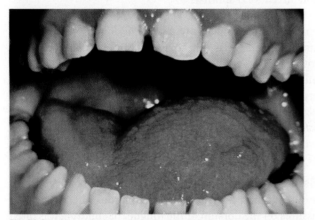

Fig. 56.3. Macroglossia: congenital hemihypertrophy.

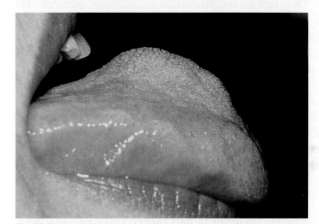

Fig. 56.4. Macroglossia: caused by a hemangioma.

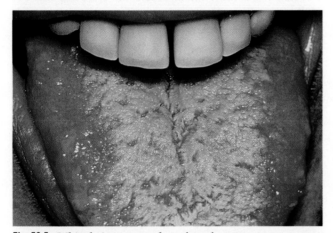

Fig. 56.5. White hairy tongue: from drug therapy.

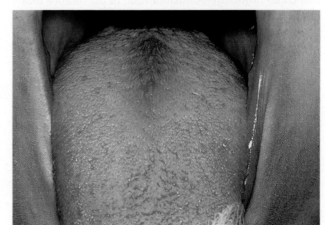

Fig. 56.6. Brown hairy tongue: after antibiotics.

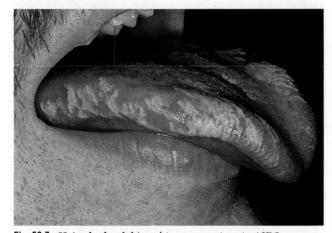

Fig. 56.7. Hairy leukoplakia: white corrugations in AIDS.

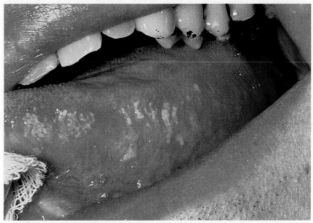

Fig. 56.8. Hairy leukoplakia: seen during dental treatment.

8

Geographic Tongue (Benign Migratory Glossitis, Erythema Migrans) (Figs. 57.1–57.4) is a benign inflammatory condition characterized by irregular bald patches found mainly on the dorsum of the tongue. The irregular pattern of patches gives the surface of the tongue a maplike appearance, thus the term *geographic*. It occurs in about 1% of the population. Women and young adults are most frequently affected. The cause is unknown, but allergies, stress, nutritional deficiencies, and hormonal and hereditary factors may be relevant. The condition classically occurs on the dorsal and lateral surfaces of the anterior two thirds of the tongue, affecting only the filiform and leaving the fungiform papillae intact.

Geographic tongue manifests in three patterns: (1) patchy areas of desquamated filiform papillae; (2) patchy desquamated areas delineated by raised, white, circinate (ring-shaped) borders; and (3) patchy areas of desquamated filiform papillae bordered by an erythematous band of inflammation. Mixtures of these patterns may be present, and the pattern on the surface of the tongue may change in size and location from day to day. Symptoms are uncommon in the first two patterns, but presence of the red inflammatory band is often associated with irritation by spicy foods and reports of burning. The condition is generally recurrent. It may appear suddenly and persist for months or years and can spontaneously disappear.

Geographic Stomatitis (Areata Erythema Migrans) (Figs. 57.5 and 57.6) Stomatitis is inflammation of the mucous lining of any of the soft tissues of the mouth. Geographic tongue is occasionally seen in association with geographic stomatitis and often with fissured tongue. Geographic stomatitis produces red annular patches of the labial and buccal mucosa, soft palate, and occasionally floor of the mouth. The patches are mild erosions of the mucosa. When asymptomatic, geographic tongue or stomatitis requires no treatment. Symptomatic lesions generally respond to topical anesthetics or topical steroids, in combination with stress reduction.

Anemia (Fig. 57.7) is a condition characterized by impaired oxygen delivery to body tissue as a result of a reduction in the number of erythrocytes, hemoglobin (the protein within the red blood cells that carries oxygen), or total blood volume. Underlying causes of anemia include *decreased production of erythrocytes* caused by a nutritional deficiency state or bone marrow suppression, *increased destruction of erythrocytes*, or *increased blood loss* as a result of hemorrhage. Iron deficiency is the most common type of anemia, frequently affecting middle-aged women and young teenagers. It produces a microcytic (small red blood cells) anemia. Deficiencies in vitamin B_{12} and folic acid cause macrocytic anemia (large red blood cells).

Anemia is a sign of an underlying disease. Thus, the cause of anemia must always be sought. Anemia produces changes in the oral mucosal membranes, but these alterations are not helpful in distinguishing the type of anemia. Analysis of erythrocyte indices is required for an accurate diagnosis. Intraoral manifestations of anemia are most prominent on the tongue. The dorsum of the tongue initially appears pale, with flattening of the filiform papillae. Continued atrophy of the papillae results in a surface that is devoid of papillae and appears smooth, dry, and glazed. This condition is commonly called bald tongue. In the final stage, a beefy or fiery red tongue is seen, sometimes with concurrent oral aphthae.

Anemia may produce a sore, painful (**glossodynia**), or burning tongue (**glossopyrosis**). The lips may be thinned and taut, and the width of the mouth may develop a narrowed appearance. Other clinical signs associated with anemia include angular cheilitis, aphthae, dysphagia, mucosal erythema and erosions, pallor, shortness of breath, fatigue, dizziness, a bounding pulse, tingling of the extremities, or difficulty walking. Therapy should be directed toward correcting the underlying cause. After therapy, the appearance of the oral tissue improves.

Fissured (Plicated) Tongue (Fig. 57.8) is a relatively common condition that presents as numerous linear groves or fissures on the dorsum of the tongue. In children, it is often associated with inherited disorders and is a component of **Melkersson-Rosenthal syndrome** (fissured tongue, swollen lips, and facial paralysis; Figs. 61.4–61.6). In adults, **fissured tongue** is most commonly associated with **hyposalivation**. Many therapeutic drugs—primarily antidepressant agents, antihistamines, antihypertensive and cardiac agents, decongestants, ganglionic blocking agents, and tranquilizers—produce hyposalivation and thus fissured tongue.

Fissured tongue can have a varied appearance. Many cases have a prominent midline groove and several branching lateral grooves. Others have multiple irregular, wavy grooves. The fissures are often 2 to 5 mm deep and have varying widths that narrow toward the periphery. Interspersed between the fissures are islands of papillae that may appear dry, atrophic, or geographic. There is a strong association with geographic tongue. Most patients are asymptomatic, although some may report mild discomfort or burning. The condition is benign and does not require treatment, although some patients may complain of **xerostomia**. Clinicians should measure the patient's salivary flow and those affected should be encouraged to brush the tongue to minimize food and bacterial accumulations.

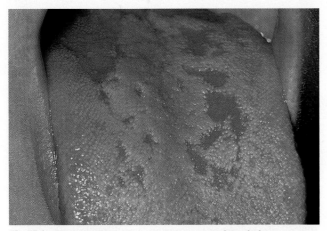

Fig. 57.1. Geographic tongue: asymptomatic denuded areas.

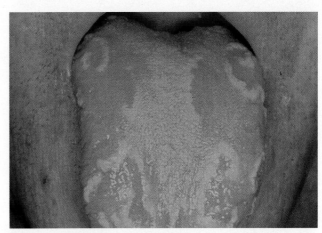

Fig. 57.2. Geographic tongue: asymptomatic white regions.

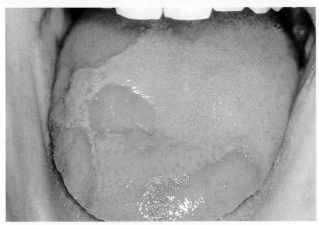

Fig. 57.3. Geographic tongue: red and painful.

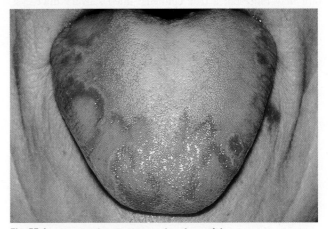

Fig. 57.4. Geographic tongue: red and painful.

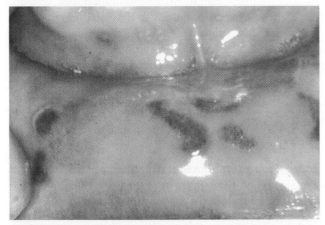

Fig. 57.5. Geographic stomatitis: symptomatic labial mucosa.

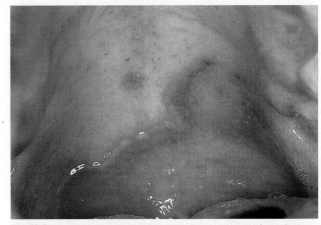

Fig. 57.6. Geographic stomatitis: annular pattern on the palate.

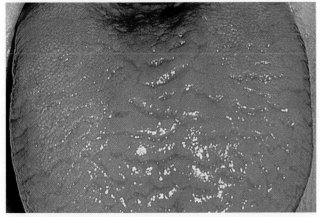

Fig. 57.7. Iron deficiency anemia: bald, burning tongue.

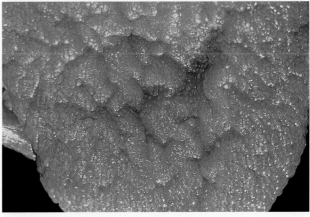

Fig. 57.8. Fissured tongue: dry, fissured, and atrophic.

129

Cyst of Blandin-Nuhn (Lingual Mucus Retention Phenomenon) (Fig. 58.1)

The glands of **Blandin-Nuhn** are accessory salivary glands on the ventral surface of the tongue composed of mixed serous and mucous elements. The cyst develops when trauma to the ventral tongue induces leaking of saliva into the surrounding tissues. It appears as a small, painless, pink-red fluid-filled swelling with raised and well-demarcated borders. The lesion is soft and fluctuant and generally located near the midline of the ventral tongue. When superficial, the cyst has balloonlike features and a pedunculated base. Deeper lesions have sessile bases. Although usually induced by trauma, the cyst of Blandin-Nuhn may be congenital. The congenital variant may represent a true epithelial-lined salivary duct cyst. These cysts rarely exceed 1 cm in diameter. Treatment is excisional biopsy.

Median Rhomboid Glossitis (Figs. 58.2–58.4)

was once thought to be a developmental defect of incomplete descent of the tuberculum impar. This theory is no longer valid. It is now accepted that **median rhomboid glossitis** is an asymptomatic rhomboid- or ovoid-shaped red area on the tongue that results from a chronic *C. albicans* infection. The most common location is the midline of the dorsum of the tongue, just anterior to the circumvallate papillae. The size and shape vary, but frequently, it appears as a well-defined, 1- to 2.5-cm red lesion with irregular but rounded borders. It affects middle-aged persons and rarely affects children. There is no racial predilection. The prevalence is often higher in patients who have diabetes, are immunosuppressed, or have completed a course of broad-spectrum antibiotics.

Median rhomboid glossitis presents early in its course as a smooth, denuded, beefy red atrophic patch devoid of filiform papillae. With time, the lesion becomes granular and lobular. An erythematous palatal candidal "kissing" lesion is sometimes observed directly over the lesion of the tongue. In this case, the condition is termed **chronic multifocal candidiasis** (Figs. 58.3 and 58.4), and immunosuppression should be suspected.

Median rhomboid glossitis is easily recognized by its clinical appearance, characteristic location, and asymptomatic nature. Early recognition and treatment with antifungal agents usually leads to resolution. End-stage median rhomboid glossitis is usually asymptomatic and refractory to antifungal treatment as the lesion becomes fibrotic and hypovascular.

Granular Cell Tumor (Figs. 58.5 and 58.6)

is a rare, benign, soft tissue tumor composed of plump polygonal cells that have an eosinophilic granular cytoplasm. This tumor may occur in cutaneous, mucosal, and visceral sites, but about 50% of cases occur in the dorsolateral surface of the tongue. Most experts believe that it is a benign proliferation of neural or neuroendocrine cells.

The **granular cell tumor** can occur at any age and in any race, but it has a slight predilection for women. Usually, the lesion consists of an asymptomatic, solitary, dome-shaped submucosal nodule covered clinically by normal, yellow, or white tissue. The surface is generally smooth but may be ulcerated if traumatized. The tumor is often sessile, well circumscribed, and firm to compression. Growth is very slow and painless; some tumors grow to several centimeters in size. Larger lesions may demonstrate a slightly depressed central area. In rare cases, these lesions are found on the ventral surface of the tongue or buccal mucosa. Approximately 10% of affected patients experience multiple lesions.

This tumor is characterized by pseudoepitheliomatous hyperplasia overlying the granular neoplastic cells. In some cases, this hyperplasia may mistakenly resemble epidermoid carcinoma. Conservative local excision is the preferred treatment. These lesions do not tend to recur.

Lingual Thyroid (Fig. 58.7)

is an uncommon nodule of thyroid tissue found just posterior to the foramen cecum on the posterior third of the tongue. It occurs when embryonic tissue from the thyroid gland fails to migrate to the anterolateral surface of the trachea. Persistent thyroid tissue occurs much more frequently in women than in men (the ratio is 4:1) and may appear at any age. If the remnant tissue becomes cystic, the condition becomes a **thyroglossal duct cyst**.

Lingual thyroid is a raised asymptomatic mass that is usually about 2 cm in diameter. Increased surface vascularity is a prominent feature. Symptoms of dysphagia, dysphonia, or hypothyroidism most often develop during puberty, pregnancy, or menopause. Clinicians can differentiate this lesion from similar lesions by confirming its distinctive location, which is posterior to the circumvallate papillae, and by using uptake studies of radioactive iodine. Biopsy should be deferred until it is ascertained that the rest of the thyroid gland is present and functioning. In more than 50% of patients with ectopic thyroid, the lingual thyroid is the only active thyroid tissue present.

Body Piercing (Oral Jewelry) (Fig. 58.8)

is the placement of a foreign object through tissue of the body. Common extraoral locations include the ears, eyebrows, ala of the nose, and belly button. Intraorally, the mucobuccal fold of the lower lip and the tongue are common sites. A popular object placed in the pierced tongue is the metallic barbell. Body piercing may be performed without anesthesia and minor regard for infection control. Common adverse events associated with the surgical piercing procedure include infection, swelling, and bleeding. Late adverse events include allergic reactions, tooth fractures, and mucogingival defects. Oral jewelry needs to be removed before taking radiographs, and patients should be advised of the potential oral health problems associated with these objects.

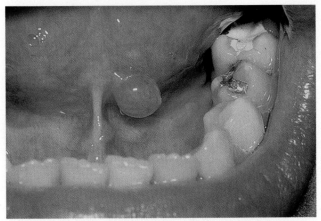

Fig. 58.1. **Cyst of Blandin-Nuhn:** variant of a mucocele.

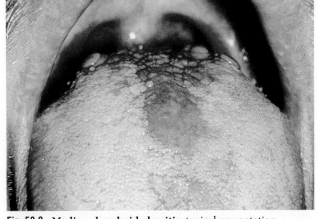

Fig. 58.2. **Median rhomboid glossitis:** typical presentation.

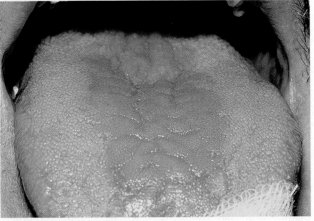

Fig. 58.3. **Median rhomboid glossitis:** smooth denuded patch.*

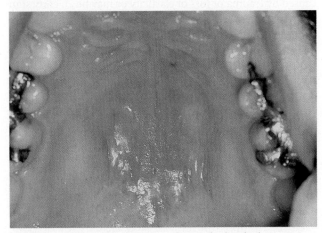

Fig. 58.4. **Contact palatal lesion:** red irregular border.*

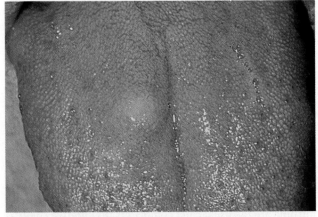

Fig. 58.5. **Granular cell tumor:** pink tongue nodule.‡

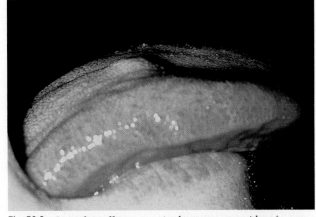

Fig. 58.6. **Granular cell tumor:** raised appearance evident.‡

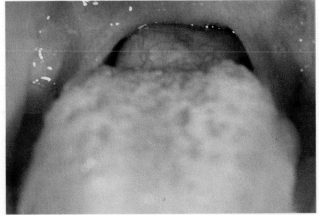

Fig. 58.7. **Lingual thyroid:** vascular midline mass tongue.

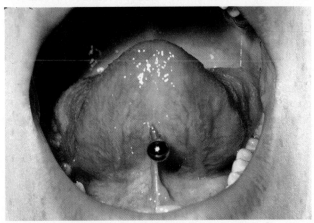

Fig. 58.8. **Body piercing:** tongue barbell.

8

131

CONDITIONS OF THE LIP

Actinic Cheilitis (Actinic Cheilosis, Solar Cheilitis) (Figs. 59.1 and 59.2) is a degenerative and premalignant lesion of the vermilion portion of the lower lip caused by chronic exposure to sunlight. Older, fair-skinned men with outdoor occupations are typically affected. In early stages, the lower lip is red and atrophic with subtle blotchy intervening pale areas and loss of the vermilion border of the lip. With increased sun exposure, irregular scaly areas develop that may thicken and contain focal white patches that can be peeled off. The lip slowly becomes firm, slightly swollen, fissured, and everted. Ulceration with a thin yellow surface crust is typical of the chronic condition. The ulcers may be caused by trauma or loss of elasticity or may be an early sign of dysplastic or carcinomatous transformation. Histologic features include epithelial atrophy, subepithelial basophilic degeneration of collagen, and increased elastin fibers. Biopsy is recommended to rule out similar sun-related diseases, such as epithelial dysplasia, carcinoma in situ, basal cell carcinoma, squamous cell carcinoma, malignant melanoma, keratoacanthoma, cheilitis glandularis, and herpes labialis.

Up to 10% of **actinic cheilitis** cases develop into cancer. Clinicians should warn the patient of the likelihood of disease progression, if sunscreen protective agents are not used when exposed to the sun. Dysplastic changes should be treated surgically or with topical applications of 5-fluorouracil.

Candidal Cheilitis (Figs. 59.3 and 59.4) is an inflammatory condition of the lips caused by *C. albicans* (a fungal infection) and a lip-licking habit. In its typical presentation, candidal organisms obtain access to and invade the surface layers of the lip after mucosal breakdown, which is caused by repeated wetting and drying of the labial tissues. Desquamation and fissuring of surface epithelium result, and a fine whitish scale consisting of dried salivary mucus may be seen. In children, the affected perilabial skin appears red, atrophic, and fissured. Chapped, dry, itchy, burning lips and the inability to eat hot spicy foods are frequent symptoms. The chronic phase of this infection is characterized by painful vertical fissures that ulcerate and are slow to heal. Antifungal ointments are helpful in resolving the condition, but ultimate resolution requires elimination of the lip-licking habit. In persistent cases, an underlying condition (e.g., chronic use of corticosteroids) or systemic problem (e.g., diabetes mellitus or HIV infection) should be ruled out. A hypersensitivity reaction to ingredients contained in lip balms or lipsticks may clinically mimic this condition.

Angular Cheilitis (Perlèche) (Figs. 59.5 and 59.6) is a painful condition consisting of erythematous fissures at the corners of the mouth that radiate angularly downward. The condition is most commonly seen after the age of 50 years and is usually encountered in women and denture wearers.

Infection by *C. albicans*, *Staphylococcus aureus*, or both is causative. These pathogens are carried to the corners of the mouth from repeated pooling of saliva and frequent licking of the corners of the mouth (perlèche: from the French "Per Lecher" meaning "thoroughly + to lick"). Patients often perform this unconscious habit in an effort to provide relief to the area.

Angular cheilitis initially produces soft, red, and ulcerated mucocutaneous tissue at the corners of the mouth. With time, the erythematous fissures become deep and extend several centimeters from the commissure onto the perilabial skin or ulcerate and involve the labial and buccal mucosa. The ulcers frequently develop crusts that split and reulcerate during normal oral function. Small yellow-brown granulomatous nodules may eventually appear. Bleeding is infrequent.

Angular cheilitis is chronic and usually bilateral and is often associated with denture stomatitis or glossitis. Predisposing conditions include anemia, poor oral hygiene, frequent use of broad-spectrum antibiotics, decreased vertical dimension, high sucrose intake, dry mouth, accentuated perioral folds, and vitamin B deficiency. Treatment should include preventive measures (such as elimination of traumatic factors, meticulous oral hygiene, re-establishment of the correct vertical dimension and salivary flow) combined with topical antifungal and antibiotic therapy. Vitamin supplementation may also prove beneficial. Elimination of any lip-licking habit is also part of the management protocol.

Exfoliative Cheilitis (Figs. 59.7 and 59.8) is a persistent condition affecting the lips that is characterized by fissuring, desquamation, and the formation of hemorrhagic crusts. *C. albicans*, oral sepsis, stress, habitual lip-licking and biting, and contact allergens are etiologic agents. An association with psychological and thyroid disorders has been reported. This condition usually begins as a single fissure near the midline of the lower lip and spreads to produce multiple fissures. The fissures may ultimately develop a yellow-white scale that peels off or ulcerate and forms hemorrhagic crusts over the entire lip. The condition is often bothersome and unsightly, with the lower lip demonstrating more prominent signs. When the condition is symptomatic, dryness and burning are the usual chief complaints. **Exfoliative cheilitis** has a predisposition for teenage girls and young women, and stress has been reported to cause acute exacerbations. Because the cause of the condition may fluctuate and appears to be multifactorial, exfoliative cheilitis is difficult to manage and may persist for many years. Treatment is best rendered through the elimination of predisposing systemic or psychological factors together with topical application of antifungal ointments, topical steroids, moisturizing agents, or tacrolimus.

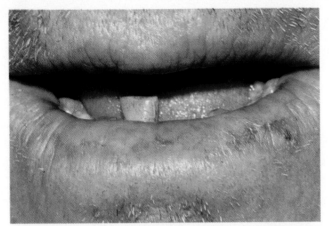

Fig. 59.1. Actinic cheilosis: vermilion border lost and scaly.

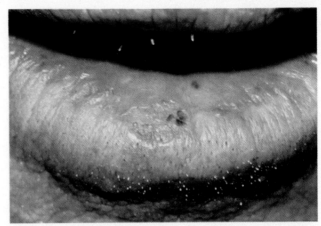

Fig. 59.2. Actinic cheilosis: everted, thickened with crusts.

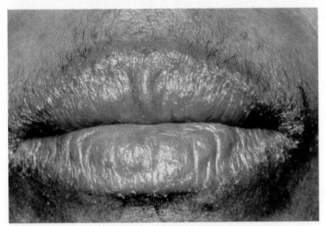

Fig. 59.3. Candidal cheilitis: whitish scale is dried mucin.

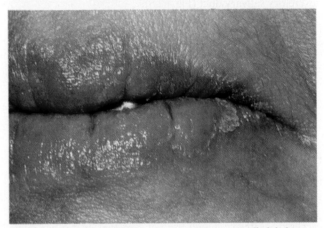

Fig. 59.4. Candidal cheilitis in a patient with uncontrolled diabetes.

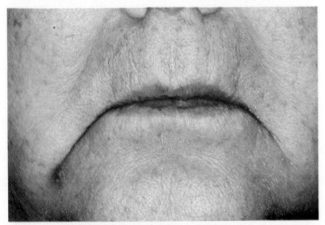

Fig. 59.5. Angular cheilitis: flaccid perioral folds.*

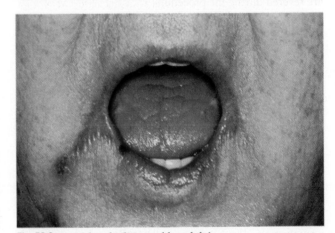

Fig. 59.6. Angular cheilitis in older adult.*

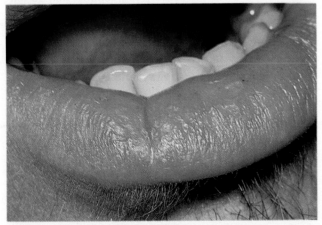

Fig. 59.7. Exfoliative cheilitis: early lesion; single fissure.

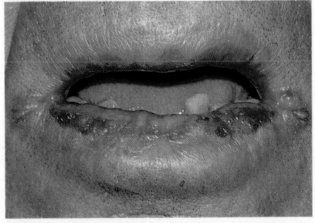

Fig. 59.8. Exfoliative cheilitis: hemorrhagic crusts.

8

Mucocele (Mucus Extravasation Phenomena) (Figs. 60.1 and 60.2) is a dome-shaped swelling of the lip or mucosa that forms when a salivary gland duct is severed and salivary secretions (mucin) leak into the soft tissue. Most **mucoceles** occur in mandibular labial mucosa. They lack an epithelial lining (so they are not a true cyst) and are surrounded by granulation tissue. A **ranula** is a variant large mucocele of the floor of the mouth caused by trauma to a sublingual gland (Bartholin) duct or, rarely, Wharton duct of the submandibular gland (Figs. 62.3 and 62.4). Mucoceles are distinguished from the rare **salivary duct cyst (sialocyst)**—a true epithelial-lined cyst caused by an obstruction that results in a dilated excretory salivary duct (Fig. 62.5).

Mucoceles are the most common nodular swelling of the lower lip. These swellings are asymptomatic, soft, fluctuant, bluish gray, and usually less than 1 cm in diameter. Swelling coincident with eating may be an occasional finding. The most common location is the lower lip midway between the midline and commissure, but other locations include the buccal mucosa, palate, floor of the mouth, and ventral tongue. Children and young adults are most frequently affected. Trauma is the cause.

Superficial mucoceles often regress spontaneously, whereas deep-seated mucoceles tend to persist and exacerbate with repeated trauma. Persistent mucoceles are treated by surgical excision. Recurrence is possible if the injured accessory salivary glands are not removed or if other ducts are severed during the procedure.

Accessory Salivary Gland Tumor (Figs. 60.3 and 60.4) Nodular swellings of the upper lip are infrequent and are usually caused by **benign minor salivary gland tumors**. About 90% of salivary tumors affect the major glands, and only 10% affect the minor glands. The most common types of benign salivary gland tumors are the **canalicular adenoma** and **pleomorphic adenoma**. These tumors are characterized by encapsulation, slow growth, and long duration (several months). Persons older than age 30 years are more commonly affected. Clinically, the pleomorphic adenoma is a pink to purple dome-shaped or multinodular lesion that protrudes from the inner aspect of the lip or vestibule. It is usually semisolid, freely movable, painless, and especially firm on palpation. The border is well circumscribed. Although it has unlimited potential for growth, the tumor generally remains less than 2 cm in diameter. Fluctuance and surface ulceration are not usual clinical features.

Malignant salivary gland tumors, such as **mucoepidermoid carcinoma** and **adenocarcinoma**, are rare in the upper lip and may be distinguished from benign neoplasia by their rapid and aggressive growth, short duration, and tendency to ulcerate and cause neurologic symptoms. Treatment of salivary gland neoplasia consists of surgical excision. If the excision is incomplete, recurrences are possible.

Nasolabial Cyst (Nasoalveolar Cyst) (Figs. 60.5 and 60.6) is a developmental cyst of soft tissue located in the cuspid-lateral incisor region of the upper lip. The cause is uncertain, and two theories have been suggested. One theory is that it is an embryonic fissural cyst arising from epithelial remnants that become entrapped during the embryologic fusion of the lateral nasal, globular, and maxillary processes. A more recent theory suggests that the tissue originates from the nasolacrimal duct. Proliferation and cystic degeneration of the entrapped tissue usually do not become clinically evident until after age 30 years, even though the tissue has been entrapped since birth. The condition has a female predilection.

The **nasolabial cyst** is a palpable swelling of the upper lip often extending to the mucobuccal fold that can cause elevation of the upper lip and ala of the nose, dilatation of the nostril, and disappearance of the nasolabial fold. The intraoral cyst may be tense or fluctuant, depending on size, and can affect the fit of a maxillary denture. Aspiration yields a yellowish or straw-colored fluid. The cyst is most often unilateral and is generally not in contact with the adjacent bone. Thus, the maxillary teeth remain vital. Infrequently, if the nasolabial cyst applies pressure to the adjacent bone, local resorption of osseous structures can result. Treatment is simple excision.

Implantation Cyst (Epithelial Inclusion Cyst) (Fig. 60.7) is an unusual cyst arising from a foreign body reaction to surface epithelium that is implanted within epidermal structures after a traumatic laceration. The cyst can occur intraorally or extraorally, at any age, and in any race or sex. Within the mouth, the lesion appears as a firm, dome-shaped, freely movable nodule located at the site of impetus, which is often the lip. Implantation cysts are usually small, solitary, and asymptomatic. Growth appears to remain constant, and the overlying mucosa appears smooth and pink. There is no swelling at mealtimes, nor is there spontaneous drainage of mucin as seen with a mucocele. A history of trauma should also lead the clinician to suspect this lesion. Surgical excision and histopathologic examination are recommended.

Mesenchymal Nodules and Tumors (Fig. 60.8) A variety of **mesenchymal tumors**, such as the fibroma, lipofibroma, and neuroma, can cause nodular swellings of the lip. The example shown here is a **neurofibroma**. Neurofibromas may be solitary or found in conjunction with von Recklinghausen disease (Figs. 81.7 and 81.8). When solitary, the neurofibroma is usually an asymptomatic, sessile, smooth-surfaced nodule of the buccal mucosa, gingiva, palate, or lips. Histologic examination of the tumor shows connective tissue and nerve fibrils. The discovery of a solitary neurofibroma requires close examination for multiple neurofibromatosis because the latter condition is associated with a marked tendency toward malignant transformation.

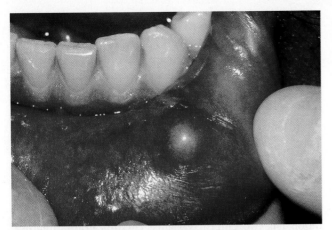
Fig. 60.1. Mucocele: small bluish superficial swelling.

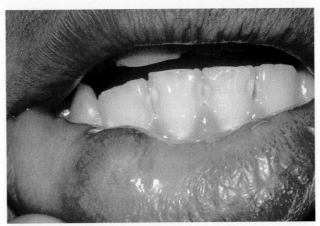
Fig. 60.2. Mucocele: bluish larger and deeper lesion.

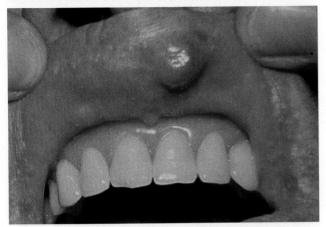
Fig. 60.3. Pleomorphic adenoma: a firm bluish nodule.

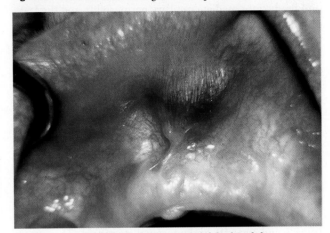
Fig. 60.4. Canalicular adenoma: purplish labial nodule.

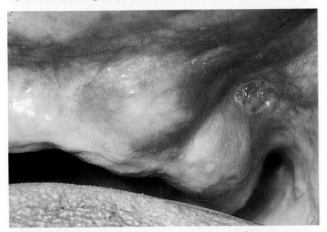
Fig. 60.5. Nasolabial cyst: a fluctuant nodule on palpation.

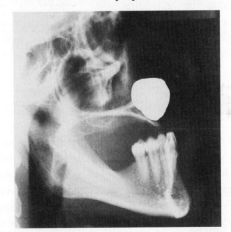
Fig. 60.6. Nasolabial cyst: injected with contrast medium.

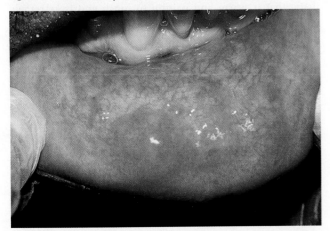
Fig. 60.7. Implantation cyst: from trauma.

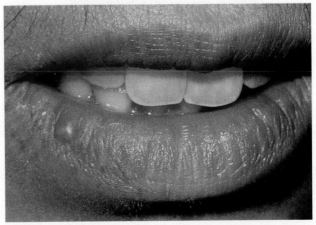
Fig. 60.8. Neurofibroma: sessile base, normal color.

8

135

SWELLINGS OF THE LIP

Angioedema (Figs. 61.1 and 61.2) is a swelling of fluid beneath the skin that is usually the result of an allergic (hypersensitivity) reaction. It occurs in *hereditary* and *acquired* forms and may be generalized or localized. Most cases are acquired and result from exposure to an allergen (such as food, cosmetics, latex, or stress) that attracts mast cells that degranulate and release histamine. Infections and autoimmune disease can induce **angioedema** by triggering capillary permeability via the formation of antigen-antibody complexes or by elevating numbers of eosinophils. Angiotensin-converting enzyme drugs used in the treatment of hypertension can also cause angioedema by increasing bradykinin levels. Histamine and bradykinin mediate capillary permeability and the leakage of plasma into the soft tissues.

The swelling develops within minutes or gradually over a few hours. When swelling affects the lips, it is usually uniform and diffuse but may be asymmetrical. The vermilion appears stretched, everted, pliable, and less distinct; the surface epithelium remains normal in color or is slightly red. Swellings of the tongue, floor of the mouth, eyelids, face, and extremities may accompany the condition. Acquired angioedema is usually recurrent and self-limiting and poses little threat to the patient. Symptoms are limited to burning or itching. Management involves prescription of antihistamines, identification and withdrawal of the allergen, and stress reduction.

The two types of rare hereditary form of angioedema (type I and type II) are autosomal dominant. They cause angioedema by activating the complement pathway. Pharyngeal and laryngeal swelling are usual along with abdominal cramping. Hereditary angioedema may be life threatening and responds poorly to epinephrine, corticosteroids, and antihistamines. Management involves avoidance of violent physical activity, trauma, and surgery. Androgenic drugs, such as Danocrine (danazol), and complement 1 (C1) inhibitor help to prevent and abort attacks.

Cheilitis Glandularis (Fig. 61.3) is a chronic inflammatory disorder of the labial salivary glands that most frequently affects older men. The lower lip is particularly susceptible and is characterized by diffuse enlargement and eversion of the lip. Although the cause remains poorly understood, the condition is associated with chronic exposure to the sun and wind and, less frequently, with smoking, poor oral hygiene, bacterial infection, and hereditary factors.

Clinical manifestations of **cheilitis glandularis** include a symmetrically enlarged, everted, and firm lower lip. With time, the inflamed labial salivary glands enlarge, and the ductal openings become dilated and appear as multiple small red spots. From these openings, a viscous, yellowish, mucopurulent exudate is secreted that makes the lip sticky. Progression of the condition causes the lip to appear atrophic, dry, fissured, and scaly and to become painful. Distinction of the vermilion border is eventually lost, and secondary infection of a deep labial fissure often results in fistulation and scarring. Emollients and sunscreens afford protection. Severe cases require vermilionectomy (lip shave), which produces an excellent esthetic result. Affected persons are at an increased risk for malignant transformation to squamous cell carcinoma.

Orofacial Granulomatosis (Cheilitis Granulomatosa) (Figs. 61.4–61.6) is a condition that results in nonpainful swelling of the orofacial tissues with a histologic finding of granulomatous inflammation in the tissues. The condition has two clinical variants: **cheilitis granulomatosa**, which involves only the lips, and **Melkersson-Rosenthal syndrome**, which has the features of unilateral facial paralysis, fissured pebbly tongue, and persistent labiofacial swelling. The condition produces noncaseating granulomas and appears to represent an abnormal immune reaction to infection or a foreign material/allergen or be a manifestation of Crohn disease or sarcoidosis. There is no sex predilection. The labial swelling develops slowly at a young age. Both lips may be firm and swollen, but symmetric enlargement of the lower lip is more common. The diffuse enlargement is asymptomatic and does not affect the color of the lip, but discrete nodules can often be palpated. The tongue, buccal mucosa, gingiva, palatal mucosa, and face can be affected. Patients respond to elimination of the allergen or odontogenic infection, as well as intralesional steroid injections and immunosuppressants. Spontaneous regression is possible.

Trauma (Fig. 61.7) to the lips often results in edema that is fluctuant, irregular, and exquisitely painful. **Trauma** may originate from an external source or may be self-induced and may cause damage (laceration or hemorrhage) to the soft tissue of the lip. Tooth fracture may accompany the condition. Traumatic enlargement of the lip is often a problem of children and mentally disabled patients who inadvertently chew their lip while under local anesthesia. For lip injuries, it is best to limit traumatic influences, apply ice compresses, and treat any lacerations or hemorrhage promptly.

Cellulitis (Fig. 61.8) means inflammation of cellular tissue. This degenerative process is caused by a bacterial infection in which the localization of pus has yet to occur. When of dental origin, cellulitis typically produces grossly swollen facial tissue that is warm and painful to touch and is extremely hard to palpation. A firm, diffusely swollen lip may be the first sign of cellulitis of odontogenic origin in the anterior region. A nonvital tooth is usually the root of the problem. Failure of host defense mechanisms to control the infection can result in an abscess or spread of infection. Treatment involves removal of necrotic pulpal tissue, drainage of the infection, culture, antibiotic sensitivity testing, and antibiotic therapy. Injection of local anesthetic into the swollen region should be avoided to minimize spread of the infection.

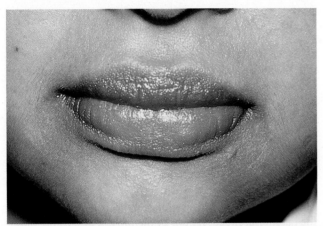
Fig. 61.1. **Angioedema:** both lips swollen and everted.

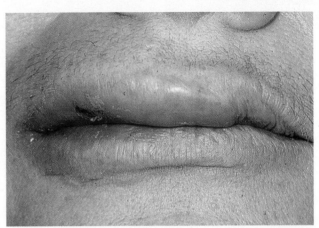
Fig. 61.2. **Angioedema:** unilateral upper and lower lip swelling.

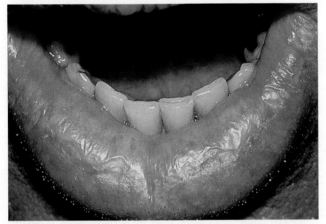
Fig. 61.3. **Cheilitis glandularis:** everted lip; red spots.

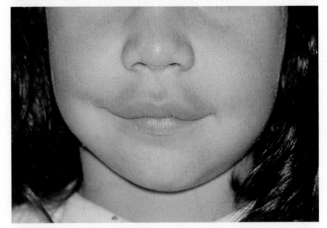
Fig. 61.4. **Orofacial granulomatosis:** facial paralysis.*

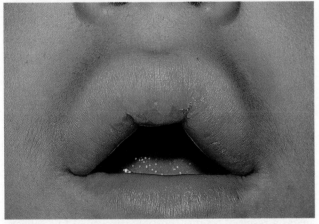
Fig. 61.5. **Orofacial granulomatosis:** lip involvement.*

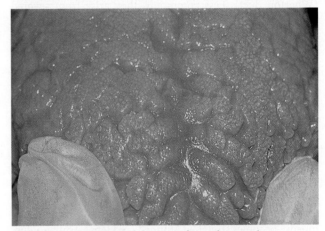
Fig. 61.6. **Orofacial granulomatosis:** fissured tongue.*

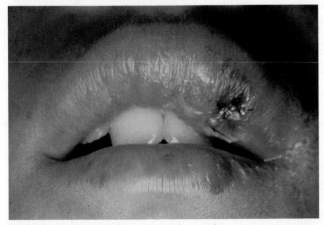
Fig. 61.7. **Trauma:** swollen, ulcerated upper lip.

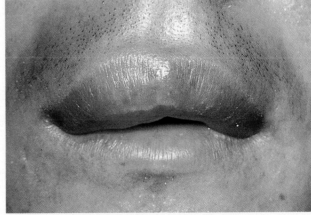
Fig. 61.8. **Cellulitis:** lip swelling; abscessed incisor.

8

SWELLINGS OF THE FLOOR OF THE MOUTH

Dermoid Cyst (Figs. 62.1 and 62.2) is a developmental cyst, usually present at birth, that develops from all three germ layers (teratoma) and is lined by epidermal cells. It may occur anywhere on the skin but has a propensity for the floor of the mouth. Few appear early in life, and most occur before age 35 years. There is no sex predilection. Those arising above the mylohyoid muscle appear as a painless midline, dome-shaped floor of the mouth swelling. The overlying mucosa is a natural pink, the tongue is slightly elevated, and palpation yields a doughlike consistency. Patients may report difficulties in eating and speaking. Growth is slow, but diameters in excess of 5 cm may be seen. **Dermoid cysts** may appear below the floor of the mouth if the original site of development is inferior to the mylohyoid muscle. In this instance, a submental swelling is noted. The lesion is histologically distinguished from an epidermoid cyst by the presence of adnexal structures, such as sebaceous glands, sweat glands, and hair follicles in the fibrous wall. The lumen contains semisolid keratin and sebum, which accounts for the doughy consistency and makes aspiration difficult. Surgical removal is the preferred treatment.

Ranula (Figs. 62.3 and 62.4) refers to a large mucocele of the floor of the mouth. Like other mucoceles, a **ranula** is caused by pooling of saliva within submucosal tissue and arises from a sialolith or after trauma to a salivary gland duct. Most involve the major excretory duct of the sublingual gland (ducts of Bartholin) or submandibular gland (Wharton duct). Less commonly, they arise from severed ducts of accessory salivary glands in the floor of the mouth. No sex predilection is apparent, and persons younger than 40 years of age are most commonly affected. Ranula also occurs in association with HIV infection.

There are two types of ranulas: (1) the more common **superficial ranula** that appears as a soft compressible swelling rising up from the floor of the mouth and (2) the dissecting or **plunging ranula** that penetrates below the mylohyoid muscle to produce a submental swelling. The plunging ranula can expand posteriorly or dissect its way downward into the neck spaces. The superficial ranula is characteristically dome shaped, translucent or bluish, fluctuant, and lateral to the midline. As the asymptomatic lesion enlarges, the mucosa becomes stretched, thinned, and tense. Unlike a dermoid cyst, digital pressure does not cause the lesion to pit. However, it can rupture, causing mucus to escape. The entire floor of the mouth may be filled by the swelling, which elevates the tongue and hinders movement. This impairs mastication, swallowing, and speech.

A ranula should be differentiated from other swellings by use of sialography, magnetic resonance imaging, or biopsy. Initial treatment is excision or marsupialization (Partsch operation), which consists of excising the overlying mucosa and suturing the remaining cystic lining to the floor of the mouth along the margins of the incision. Incision and drainage are not the treatments of choice, as they may reaccumulate fluid. Removal of the affected major salivary gland is required for recurrent and plunging ranulas.

Salivary Duct Cyst (Fig. 62.5) is an epithelium-lined recess that arises within salivary gland ductal tissue, either the major or minor glands, as a result of an obstruction or developmental defect. **Salivary duct cysts** are slow-growing and asymptomatic fluctuant swellings that frequently develop in the lip, buccal mucosa, floor of the mouth, or parotid gland. When superficial, they are blue or amber in color. Deep lesions do not alter the color of the mucosa. Treatment is excision.

Sialolith (Fig. 62.6) or salivary stone (calculus) is a calcified complex within a salivary gland or duct that may obstruct salivary flow and cause floor of the mouth swelling. They are usually round or oval and smooth or rough surfaced. Concentric laminations of different densities are often seen. **Sialoliths** occur most frequently after age 25 years, twice as often in men as in women, and usually in the excretory (Wharton) duct of the submandibular gland. The ascending and tortuous course of the excretory duct, along with high mucous content and alkaline pH of the saliva, are significant factors in stone formation.

Obstruction of salivary flow by a sialolith in Wharton duct results in a floor of the mouth swelling that contains a firm-to-hard nodule. Acute symptoms, such as pain and tenderness, often recur at mealtime. Swelling may extend along the course of the excretory duct and last for hours or days, depending on the blockage. The overlying mucosa usually remains pink, unless secondarily infected. In this case, the mucosa may turn red, and pus may emanate from the ductal opening. A sialolith can also cause a **salivary duct cyst** by increased intraductal pressure (see Fig. 62.5). Management involves appropriate radiographic imaging, and surgical removal of the sialolith. Localized cellulitis and fever require the use of antibiotics before invasive procedures.

Mucocele (Figs. 62.7 and 62.8) is a soft fluctuant lesion involving the retention of mucus in subepithelial tissue, usually as a result of trauma (possibly iatrogenic) to a salivary gland duct. These clear or bluish dome-shaped swellings may occur on the lip (Fig. 60.1), floor of the mouth, ventral tongue, palate, or buccal mucosa. They are asymptomatic and less than 1 cm in diameter. The base of the lesion is usually sessile, although pedunculated bases are possible. Children and young adults are most frequently affected. Superficial lesions may heal spontaneously, whereas persistent lesions should be excised and examined microscopically. If the condition is managed properly, recurrences are rare.

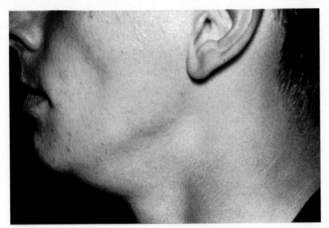

Fig. 62.1. **Dermoid cyst:** below mylohyoid muscle.

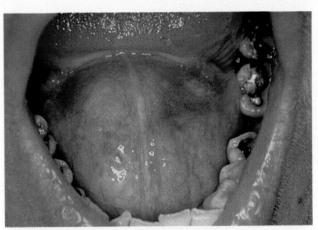

Fig. 62.2. **Dermoid cyst:** above mylohyoid muscle.

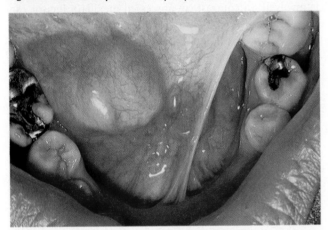

Fig. 62.3. **Ranula:** typical size, color, and translucency.

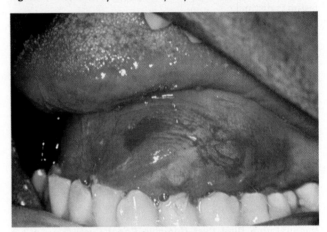

Fig. 62.4. **Ranula:** rare large lesion; impairs eating.

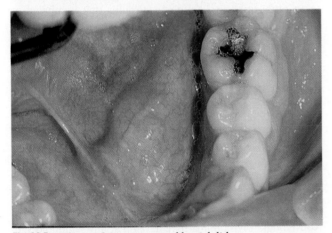

Fig. 62.5. **Salivary duct cyst:** caused by sialolith.

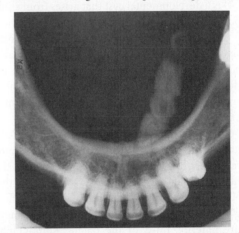

Fig. 62.6. **Sialoliths:** concentric laminations of several calculi.

8

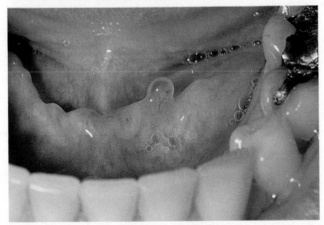

Fig. 62.7. **Mucocele:** superficial translucent lesion.

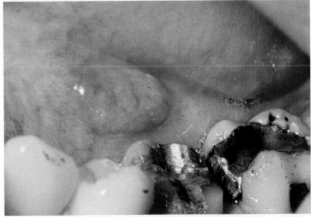

Fig. 62.8. **Mucocele:** from trauma during crown preparation.

Palatal Torus (Torus Palatinus) (Fig. 63.1) is a bony exostosis (outgrowth) located in the midline of the hard palate posterior to the bicuspid teeth (Fig. 34.2). It affects approximately 20% of adults. **Tori** are frequently inherited, with a higher incidence in women than in men. After puberty, there is a tendency for slow growth.

Tori vary in size and shape. The flat torus sits on a broad base; the surface is smooth and minimally convex. The spindle torus is an enlarged, narrow, bony ridge along the midline of the palate. The lobular torus sits on a single base and is divided into lobules by one or several grooves. The covering mucosa is pale pink, thin, and delicate. The boundary of the lesion is distinct.

The **palatal torus** is frequently asymptomatic unless traumatized, with some patients unaware of the torus until after the traumatic episode. Palatal tori should be removed if they interfere with eating, speaking, playing a musical instrument, or a prosthetic appliance.

Lipoma (Figs. 63.2 and 81.3) is a common benign mesenchymal tumor, but an uncommon intraoral finding. It is composed of adipocytes (fat cells) and appears as a well-circumscribed, dome-shaped yellowish submucosal mass. The buccal mucosa, tongue, floor of the mouth, and alveolar fold are common sites. The palate is a rare site of involvement. Treatment is excision.

Nasopalatine Duct Cyst (Incisive Canal Cyst) (Figs. 63.3 and 63.4) is a developmental cyst that arises from entrapped squamous or respiratory epithelial remnants of the nasopalatine duct within the incisive canal. It is the most common nonodontogenic cyst in the oral cavity. It may occur at any age and anywhere along the course of the incisive canal. However, the cyst is generally confined to palatal bone between the maxillary central incisors at the height of the incisive canal (see Fig. 38.4).

This cyst is usually asymptomatic and discovered as an incidental finding during routine examination. Symptomatic cysts are usually bacterially infected. Infrequently, the cyst of the incisive papilla arises entirely in soft tissue of the incisive papilla, where it appears as a small, superficial, fluctuant swelling (Fig. 38.5). A mature incisive canal cyst may swell the entire anterior third of the palate. Radiographically, the cyst appears as a well-delineated, midline, symmetrically oval or heart-shaped radiolucency located between the roots of vital maxillary central incisors. The margin is sclerotic and contiguous with the incisive canal. Root divergence and root resorption of the central incisors are occasional findings associated with large lesions. A similar cyst that is located more posteriorly in the palate has been called the **median palatal cyst** (Fig. 38.5). Current beliefs are that both cysts represent the same entity found in slightly different locations. All three conditions are treated by surgical enucleation.

Periapical Abscess (Figs. 63.5 and 63.6) is a fluctuant, soft tissue swelling consisting of necrotic material and pus resulting from bacterial infection and necrosis of the pulp. It appears at the periapex of a diseased tooth that is often tender to percussion, mobile, and slightly high in occlusion. Regional lymphadenopathy, fever, malaise, and trismus are common accompanying features. Examination of the teeth and supporting tissues along with diagnostic testing reveal the offending nonvital tooth. Radiographs often show a periapical radiolucency (Fig. 37.5).

Any abscessed maxillary tooth may produce a swelling of the palate. Generally, the swelling is red-purple, soft, tender, and lateral to the midline if a maxillary posterior tooth is involved. In contrast, an abscessed maxillary incisor can cause a midline swelling in the anterior third of the palate or lip. Aspiration or incision releases creamy yellow or yellow-green pus. Drainage, root canal therapy, or extraction is indicated to prevent spread of the infection. Antibiotics, analgesics, and antipyretic agents may also be needed.

Periodontal Abscess The differential diagnosis for a unilateral palatal swelling should include periodontal abscess—a localized infection involving the periodontium (refer to Figs. 51.7 and 51.8).

Lymphoid Hyperplasia (Fig. 63.7) is a rare, benign, reactive process that involves proliferation (rapid growth) of normal lymphoid tissue of the oropharynx (tonsils), tongue, floor of the mouth, soft palate, or lymph node in response to an often unknown antigenic stimulus that is inhaled or ingested. Persons older than 30 years are most often affected. Clinical examination reveals a soft to firm swelling arising at the posterior extent of the hard palate that grows slowly (up to 3 cm), either unilaterally or bilaterally. The surface of the mature lesion is pink to purple, nonulcerated, and dome shaped or lumpy. Patients rarely report pain. Biopsy is recommended. However, the condition resolves spontaneously.

Lymphoma (Fig. 63.8) is a malignant neoplastic growth of lymphocytes. They are classified into **Hodgkin** or **non-Hodgkin lymphoma** and subdivided by cell type and into nodal and extranodal disease. Epstein-Barr virus is often a factor in inducing malignant transformation of the lymphocytes. Non-Hodgkin lymphoma may develop at any lymphoid site, including cervical lymph nodes, mandible, palate, and, rarely, the gingiva. Primary lymphomas of the palate occur most commonly in patients older than 60 years but may be seen in younger patients, especially those with acquired immunodeficiency syndrome (AIDS). The tumor arises at the junction of the hard and soft palates as a soft, spongy, nontender, nonulcerated swelling. The surface is often lumpy and purplish. Rarely does it affect the underlying palatal bone. Early recognition and biopsy are important so that treatment may be initiated when the lesion is confined entirely to the palate. Irradiation and chemotherapy are used to treat palatal lymphomas.

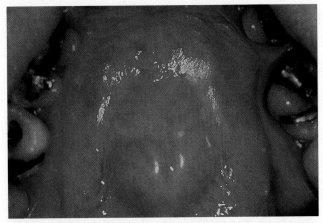

Fig. 63.1. Torus palatinus: flat, slight lobulation.

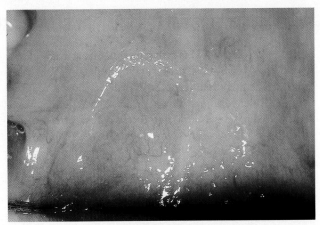

Fig. 63.2. Lipoma: palatal nodule; hypervascular surface.

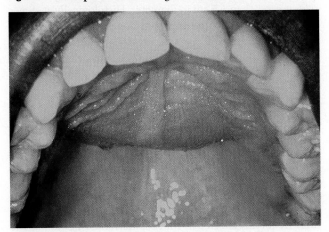

Fig. 63.3. Nasopalatine duct cyst: anterior palate swelling.

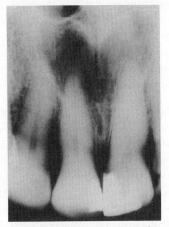

Fig. 63.4. Nasopalatine duct cyst: classic heart shape.

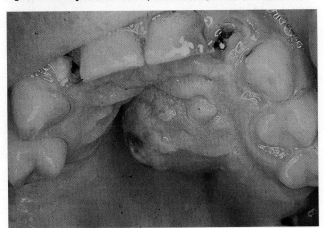

Fig. 63.5. Periapical abscess: from nonvital lateral incisor.

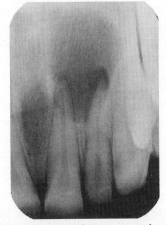

Fig. 63.6. Periapical abscess: large periapical radiolucency.

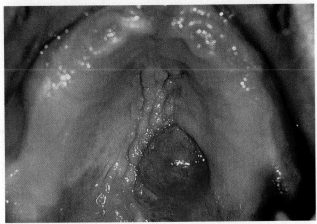

Fig. 63.7. Lymphoid hyperplasia: at posterior palate.

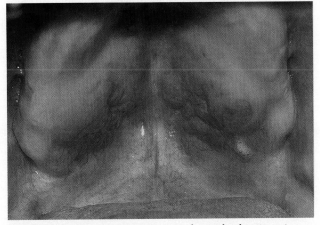

Fig. 63.8. Lymphoma of palate: nontender, with telangiectasia.

Sialadenitis (Fig. 64.1) is inflammation of a salivary gland. It is often caused by obstruction and bacterial infection (bacterial sialadenitis) that occurs when salivary flow is reduced because of dehydration, illness, or an obstruction. Salivary stasis allows pathogens (*Staphylococcus aureus*, *Streptococcus viridans*, and *Streptococcus pneumoniae*) to travel up the duct system and replicate. Viruses (mumps, coxsackie, echo) also can be causative. The parotid and submandibular glands are most often affected. Treatment is directed toward eliminating the cause and involves use of antibiotics, sialendoscopy, and agents that stimulate salivary flow.

A distinct type of sialadenitis, **subacute sialadenitis**, affects the minor salivary glands of the palate of young men. It appears as a painful, rapid-appearing, reddish nodular swelling (up to 1 cm) that has an intact, nonulcerated surface. The cause is unknown. Biopsy reveals acinar atrophy and necrosis and a diffuse inflammatory infiltrate. Healing occurs within three weeks with or without treatment.

Necrotizing Sialometaplasia (Figs. 64.2 and 64.3) is a benign, self-healing lesion of the accessory palatal salivary glands that can be confused clinically and histologically with carcinoma. This destructive inflammatory lesion begins after trauma and presents as a rapidly growing swelling on the lateral aspect of the hard palate, particularly in men older than 40 years. Tissue infarction as a result of vasoconstriction and ischemia caused by trauma or dental injection appears causative. Rarely, the soft palate or buccal mucosa is involved. Bilateral cases have been reported. The initial presentation is a small painless nodule that enlarges and causes pain. Within a few weeks, it ulcerates, and the pain diminishes. The size of the swelling varies, and growth to a diameter of 2 cm is possible. A deep central ulcer with a grayish pseudomembrane is characteristic. The ulcer is irregular and pebbly; the border is often rolled. Healing occurs on its own over 4 to 8 weeks or after a biopsy. Biopsy is recommended to rule out similar-appearing lesions, such as salivary gland tumors and malignant lymphoma. Histologically, it demonstrates squamous metaplasia of ductal epithelium, which may be misdiagnosed as mucoepidermoid carcinoma.

Benign Accessory Salivary Gland Neoplasm (Figs. 64.4 and 64.5) There are more than 10 types of benign salivary gland tumors. As many as 80% occur within the parotid gland, 10% in the submandibular gland, and about 10% to 20% in minor salivary glands. Most are pleomorphic adenoma, Warthin tumor, oncocytoma, or basal cell adenoma. Two of the more common types are discussed.

The **basal cell (monomorphic) adenoma** is a benign tumor that can develop in the accessory salivary glands of the palate, most commonly in older women. It appears as a slow-growing dome-shaped mass. The tumor is encapsulated and consists of a regular glandular pattern and usually only one cell type. It lacks a mesenchymal component as seen in pleomorphic adenoma. Treatment is surgical excision.

The **pleomorphic adenoma** (benign mixed tumor) is the most common benign neoplasm of accessory salivary glands. It occurs more often in major than minor salivary glands. When the minor glands are affected, the palate is the most common location. These neoplasms are most frequent in adult women and tend to occur lateral to the midline and distal to the anterior third of the hard palate.

The clinical presentation of the pleomorphic adenoma is a painless, firm, slow-growing, nonulcerated, dome-shaped swelling. Palpation reveals isolated softer areas and a smooth or lobulated surface. Slow persistent enlargement over a period of years is typical, and lesions may achieve sizes greater than 1.5 cm in diameter. Histologically, it shows myoepithelial cells in a nestlike arrangement, with pools of myxoid, chondroid, and mucoid material. A distinct fibrous connective tissue capsule containing tumor cells surrounds and usually limits the extension of the tumor. Thorough excisional biopsy is recommended to limit recurrence. Tumorous involvement of the capsule may play a role in recurrence.

Malignant Accessory Salivary Gland Neoplasm (Figs. 64.6– 64.8) There are more than 15 different types of malignant salivary gland tumors. **Adenoid cystic carcinoma** (cylindroma) and **mucoepidermoid carcinoma** are the two most common intraoral malignant neoplasms of the accessory salivary glands. Persons between the ages of 20 and 50 years are most frequently affected by mucoepidermoid carcinoma. The adenoid cystic carcinoma usually occurs after age 50 years. The adenoid cystic carcinoma occurs also in respiratory, gastrointestinal, and reproductive tissues, whereas mucoepidermoid carcinoma may occur in the skin, respiratory tract, or centrally within bone, particularly the mandible.

Malignant accessory salivary gland neoplasms occur frequently in the posterior palate. These neoplasms are usually asymptomatic, firm, dome-shaped swellings that occur lateral to the midline. The overlying tissue appears normal in the early stages, but the mucosa later becomes erythematous, with several small telangiectatic surface vessels. These neoplasms grow more quickly and are more painful than benign salivary gland tumors. Induration and eventual spontaneous ulceration are common. A bluish appearance or a mucous exudate emanating from the ulcerated tumor surface as well as pools of necrotic fluid within the tumor visible radiographically are distinctive features of mucoepidermoid carcinoma.

Treatment is radical excision. The prognosis varies, depending on the histologic grade, and presence of metastasis. Adenoid cystic carcinoma rarely metastasizes but is an infiltrating malignancy with a propensity for distant spread by perineural invasion. Thus, lifetime follow-up is necessary. In contrast, the mucoepidermoid carcinoma infrequently metastasizes and is more easily cured by surgical means. Other malignant accessory salivary gland neoplasms include the acinic cell adenocarcinoma, polymorphous low-grade adenocarcinoma, carcinoma ex pleomorphic adenoma, carcinosarcoma, and malignant mixed tumor.

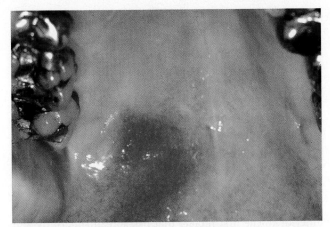

Fig. 64.1. Subacute sialadenitis: in young man.

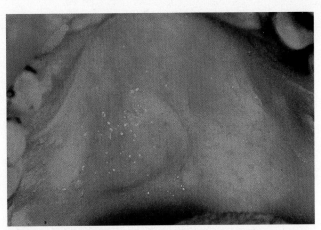

Fig. 64.2. Necrotizing sialometaplasia: painful swelling.

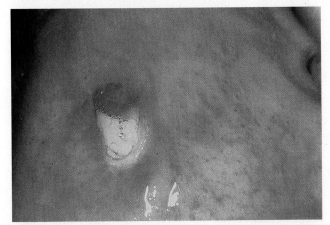

Fig. 64.3. Necrotizing sialometaplasia: ulcerative phase.

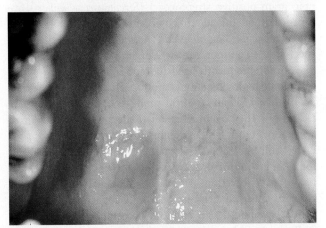

Fig. 64.4. Basal cell adenoma: painless nodule.

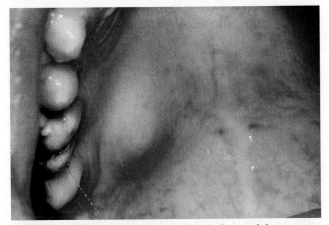

Fig. 64.5. Pleomorphic adenoma: strikingly firm nodule.

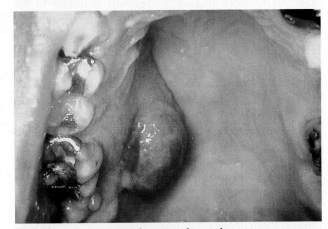

Fig. 64.6. Malignant mixed tumor: ulcerated.

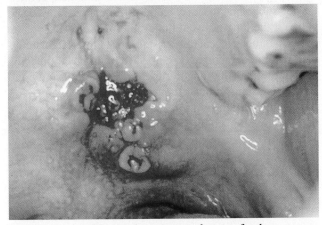

Fig. 64.7. Mucoepidermoid carcinoma: draining fistulas.

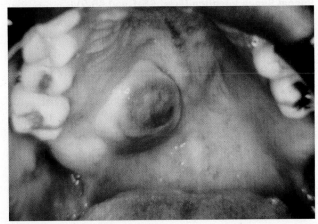

Fig. 64.8. Adenoid cystic carcinoma: surface ulceration.

143

SWELLINGS OF THE FACE

Odontogenic Infection (Figs. 65.1–65.8) Orofacial infections arise when microbes invade tissue, replicate, and overwhelm the local immune response. Infections are promoted by poor health and systemic disease, poor oral hygiene, and traumatic surgery. Oral infections are called odontogenic when they are tooth related. Most **odontogenic infections** arise as a consequence of pulpal necrosis, apical periodontitis, and pericoronitis. Almost all odontogenic infections are polymicrobial, consisting of anaerobic (65%) and aerobic (35%) bacteria. Obligate gram-negative anaerobes (*Prevotella*, *Fusobacterium*, *Bacteroides* species), anaerobic gram-positive organisms (*Peptostreptococcus* species), and facultative anaerobic gram-positive streptococci (*Streptococcus milleri*) are the most frequently identified organisms. Other contributors are *lactobacillus*, *diphtheroids*, *Actinomyces*, and *Eikenella* species. It is common for these organisms to be resistant to one or more frequently used antibiotics.

Odontogenic infections produce four classic features: *calor (heat)*, *dolor (pain)*, *rubor (redness)*, and *tumor (swelling)*. They begin as a soft tissue swelling adjacent to a necrotic tooth. The swelling slowly enlarges and produces dull pain and a bad taste. It may remain localized for a long time or progress to an abscess, parulis, cellulitis, or space infection. An **abscess** is an acute swelling that contains pus and necrotic debris. It appears as a well-localized swelling that is soft and occasionally pointed (Fig. 51.7). It is visible in or outside the mouth and drains spontaneously or when incised. The **parulis** is similar to the abscess, but the bacterial infection drains through a sinus tract onto the mucosal surface as a yellow-red papule (Figs. 50.1 and 50.2). In most cases, the parulis represents chronic infection and is asymptomatic. **Cellulitis** is an early feature of a spreading odontogenic infection; it represents a diffuse inflammatory response that has not yet localized. Cellulitis produces a diffuse, red, warm, hard swelling (generally over the cheek or mandible) that is firm and tender to palpation (Fig. 61.8). It may mature into an abscess and drain or become aggressive and spread. Spread of infection beyond anatomic boundaries through fascial planes (spaces) is called a **space infection**. There are more than 10 fascial spaces in the face, and a few examples that cause swelling because of infected tooth or jaw are provided below.

Buccal Space Infection (Figs. 65.1 and 65.2) is most often caused by an odontogenic infection that has spread beyond the cortical plate, lateral to the buccinator muscle and anterior to the masseter muscle. It frequently arises from lateral migration of pathogenic bacteria that infect the periapex of a maxillary or mandibular molar. Entry into the space is usually gained at the posterior insertion of the buccinator muscle. Pain, swelling, fever, and chronic inflammation of a mandibular molar are the most prominent features.

Masseteric (Submasseteric) Space Infection (Figs. 65.3 and 65.4) is generally the result of an odontogenic infection that has spread posteriorly from an infected mandibular molar or buccal space to a region located under the masseter muscle and over the lateral aspect of the ramus. The swelling is firm and nonfluctuant and overlies the angle of the mandible. Masseteric muscle involvement produces marked trismus (difficulty in opening). Computed tomography and magnetic resonance imaging are useful in defining this condition.

Infraorbital Space Infection (Figs. 65.5 and 65.6) is the result of an infected maxillary tooth (usually a tooth anterior to the first molar) that has spread superiorly and involves the region lateral to the nasal ala and below the eye. Grave concern is raised when the infection encroaches on the eyelid or affects vision, because the ophthalmic (angular) veins lack valves and spread of infection to the brain is possible. **Cavernous sinus thrombosis** is a severe infection resulting from spread of infection via the angular veins to the brain.

Treatment of odontogenic infection involves four steps: (1) removal of the source of the infection, (2) establishment of drainage, (3) provision of antibiotics when needed, and (4) provision of supportive care. The infection is often controlled by instituting root canal therapy or extraction of the offending tooth when the infection is localized (e.g., parulis, apical periodontitis). These treatments provide a pathway for drainage and reduce the bacterial load. Alternatively, incision and drainage can be performed to drain an abscess. If the condition is diffuse, as in cellulitis or pericoronitis, incision and drainage are generally unsuccessful and not recommended. Root canal therapy or extraction is used to treat cellulitis caused by a nonvital tooth, whereas pericoronitis is generally managed first with irrigation and antibiotics. When the pain of pericoronitis remits, extraction is performed. Guidelines for prescribing antibiotics include the presence of a spreading infection (regional lymphadenopathy, fever, malaise, swelling beyond anatomic boundaries) in combination with inability to establish drainage or immune compromise. Penicillin VK is the drug of choice, generally prescribed as 1,000 mg at first dose and then 500 mg orally four times daily for 7 days.

Ludwig Angina (Figs. 65.7 and 65.8) is a severe and rapidly spreading cellulitis that involves the submandibular, submental, and sublingual spaces bilaterally. These spaces are located between the tongue, hyoid bone, and lingual cortical plates of the mandible. It generally arises from an infected mandibular molar or a fractured (and infected) mandible. Spreading infection forces the tongue superiorly and posteriorly and forces the submandibular tissues apically. This impinges on the airway and can result in airway obstruction. Aggressive use of antibiotics, culture, sensitivity, and multiple incisions and drains may be required to control the infection. In some patients, emergency procedures, such as a tracheostomy, are needed to sustain life.

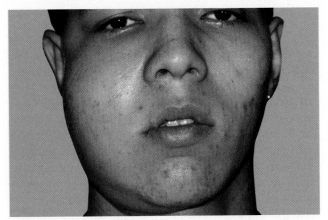

Fig. 65.1. Buccal space infection: infected mandibular molar.

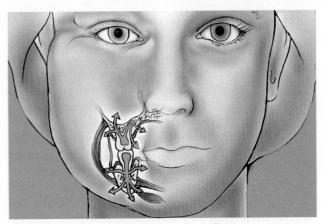

Fig. 65.2. Buccal space infection: anatomic illustration.

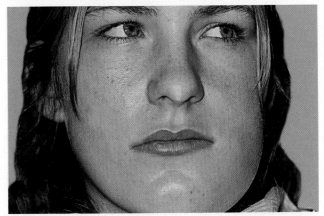

Fig. 65.3. Masseteric space infection: infected left mandibular first molar.

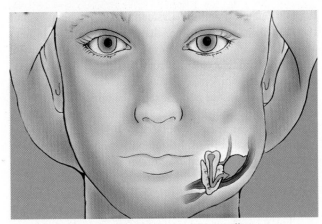

Fig. 65.4. Masseteric space infection: anatomic illustration.

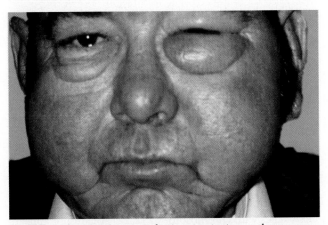

Fig. 65.5. Infraorbital space infection: impinging on the eye.

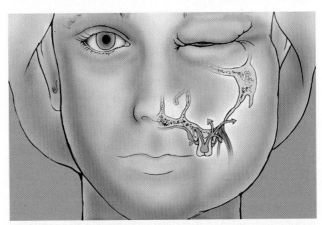

Fig. 65.6. Infraorbital space infection: anatomic illustration.

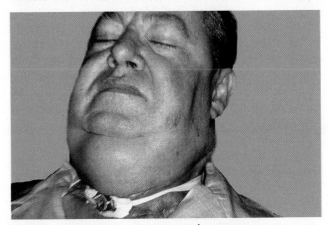

Fig. 65.7. Ludwig angina: requiring tracheostomy.

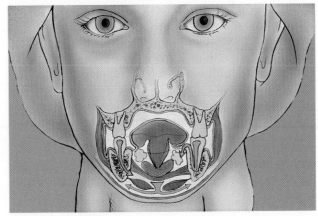

Fig. 65.8. Ludwig angina: anatomic illustration.

8

Sialadenosis (Fig. 66.1) is a painless noninflammatory swelling of major salivary glands. The condition indicates an underlying systemic disorder, such as alcoholism, anorexia nervosa, bulimia, diabetes, drug reaction, malnutrition, or HIV infection. It arises when acinar cells swell, probably because of dysregulation of autonomic innervation of the gland. Most cases begin as slow-growing, painless swellings of the parotid gland. It is often bilateral but can be unilateral. Salivary flow may be reduced. Microscopy shows hypertrophied acinar cells engorged with secretory granules and fat infiltration. Treatment attempts to control the systemic disease.

Warthin Tumor (Papillary Cystadenoma Lymphomatosum) (Fig. 66.2) is a benign tumor that is more common in men after age 60 and occurs almost exclusively in the parotid gland. It is thought to arise from entrapped glandular elements or proliferation of ductal epithelium. Smokers have eight times the risk as nonsmokers. The tumors arise mostly in the tail of the parotid gland as a painless, slow-growing, doughy, nodular mass. About 5% to 10% occur in parotid glands bilaterally. The submandibular and minor salivary glands are rarely affected. The tumor is composed of bilayered, oncocytic ductal epithelium that forms uniform rows and papillae surrounding cystic spaces. A lymphoid stroma surrounds the epithelium. Biopsy and excision are recommended. Recurrence and malignant transformation are rare.

Sjögren Syndrome (Fig. 66.3) is a chronic autoimmune disease in which the mouth and eyes become extremely dry. It is characterized by progressive lymphocytic infiltration that results in exocrine gland dysfunction. The cause of the disease remains unknown. It affects 1 in 2,000 persons, women in 90% of cases, and usually manifests between 35 and 50 years of age. The primary form, sicca syndrome, is limited to the salivary and lacrimal glands, producing dry eyes (xerophthalmia) and dry mouth (xerostomia). Oral and ocular disease accompanied by systemic disease (i.e., rheumatoid arthritis, systemic lupus erythematosus, and infiltrative disease of gastrointestinal and pulmonary exocrine glands) is known as secondary Sjögren syndrome. The syndrome develops slowly and involves progressive enlargement of the major salivary glands, particularly the parotid glands bilaterally. The glands become firm but not painful. Involvement of the pancreas or gall bladder results in abdominal symptoms. Labial salivary gland biopsy shows multiple lymphocyte aggregates adjacent to salivary acini. Serum markers, that is, autoantibodies (anti-SS-A and anti-SS-B) and rheumatoid factor, together with ocular and oral dryness help confirm the diagnosis. Management of dryness is attempted with artificial tears and saliva. Pilocarpine, cevimeline, fluoride, and chlorhexidine are useful. Patients are at increased risk for caries and the development of lymphoma.

Cushing Disease and Syndrome (Fig. 66.4) Cushing disease (hyperadrenocorticism) is a condition that results from excess corticosteroid secretion from the adrenal gland. It is usually induced by a pituitary adenoma. Cushing syndrome, in contrast, results from chronic corticosteroid use. High serum cortisol levels cause fluid retention, hypertension, and hyperglycemia as well as truncal obesity, a round (moon-shaped) face with plethora (red), facial and truncal acne, a buffalo hump at the back of the neck, and purple abdominal striae. These features are caused by collagen wasting, dermal weakening, capillary fragility, and fluid accumulation. Treatment is directed toward eradicating tumors and correcting daily cortisol levels.

Masseter Hypertrophy (Fig. 66.5) is an increase in the size of the masseter muscle because of increased size of the cells. It occurs as a result of chronic muscle activity induced by tooth clenching, gum chewing, or bruxism. The masseter muscles are firm and nontender. Enlargement is most prominent over the angle of the mandible.

Neurofibromatosis (von Recklinghausen Disease) (Fig. 66.6) is an inherited (autosomal dominant) disorder caused by a loss of a tumor suppressor gene (NF1 or NF2) that results in multiple neurofibromas (tumors involving nerve tissue) of the skin, mouth, bone, nervous system, and gastrointestinal tract. Accompanying skin pigmentations include café au lait spots, axillary freckling (Crowe sign), as well as Lisch nodules in the iris. The tumors appear after puberty as papules, nodules, or pendulous growths and can affect the cranial or spinal nerves, causing vision or hearing loss. In the mandible, they can expand the mandibular canal and cortical plates, produce facial swelling, or, rarely, undergo malignant transformation.

Cystic (Lymphangioma) Hygroma (Fig. 66.7) is a benign growth or hamartoma of lymphatic vessels (lymphangioma) that fail to drain lymph properly. As a result, lymph collects within the numerous dilated vessels. Most appear in the head, neck, and axilla as soft, compressible swellings. Airway obstruction may be a concern. Excision is generally successful.

Ewing Sarcoma (Fig. 66.8) is a small, round cell malignancy caused by a chromosomal translocation (i.e., chromosome 11 switches with chromosome 12 or 22). The tumor appears to have a neuroectodermal origin. Persons younger than 25 years are most often affected. Most sarcomas arise in the femur, pelvis, and ribs; less than 5% arise in jaws. Some arise in soft tissue without bony involvement. In the jaws, the mandible is most often involved. Patients present with swelling, pain, paresthesia, loose teeth, fever, leukocytosis, and an elevated sedimentation rate. The mass is soft when the tumor has penetrated the bony cortical plate. Radiographs show displaced teeth and a destructive radiolucent mass with ill-defined margins. Metastasis to lung, liver, and lymph nodes occurs frequently. Survival rates of 55% to 75% have been achieved with the combined use of radiation, surgery, and chemotherapy.

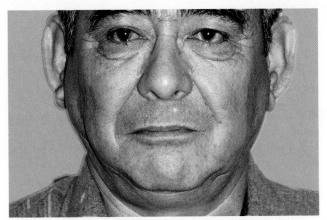

Fig. 66.1. **Sialadenosis:** of the parotid glands in a diabetic patient.

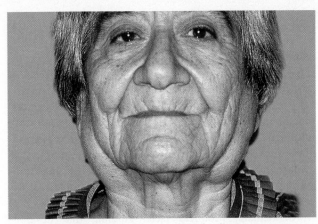

Fig. 66.2. **Warthin tumor:** bilateral parotid enlargement.

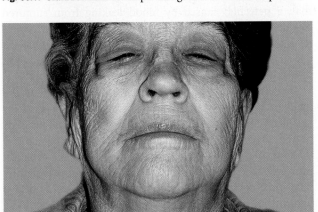

Fig. 66.3. **Sjögren syndrome:** dry eyes, parotid enlargement.

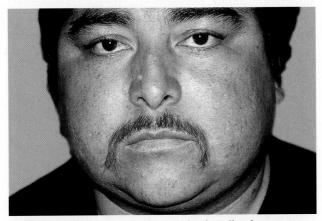

Fig. 66.4. **Cushing syndrome:** acne and red swollen face.

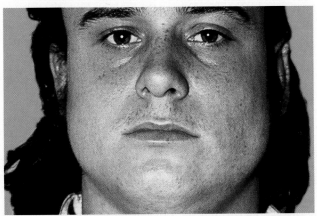

Fig. 66.5. **Masseter hypertrophy:** in a clench.

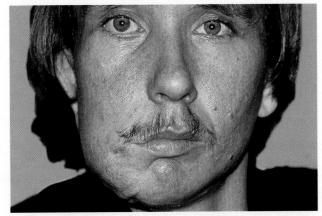

Fig. 66.6. **Neurofibromatosis:** asymmetrical enlargement.

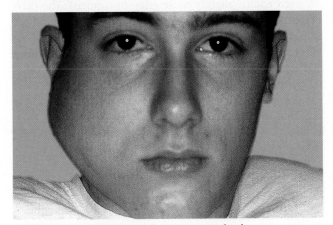

Fig. 66.7. **Cystic hygroma:** soft, present since birth.

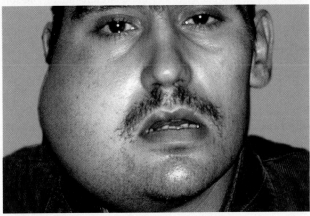

Fig. 66.8. **Ewing sarcoma:** rapidly growing malignancy.

8

147

Angioedema (Fig. 67.1) is a hypersensitivity reaction characterized by accumulation of fluid within cutaneous or mucosal tissues. The resulting tissues are soft, swollen, and itchy. It can be triggered by mechanical trauma, stress, infection, or an allergen. Most cases are acquired and result from IgE-mediated mast cell degranulation and release of histamine after exposure to an allergen (such as food) or physical contact. Histamine mediates capillary leakiness. Infections and autoimmune disease are less common triggers of the condition.

Angioedema produces facial swelling that develops within minutes or over a few hours. The swellings are usually uniform, diffuse, and symmetric. The lips are commonly affected, producing overly full, stretched, pliable swellings. Generally, the skin tone remains normal in color or is slightly red. The tongue, floor of the mouth, eyelids, face, and extremities may also be affected. **Acquired angioedema** is usually recurrent and self-limiting and poses little threat to the patient. Symptoms are limited to burning or itching. Management involves use of antihistamines, identification and withdrawal of allergenic stimuli, and stress reduction.

In the rare autosomal dominant **hereditary (nonallergic) form**, angioedema is caused by an enzyme deficiency (type I) or a dysfunctional enzyme (type II) that results in activation of the complement pathway. Prophylactic treatment involves avoidance of trauma and violent physical activity and use of androgenic drugs, such as Danocrine (danazol). In emergencies or before surgery, the following can be used: fresh frozen plasma, complement (C1) inhibitor, or kallikrein inhibitors. Lymphoproliferative disorders or use of angiotensin-converting enzyme (ACE) drugs (for high blood pressure) and nonsteroidal anti-inflammatory drugs can also cause angioedema. These entities can induce angioedema by increasing bradykinin levels, not by the release of histamine. Thus, proper patient evaluation and the correct diagnosis are imperative for proper management of angioedema.

Emphysema (Fig. 67.2) is defined as the abnormal presence of air in tissue. Although rare in dentistry, it most often occurs during a surgical procedure when compressed air from an air-driven handpiece or syringe is forced under a mucoperiosteal flap, through an open pulp chamber, or intra-alveolarly. The air becomes entrapped in subcutaneous tissue or a fascial plane. Under these circumstances, the soft tissues adjacent to the surgical site distend within minutes of the procedure. The swelling is soft or mildly firm and yields a distinctive crackling sound (crepitus) on palpation. The entrapped air can migrate along fascial planes through the neck to the sternum, into the prevertebral fascia and mediastinum, toward the temporal and orbital regions, or into the vascular system. **Emphysema** is associated with risks for infection, air embolism, and death. Broad-spectrum antibiotics are recommended to prevent infection. Signs suggestive of embolic sequelae, such as sudden vision changes, dyspnea, altered heart rate, or loss of consciousness, warrant immediate emergency care.

Postoperative Bleeding (Figs. 67.3–67.6) Facial swelling can result from orofacial bleeding when excess bleeding or blood pools below the epithelium. The end result is **purpura**, the accumulation of blood within the subcutaneous or submucosal tissues. Purpura is classified according to the size of the lesion produced. **Petechiae** are pinpoint, flat, round red spots under the skin surface caused by hemorrhage from the capillaries (bleeding into the skin). A small bruise, larger than a petechia, caused by blood leaking from ruptured blood vessels into the surrounding tissues is called an **ecchymosis**. A **hematoma** is a large localized collection of blood in a tissue, organ, or body space resulting from a broken blood vessel.

In dentistry, hematomas are commonly caused by the inadvertent needle penetration into the posterior superior alveolar vein. Swelling occurs without pain within seconds or minutes of the trauma. The swelling grows uniformly and without color change in the posterior cheek region, over and in front of the mandibular ramus. The hematoma is slightly firm and compressible. It may cause tissue tenderness, nerve paresthesia, and muscle trismus. Pressure and ice should be applied to the hematoma during the first 24 hours. Thereafter, heat should be applied to dissipate the blood. Depending on its size, the lesion may take more than 1 week to resolve and may discolor the skin. During the healing phase, the color of the skin fades from purple to brown, then tan and yellow as the lesion migrates downward toward the chest. Antibiotics should be considered if the hematoma is caused by severance of a vessel with a contaminated instrument.

Bell Palsy (Figs. 67.7 and 67.8) is a sudden weakness and paralysis of cranial nerve VII on one side of the face. The condition results in the inability to move the muscles of facial expression on the affected side. Events that damage or traumatize the facial nerve are most frequently causative and include surgery, tooth extraction, infection, or exposure to cold. About one third of cases are linked to reactivation of herpesvirus within the geniculate ganglion. All persons are susceptible, but the condition is seen most often in middle-aged adults (slightly more often in women). The palsy presents with abrupt onset of inability to raise the forehead skin, close the eye, and lift the corner of the mouth of the affected side. Eye watering (crocodile tears), mouth drooling, and loss of taste are common consequences. Without treatment, the palsy may be temporary or permanent. Steroid (prednisone) therapy and antivirals (valacyclovir) have proven to be effective in treating Bell palsy, especially if given within 72 hours of outbreak. Palliative care to protect the eye from corneal ulceration should also be provided.

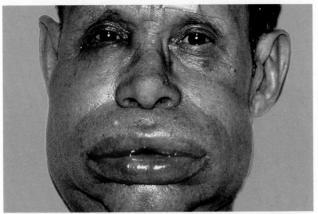

Fig. 67.1. **Angioedema:** caused by contact with latex rubber.

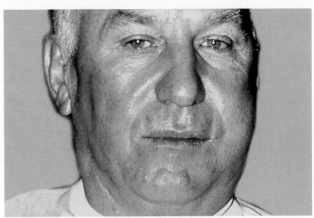

Fig. 67.2. **Air emphysema:** after flap surgery.

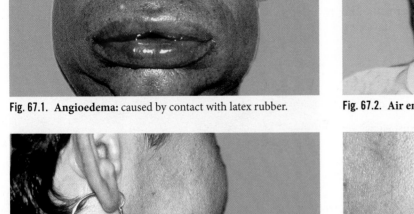

Fig. 67.3. **Hematoma:** posterior alveolar vein injured.*

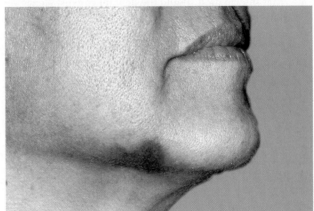

Fig. 67.4. **Hematoma:** 1 week later.*

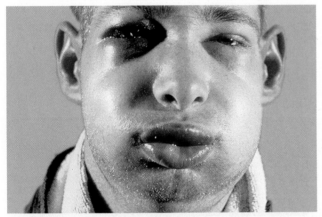

Fig. 67.5. **Surgical trauma:** swelling 2 days postoral surgery.‡

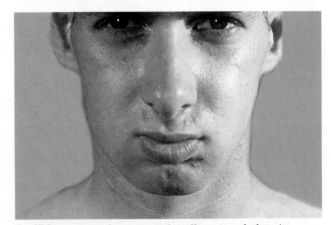

Fig. 67.6. **Healing of postsurgical swelling:** 2 weeks later.‡

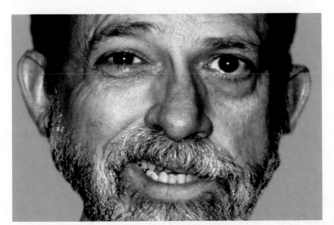

Fig. 67.7. **Bell palsy:** inability to lift left side of the face.

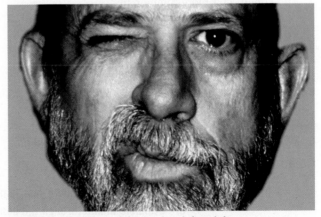

Fig. 67.8. **Bell palsy:** inability to close left eyelids.

8

149

CASE 36. (FIG. 67.9)

This 79-year-old Caucasian man was visited in a nursing home. His oral care is dependent largely on the nursing staff. During your oral exam, you notice this growth. The nursing staff believe that it was not present a few days ago.

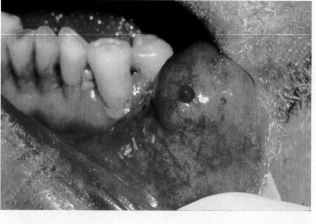

1. Describe the clinical findings.

2. What is the fluid on the surface of the lesion?

3. Is this a normal finding, a variant of normal, or disease?

4. What information should the dental hygienist elicit from the patient and the nursing staff?

5. Would a dentist expect this condition to be symptomatic?

6. List conditions you should consider in the differential diagnosis, and note which condition is most likely the correct diagnosis.

7. Why is this lesion pink and not clear or bluish in color?

8. What do you notice about the teeth and periodontium?

9. Does the presence of this soft tissue lesion prevent the provision of periodontal debridement?

10. What should a hygienist (or dentist) communicate to the patient and nursing staff?

CASE 37. (FIG. 67.10)

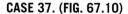

This 29-year-old man comes to your dental office for routine dental work. He has no dental symptoms and does not have a fever. The lesion does not rub off. He claims to have multiple sexual partners.

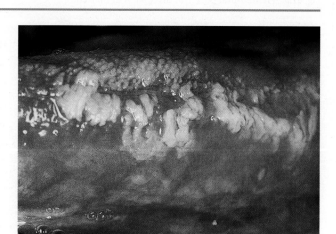

1. Describe the clinical findings. Include normal and abnormal findings.

2. What information should the dental hygienist elicit from the patient?

3. Is this a normal finding, a variant of normal, disorder, or disease?

4. What conditions should you consider in the differential diagnosis?

5. This condition is more common in:
   A. HIV-seronegative men
   B. HIV-seropositive men
   C. HIV-seropositive women
   D. HIV-seronegative women

6. True or false: This condition can occur in persons who take immunosuppressive drugs for organ transplantation.

7. True or false: This condition is limited to the tongue.

8. Why is it significant that the lesion cannot be rubbed off?

9. What should the dentist communicate to the patient?

Additional cases to enhance your learning and understanding of this section are available Online through the book's Navigate 2 Advantage Access site.

Intraoral Findings by Color Changes

Objectives

- Define and use diagnostic terms that describe white, red, and pigmented lesions of the oral mucosa.
- In the clinical setting, document the characteristics of white, red, and pigmented lesions of the oral mucosa in terms of anatomic location, color, border, and configuration.
- Recognize the causes and clinical features of white, red, and pigmented lesions of the oral mucosa.
- Use the diagnostic process to distinguish similar-appearing white, red, and pigmented lesions of the oral mucosa.
- Recommend appropriate treatment options for white, red, and pigmented lesions of the oral mucosa.
- Identify conditions discussed in this section that would (1) require the attention of the dentist, (2) affect the delivery of noninvasive and invasive dental procedures, or (3) need to be further evaluated by a specialist.

In the figure legends, *‡ denotes the same patient.

Fordyce Granules (Figs. 68.1 and 68.2) are sebaceous glands found within the oral mucosa. Technically speaking, they are sebaceous choristomas (i.e., normal tissue in an abnormal location); their normal location is within the upper layer of the dermis (skin). These asymptomatic granules consist of individual sebaceous glands that are 1 to 2 mm in diameter. Characteristically, they appear as white, creamy white, or yellow slightly raised papules on the posterior buccal mucosa and vermilion of the upper lip. They usually occur in multiples, forming discrete clusters, plaques, or patches. Enlarged clusters may feel rough to palpation and to the patient's tongue. They are sometimes an isolated finding. Less common locations include the labial mucosa, retromolar pad, attached gingiva, tongue, and frenum.

Fordyce granules arise from sebaceous glands embryologically entrapped during fusion of the maxillary and mandibular processes. They become more apparent after sexual maturity as the sebaceous system develops. Rarely, an intraoral hair may be seen in association with the condition.

Fordyce granules occur in approximately 80% of adults, and no race or sex predilection has been reported. However, the density of granules per mucosal area is greater in men than in women. Histologic examination shows rounded nests of clear cells, 10 to 30 per nest, in the lamina propria and submucosa. These cells have darkly staining, small, centrally located nuclei. The clinical appearance is adequate for diagnosis of Fordyce granules. Biopsy is not usually required.

Linea Alba (Figs. 68.3 and 68.4) translates from Latin to mean "white line." This common intraoral finding appears as a raised white wavy line of variable length and prominence. It is located at the level of the occlusion on the buccal mucosa. Generally, the linea alba is asymptomatic, 1 to 2 mm wide, and extends horizontally from the second molar to the canine region of the buccal mucosa, ending at the caliculus angularis (Fig. 1.3). The lesion is most often found bilaterally and cannot be rubbed off. It develops in response to frictional activity of the teeth, which results in thickened (hyperkeratotic) epithelial changes. The condition is often associated with crenated tongue and may be a sign of pressure, bruxism, clenching, or sucking trauma. The clinical appearance is diagnostic. No treatment is required.

Leukoedema (Figs. 68.5 and 68.6) is an opalescent, milky-white, or gray surface change of the buccal mucosa. This common mucosal variant is associated with dark-pigmented persons but may be seen infrequently in lighter-pigmented persons. The incidence of leukoedema tends to increase with age, and 50% of African American children and 92% of African American adults are affected. The labial mucosa, soft palate, and floor of the mouth are less common locations of occurrence.

Clinically, leukoedema is usually faint and bilateral. Close examination of leukoedema reveals fine white lines and wrinkles. Exaggerated and long-standing cases have overlapping folds of tissue. Prominence of the lesion is related to the degree of underlying melanin pigmentation, level of oral hygiene, and amount of smoking or use of strong oral rinses. The borders of the lesion are wavy and diffuse; they fade into adjacent tissue, which makes it difficult to determine where the lesion begins and ends. The condition is diagnosed by stretching the mucosa, which causes the white appearance to significantly diminish or disappear. Wiping the lesion fails to remove it. The cause of leukoedema is unknown, although it is more severe in smokers and diminishes with smoking cessation. Histologic examination of biopsy specimens shows increased epithelial thickness with prominent intracellular edema of the spinous (middle) layer without evidence of inflammation. No serious complications are associated with this lesion, and no treatment is required.

Morsicatio Buccarum (Figs. 68.7 and 68.8) is derived from the Latin word *morsus* (bite) and is the term used to describe the changes in the oral mucosa that are due to cheek biting or cheek chewing. Morsicatio buccarum is a common nervous habit that produces a progression of mucosal changes. Initially, slightly raised irregular white plaques appear in a diffuse pattern that cover areas of trauma. Increased injury produces a hyperplastic response that increases the size of the plaque. A linear or striated pattern is sometimes observed that contains thick corrugated areas and intervening zones of erythema. Persistent injury leads to an enlarging plaque with irregular zones of traumatic erythema and ulceration.

Chewing of the oral mucosa is usually seen on the anterior buccal mucosa and less frequently on the labial mucosa. The lesions may be unilateral or bilateral and can occur at any age. No sex or race predilection has been reported. Diagnosis requires visual or verbal confirmation of the nervous habit. Although morsicatio buccarum has no malignant potential, patients should be advised of the mucosal alterations. Because of the similar clinical appearance, speckled leukoplakia and candidiasis should be ruled out. Microscopic examination of biopsied tissue shows a normal maturing epithelial surface with a corrugated and thickened parakeratotic surface and minor subepithelial inflammation.

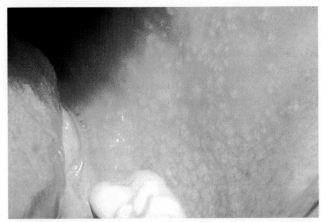
Fig. 68.1. Fordyce granules: clustered in buccal mucosa.

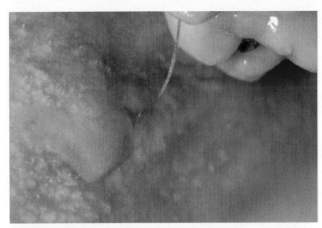
Fig. 68.2. Fordyce granules: with rare intraoral hair.

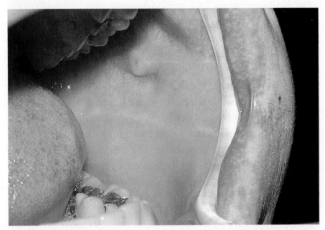
Fig. 68.3. Linea alba: on buccal mucosa.

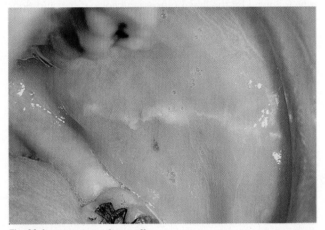
Fig. 68.4. Prominent linea alba.

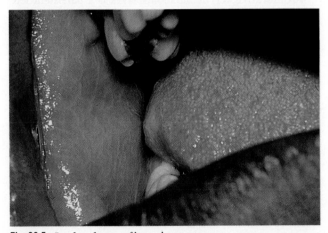
Fig. 68.5. Leukoedema: of buccal mucosa.

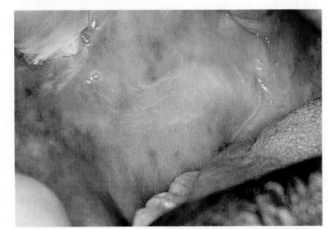
Fig. 68.6. Leukoedema: prominent in a smoker.

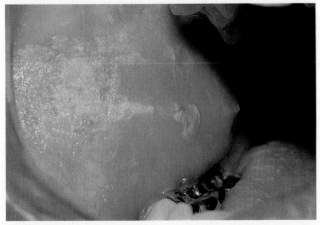
Fig. 68.7. Morsicatio buccarum: caused by cheek biting.

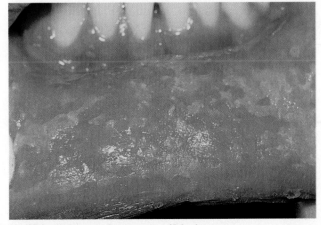
Fig. 68.8. Morsicatio buccarum: of labial mucosa.

153

WHITE LESIONS

White Sponge Nevus (Familial White Folded Dysplasia) (Figs. 69.1 and 69.2) is an inherited condition characterized by the appearance of asymptomatic, white, folded, spongy plaques. The lesions exhibit a symmetric wavy pattern. This condition is a relatively rare genodermatosis caused by point mutations in genes that regulate keratin 4 and keratin 13 production. As a result, epithelial maturation and exfoliation are altered. **White sponge nevus** appears at birth or early childhood, persists throughout life, and exhibits no race or sex predilection. Because it has an autosomal dominant pattern of transmission, several family members are typically affected.

The most common location is the buccal mucosa bilaterally, followed by the labial mucosa, alveolar ridge, and floor of the mouth. It may involve the entire oral mucosa or be distributed unilaterally as discrete white patches. The gingival margin and dorsal tongue are almost never affected, although the soft palate and ventrolateral tongue are commonly involved. The size of the lesions varies. Extraoral mucosal sites may involve the nasal cavity, esophagus, larynx, vagina, and rectum. The oral features are remarkably similar to those of **hereditary benign intraepithelial dyskeratosis**. However, eye involvement occurs with the latter. Microscopically, white sponge nevus shows prominent parakeratosis, thickening and clearing of the spinous layer, and perinuclear tangles of keratin tonofilaments. No treatment is required.

Traumatic White Lesions (Figs. 69.3 to 69.5) are caused by many physical and chemical irritants, such as frictional trauma, heat, topical use of aspirin, excessive use of mouthwash, caustic liquids, and even toothpastes. Frictional trauma is often noted on the attached gingiva. It is caused by excessive toothbrushing, movement of oral prostheses, and chewing on the edentulous ridge. With time, the mucosa becomes thickened and develops a roughened white surface that does not wipe off. Pain is absent. Histologic examination reveals hyperkeratosis.

Acute trauma can produce a white peeling or corrugated lesion if superficial layers of mucosa are damaged. Lesions usually appear as white patches with diffuse irregular borders. Underneath is a raw, red, or bleeding surface. Moveable mucosa is more susceptible to trauma than is attached mucosa. Pain relief and healing occur within days of removing the cause.

Another white lesion caused by trauma is a **scar**. It represents a fibrous healing response of the dermis. Scars are often asymptomatic, linear, whitish pink, and sharply delineated. A thorough history may reveal previous injury, recurrent ulcerative disease, seizure disorder, or previous surgery.

Leukoplakia (Figs. 69.6 to 69.8) is a clinical term for a white plaque or patch that cannot be rubbed off, cannot be classified clinicopathologically as any other disease, and cannot be attributed to a specific cause. Persons of any age may be affected, but the majority of cases occur in men between the ages of 45 and 65 years.

Leukoplakias are protective reactions against chronic irritants. Areca nut (betel), tobacco, alcohol, syphilis, vitamin deficiency, galvanism, ultraviolet radiation, immunosuppression, and candidiasis are strongly associated with these lesions. Leukoplakias vary considerably in size, location, and clinical appearance. Preferential sites are the lateral and ventral tongue, floor of the mouth, alveolar mucosa, lip, soft palate-retromolar trigone, and mandibular attached gingiva. The surface may appear smooth and homogeneous, thin and friable, fissured, corrugated, verrucoid, nodular, or speckled. Lesions can vary in color, from faintly translucent white, gray, to brown-white.

A classification system offered by the World Health Organization recommends two divisions for oral leukoplakias: **homogeneous** and **nonhomogeneous**. Homogeneous leukoplakias are uniform white lesions with a smooth, wrinkled, or corrugated surface. Nonhomogeneous leukoplakias are subdivided into **erythroleukoplakia** (white lesion with large red component), **nodular** (white lesion with raised and pebbly surface), **speckled** (white lesion with small red components), and **verrucoid** (white lesion with raised corrugated surface).

Most leukoplakias (80%) are benign; the rest are dysplastic (premalignant) or cancerous. The clinical challenge lies in determining which are premalignant or malignant, because up to 16% of leukoplakias progress to carcinoma within 25 years. High-risk sites of malignant transformation include the floor of the mouth, lateral and ventral tongue, uvulopalatal complex, and lips.

Proliferative verrucous leukoplakia is a persistent leukoplakia with a verrucoid (wartlike) appearance and a high risk for malignant transformation (Fig. 69.8). It is an unusual leukoplakia because it has a strong female predilection, an infrequent association with smoking, and an occasional association with human papillomavirus infection. It occurs at any adult age but most commonly after age 60. Lesions are multifocal and have a white, corrugated, or pebbly exophytic surface (pebbly outgrowths or wartlike outgrowths). Lesions spread slowly, rarely regress, and tend to recur after excision. About 70% of these leukoplakias developed into carcinoma.

Leukoplakias with localized red areas confer a high risk for carcinoma. Evidence indicates that nonhomogeneous leukoplakias, particularly oral **speckled leukoplakias**, represent epithelial dysplasia in 90% of the cases and have the highest rate of malignant transformation among intraoral leukoplakias. *Candida albicans*, often associated with oral speckled leukoplakias, may have a role in the dysplastic changes seen.

The initial step in the treatment of leukoplakia is to eliminate any irritating and causative factors and then observe for healing. Unexplained persistent oral leukoplakias must be biopsied. Several biopsy sites may be necessary for diffuse or multifocal lesions. Nonhomogeneous or reddish areas of the lesion should always be selected for biopsy because they are associated with a higher risk for dysplasia and malignant transformation. If dysplasia or cancer is diagnosed, complete surgical removal is recommended.

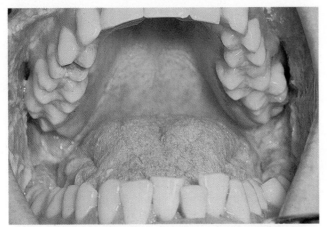

Fig. 69.1. **White sponge nevus:** buccal mucosa, soft palate.*

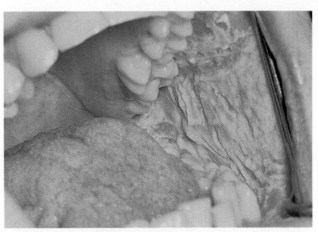

Fig. 69.2. **White sponge nevus:** of buccal mucosa.*

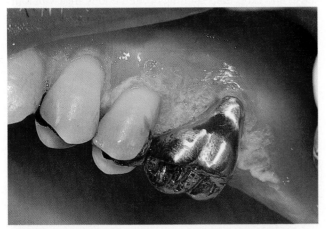

Fig. 69.3. **Traumatic white lesion:** toothbrushing associated.

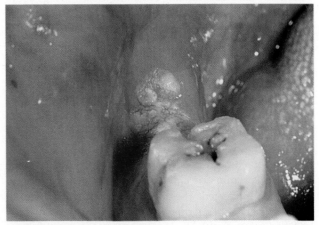

Fig. 69.4. **Traumatic white lesion:** frictional keratosis.

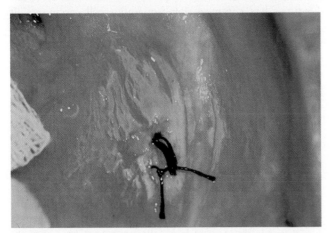

Fig. 69.5. **Traumatic white lesion:** burn from topical aspirin.

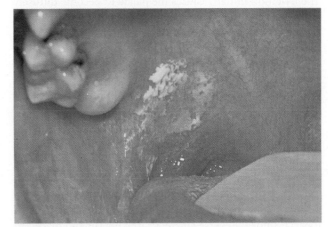

Fig. 69.6. **Leukoplakia:** hyperkeratosis of soft palate.

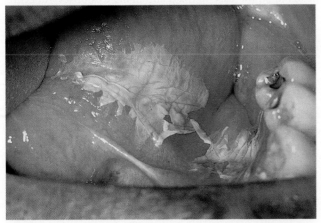

Fig. 69.7. **Leukoplakia:** of floor of the mouth and ventral tongue.

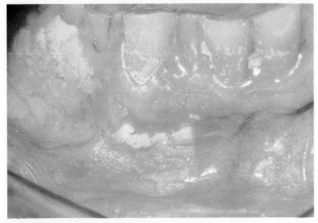

Fig. 69.8. **Proliferative verrucous leukoplakia:** spreading.

155

TOBACCO-ASSOCIATED WHITE LESIONS

Cigarette Keratosis (Figs. 70.1 and 70.2) Keratosis is a condition characterized by thickened patches on the skin. **Cigarette keratosis** is a specific reaction evident in persons who smoke nonfiltered or marijuana cigarettes to a very short length. The lesions, which approximate each other on lip closure, involve the upper and lower lips at the location of cigarette placement. These keratotic patches are about 7 mm in diameter and are located invariably lateral to the midline. Raised white papules are evident throughout the patch, producing a roughened texture and firmness to palpation. Cigarette keratoses may extend onto the labial mucosa, but the vermilion border is rarely involved. Elderly men are most commonly affected. Smoking cessation usually brings about resolution. Development of an ulcer or crust should raise suspicion of neoplastic transformation.

Nicotine Stomatitis (Smoker's Palate) (Figs. 70.3 and 70.4) is a direct response of the oral mucosa to prolonged pipe and cigar smoking. Its severity is correlated with the intensity and duration of smoke exposure. It is usually found in middle-aged and elderly men, in unprotected palatal regions (not covered by a maxillary denture) that contain minor salivary glands, that is, posterior to the palatal rugae, on the soft palate, and sometimes extending onto the buccal mucosa. The condition is symmetric and painless. Rarely, the dorsum of the tongue is affected. These tobacco-associated changes of the tongue have been termed **glossitis stomatitis nicotina**.

Nicotine stomatitis shows progressive changes with time. The irritation initially causes the palate to become diffusely erythematous. The palate eventually becomes grayish-white secondary to hyperkeratosis. Multiple discrete keratotic papules with depressed red centers develop that correspond to dilated and inflamed excretory duct openings of the minor salivary glands. The papules enlarge as the irritation persists but fail to coalesce, producing a characteristic cobblestone (parboiled) appearance of the palate. Isolated but prominent red-centered papules are common. Brown staining of the lingual surface of the posterior teeth accompanies this condition. Whether nicotine stomatitis arises as a consequence of heat or tobacco is a matter of debate. However, the lack of malignant progression suggests that the heat may be more contributory to the lesion than the chemicals in tobacco smoke. Reverse cigarette smoking (lit end placed in the mouth—common to persons from India) produces similar findings. Smoking cessation usually results in regression. Biopsy is rarely needed to confirm the diagnosis.

Snuff Dipper's Patch (Tobacco Chewer's Lesion, Snuff Keratosis) (Figs. 70.5 and 70.6) A wrinkled yellow-white area in the mucobuccal fold—or mandibular buccal or labial mucosa—suggests persistent intraoral use of unburned tobacco. The hard palate, floor of the mouth, and ventral tongue may also be affected if tobacco is placed in the maxillary vestibule or beneath the tongue. Smokeless tobacco is marketed in various forms (snuff, dip, plug, or quid) and leaves its characteristic mark at the preferential site of tobacco placement. Posterior sites are commonly used for dip, plug, or quid, whereas anterior sites are preferred for snuff. Persons who vary placement of the tobacco have multiple, less prominent oral lesions. Male teenagers are most frequently affected, largely because of intensive marketing and peer and sports associations. Higher prevalence is found in southern and Appalachian states.

Early **snuff dipper's patches** are pale pink keratoses with corrugated or wrinkled surfaces. The color may progress from white and yellow-white to yellow-brown as hyperkeratosis and exogenous staining occur. Lesions are asymptomatic and often at least 1 cm in diameter.

Long-term use of smokeless tobacco is associated with tooth abrasion, periodontal recession, caries, epidermal dysplastic changes, and possibly carcinoma. The dysplastic changes, which take many years to develop, are associated with the carcinogenic nitrosamines present in the tobacco. To achieve resolution, cessation of use is recommended. If normal appearance does not return 14 days after cessation, biopsy is necessary.

Verrucous Carcinoma (of Ackerman) (Figs. 70.7 and 70.8) appears as a warty, exophytic, white-and-red mass that is firm to palpation. Some would describe it as cauliflower-like or papulonodular tumor. It is a low-grade, nonmetastasizing, variant malignant squamous cell carcinoma and is 25 times less common than squamous cell carcinoma. It most frequently arises in association with long-term tobacco use, especially smokeless tobacco at the site of chronic placement. About 30% of **verrucous carcinomas** are associated with human papillomavirus infection.

The buccal mucosa, vestibule, mandibular gingiva, and palate are the most common oral sites of verrucous carcinoma. Men older than 60 years who have used smokeless tobacco for many years are most often affected. The disease is rare in persons younger than 40 years and in persons who do not use tobacco. Nonoral sites can also be affected.

Verrucous carcinoma has a distinctive surface appearance. A characteristic feature is a white-gray, undulating keratotic surface with pink-red pebbly papules throughout. Lateral growth, which usually exceeds vertical growth, leads to an increase in mass and diameters of several centimeters. Large lesions can be locally destructive by invading and eroding the underlying alveolar bone. Similar-appearing lesions include verrucous epithelial hyperplasia, pyostomatitis vegetans, and proliferative verrucous leukoplakia.

Recommended treatment for verrucous carcinoma is wide surgical excision. After surgery, the long-term prognosis of affected patients is better than squamous cell carcinoma and improves when the use of smokeless tobacco is discontinued.

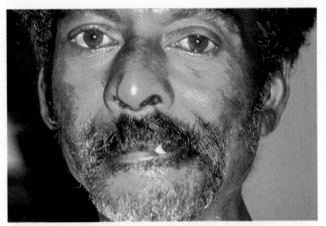

Fig. 70.1. Cigarette keratosis: user of unfiltered cigarettes.*

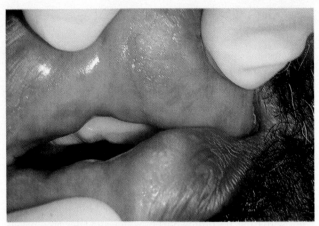

Fig. 70.2. Cigarette keratosis: on labial mucosa.*

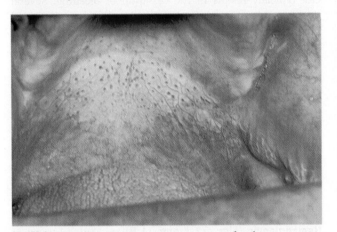

Fig. 70.3. Nicotine stomatitis: prominent on soft palate.

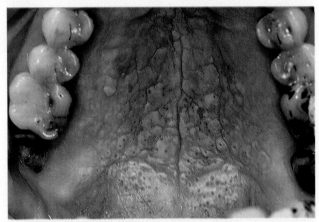

Fig. 70.4. Nicotine stomatitis: in a reverse smoker.

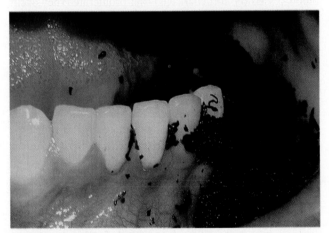

Fig. 70.5. Snuff dipper's patch: under chewing tobacco.

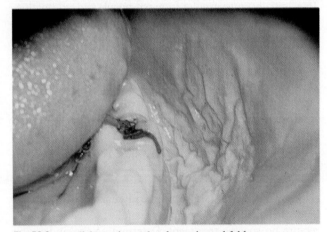

Fig. 70.6. Snuff dipper's patch: of mucobuccal fold.

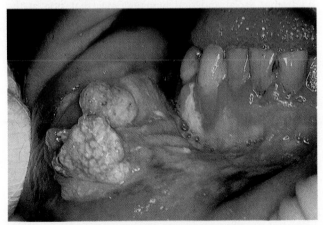

Fig. 70.7. Verrucous carcinoma: of the labial mucosa.

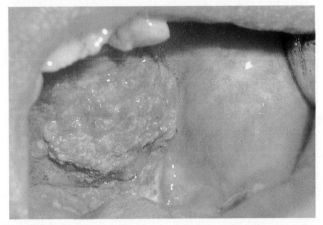

Fig. 70.8. Verrucous carcinoma: maxillary alveolar ridge.

9

Many lesions appear red because they have a vascular component. This section discusses red lesions associated with abnormalities of blood vessels and blood.

Purpura (Figs. 71.1 to 71.4) are demarcated red-purple discolorations produced by bleeding underneath the surface of the skin. They are caused by an underlying abnormality, such as a platelet or clotting disorder, capillary fragility, or infection. **Purpura** are classified by size as petechiae (less than 3 mm), purpura (3 mm to 1 cm), and ecchymoses (greater than 1 cm). Purpura initially appears bright red but tends to discolor with time, becoming purplish-blue and later brown-yellow. Because these lesions consist of extravasated blood, they do not blanch on diascopy (pressure with a glass slide).

Petechiae are pinpoint, nonraised, circular red spots. The soft palate is the most common intraoral location for multifocal petechiae. Palatal petechiae may represent an early sign of viral infection (infectious mononucleosis), scarlet fever, leukemia, platelet disorder, or coagulation disorder. They may also indicate rupture of palatal capillaries caused by coughing, sneezing, vomiting, or fellatio. Suction petechiae under a maxillary denture are not true purpura. They result from candidal infection and the resulting inflammation of the orifices of accessory salivary glands, not because of denture-created negative pressure as previously believed.

Purpura are bigger than petechiae, but smaller than an ecchymosis. **Ecchymosis** (common bruise) is an area of extravasated blood usually greater than 1 cm in diameter. They initially range in color from red-purple and fade to blue-green-brown (i.e., days later). Careful physical evaluation may reveal the cause to be trauma, hemostatic disorders, Cushing disease, amyloidosis, neoplastic disease, primary idiopathic or secondary thrombocytopenic purpura, or use of anticoagulant drugs such as aspirin, warfarin (Coumadin), heparin, direct thrombin inhibitors, or activated factor X inhibitors.

Hematomas (large bruise) are large pools of extravasated blood resulting from trauma that results in a palpable mass. They occur commonly in the oral cavity as a result of a blow to the face, tooth eruption, or damage to the posterior superior alveolar vein during administration of local anesthesia (Figs. 67.3 and 67.4). They are usually dark red-brown and tender to palpation. Hematomas generally fade with time and require no specific treatment. Determining the underlying cause of purpura and hematomas is the prime consideration.

Varicosity (Varix) (Fig. 71.5) A **varix** is a dilated vein frequently seen in elderly persons. The swelling is caused by reduced elasticity of the vascular wall as a result of aging or by an internal blockage of the vein. The ventrolateral surface of the anterior two thirds of the tongue is a common location. The floor of the mouth, lip, and labial commissure are other common sites. Varices appear dark red to blue-purple. They are usually single, round, dome shaped, and fluctuant. Palpation of the lesion disperses the blood from the vessel and causes the area to blanch. Thus, the lesions are diascopy positive.

Varices are benign and asymptomatic and require no treatment. If they are of cosmetic concern, varices can be surgically removed without significant bleeding. Varices are sometimes slightly firm because of fibrotic changes. Thrombosis is a rare complication that produces a firm nodule within the varix. When several veins on the ventral tongue are prominent, the condition is called **phlebectasia linguae**, or caviar tongue.

Thrombus (Fig. 71.6) is the formation of a blood clot in a blood vessel. The series of events that includes trauma, activation of the clotting sequence, and formation of a blood clot typically results in the cessation of bleeding. Several days later, plasminogen initiates clot breakdown, and normal blood flow resumes. In certain cases, if the clot does not dissolve, blood flow stagnates and a **thrombus** is formed.

Intraoral thrombi appear as raised red-brown or blue round nodules, typically in the labial mucosa. They are firm to palpation and may be slightly tender. No sexual predilection is evident, but thrombi are most commonly seen in patients older than 45 years. Thrombi concentrically enlarge to occlude the entire lumen of the vessel or mature and *calcify* to form a **phlebolith**. Phleboliths are rare oral findings that develop in the cheek, lips, or tongue. Radiographs show phleboliths to be doughnutlike, circular, radiopaque foci with a radiolucent center.

Hemangiomas (Figs. 71.7 and 71.8) are benign tumors of blood vessels (endothelial cells) that proliferate. They occur early in life, more commonly in women than in men, and develop in any soft tissue or bony intraoral location. They are divided into two forms: **capillary** (consisting of small fine vessels) or **cavernous** (consisting of large thin-walled vascular spaces).

Soft tissue hemangiomas occur commonly in the dorsum of the tongue, gingiva, and buccal mucosa. When situated deep within the connective tissue, they do not alter the color of the mucosal surface. Superficial hemangiomas, in contrast, are red, blue, or purple; flat or slightly elevated; smooth-surfaced; and somewhat firm. Hemangiomas are positive to diascopy and may vary in size from a few millimeters to several centimeters. The borders are usually diffuse. Lobular surfaces are infrequent. Single hemangiomas are most common, whereas multiple lesions are seen in Maffucci syndrome. Facial and oral hemangiomas that stop at the midline form a characteristic component of **Sturge-Weber syndrome**.

Congenital hemangiomas typically involute. Surgical excision, sclerosing agents, cryotherapy, and radiation therapy have been used to eliminate large and persistent lesions. The differential diagnosis should include its malignant counterpart (hemangioendothelioma) and Kaposi sarcoma (Fig. 93.7), the latter being a malignant vascular tumor associated with immune suppression (HIV), aging, and human herpesvirus 8 infection.

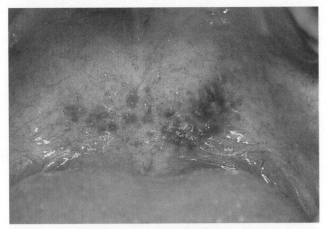

Fig. 71.1. Petechiae: caused by viral illness and coughing.

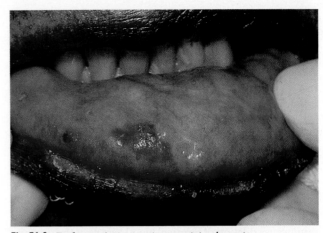

Fig. 71.2. Ecchymosis: in a patient receiving heparin.

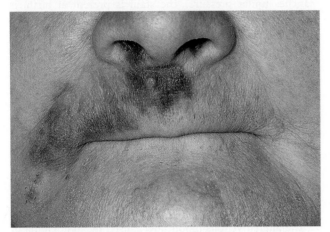

Fig. 71.3. Hematoma: after trauma from falling.*

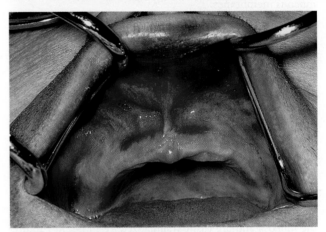

Fig. 71.4. Hematoma: of maxillary mucosa and gingiva.*

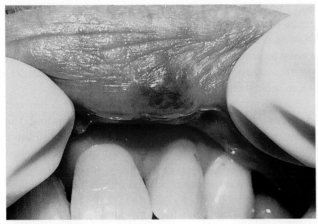

Fig. 71.5. Varix: diascopy positive.

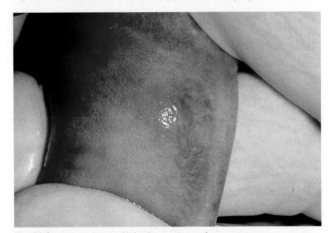

Fig. 71.6. Thrombus: of labial mucosa within a varix.

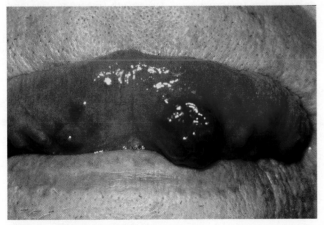

Fig. 71.7. Hemangioma: of ventral tongue.

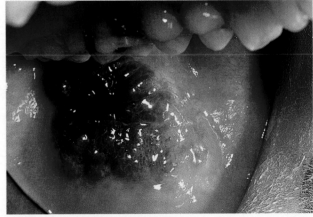

Fig. 71.8. Hemangioma: of buccal mucosa.

RED LESIONS

Hereditary Hemorrhagic Telangiectasia (Rendu-Osler-Weber Syndrome) (Figs. 72.1–72.4) is a genetic disorder that causes abnormalities of blood vessels such that some arteries flow directly into veins rather than into capillaries. These abnormalities are known as *arteriovenous malformations*. This disease is autosomal dominant and has three forms (types 1, 2, and 3) involving mutations in the ACVRL1, endoglin (ENG), and SMAD4 genes, respectively; each codes for proteins involved in the transforming growth factor-beta (TGF-β)–signaling pathway that regulates the lining and integrity of blood vessel walls. The defects that result cause dilation of terminal blood vessels of the skin and mucous membranes.

Hereditary hemorrhagic telangiectasia is characterized by numerous telangiectasias, which appear as red-purple macules of the skin, mucosa, and other tissues and organs. The lesions are usually 1 to 3 mm, lack central pulsation, and blanch on diascopy. The telangiectasias begin early in life. After puberty, the size and number of lesions tend to increase with age. Men and women are affected equally. Bleeding, such as bleeding from the nose (epistaxis), is a prominent and early feature of this disease.

History, clinical appearance, and histologic features are important in making the diagnosis of hereditary hemorrhagic telangiectasia, as the disease is asymptomatic in many victims. Clinically evident lesions are located immediately subjacent to the mucosa and are easily traumatized, resulting in rupture, hemorrhage, and ulcer formation. Skin lesions are less subject to rupture because of the overlying cornified epithelium. The most common locations on the skin are the palms, fingers, nail beds, face, and neck. Mucosal lesions can be found on the lips, tongue, nasal septum, and conjunctivae. The gingiva and the hard palate are less commonly involved. Vascular malformations also involve the lung, brain, and gastrointestinal tract, especially the liver. Complications are associated with bleeding at various sites, including epistaxis from drying or irritation of involved nasal mucosa or from nasotracheal intubation; gastrointestinal bleeding, melena, and iron deficiency anemia caused by rupture of telangiectasias of the gastrointestinal mucosa and prolonged bleeding; and hematuria caused by rupture of telangiectasia within the urinary tract. Other complications include cirrhosis of the liver, pulmonary arteriovenous fistulae leading to pulmonary hypertension, and brain abscesses and emboli. Precautions are recommended with the use of inhalation analgesia, general anesthesia, oral surgical procedures, and hepatotoxic and antihemostatic drugs. Rupture of a telangiectasia may cause hemorrhage that is best controlled by pressure packs. In patients who have pulmonary arteriovenous malformations, antibiotic prophylaxis before invasive dental treatment is recommended because of risk of cerebral abscess. Identification of this disorder warrants screening of family members by a physician.

Sturge-Weber Angiomatosis (Sturge-Weber or Encephalotrigeminal Syndrome) (Figs. 72.5–72.8) is a rare, nonhereditary disorder present at birth characterized by a port-wine birthmark and neurological abnormalities. The syndrome results from the persistence of a vascular plexus and produces four prominent features: (1) venous angiomas of the leptomeninges of the brain, (2) a port-wine stain of the face, (3) neuromuscular deficits, and (4) oculo-oral lesions.

The **port-wine stain** or nevus flammeus, a macular hemangioma, is the most striking feature of the syndrome. The facial hemangioma is well demarcated, flat or slightly raised, usually unilateral, and red to purple in color. It blanches under pressure. The stain is present at birth, is distributed along one or several branches of the trigeminal nerve, and typically extends to the patient's midline without crossing to the other side. The ophthalmic division of the trigeminal nerve is most frequently affected. No tenderness or inflammation is associated with the hemangioma, and it does not enlarge with age. In many patients with solitary congenital port-wine angiomas of the face, lesions regress spontaneously at puberty. Approximately 20% of persons with facial port-wine stains have Sturge-Weber angiomatosis. The remainder are free of the other features of the syndrome. Involvement of the ophthalmic branch of the trigeminal nerve appears to be most predictive of full involvement of the syndrome.

The altered venous blood flow caused by an angioma of the leptomeninges usually affects only one side of the brain and can result in degeneration of the cerebral cortex, seizures, mental retardation, and hemiplegia. On lateral skull radiographs, gyriform calcifications characteristically appear as double-contoured "tramlines." Approximately 30% of patients have ocular abnormalities, including angiomas, colobomas, or glaucoma.

Vascular hyperplasia involving the buccal mucosa and lips, only on one side, is the most frequent oral finding. The palate, gingiva, and floor of the mouth may also be affected. The bright red oral patches are located on areas supplied by the branches of the trigeminal nerve. Like facial lesions, these patches stop abruptly at the midline. Involvement of the gingiva may produce edematous tissue and cause difficulty with hemostasis when surgical procedures involving these tissues are performed. Abnormal tooth eruption, enlarged lips (macrocheilia), large teeth (macrodontia), and enlarged tongue (macroglossia) are sequelae of the vascular overgrowths. Gingival overgrowth may result from phenytoin therapy, which is given because these patients are subject to seizures. Careful assessment of the enlarged gingiva on the ipsilateral side, including biopsy, may be required to establish vascular involvement or drug-induced gingival overgrowth. In areas of vascular hyperplasia, oral surgery should be performed in accordance with strict hemostatic measures.

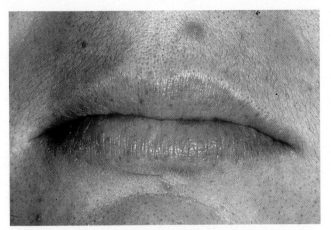
Fig. 72.1. Hereditary hemorrhagic telangiectasia: lips.*

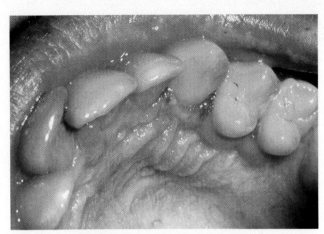
Fig. 72.2. Hereditary hemorrhagic telangiectasia: gingivae.*

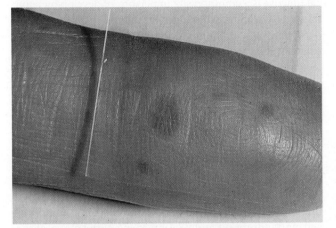
Fig. 72.3. Hereditary hemorrhagic telangiectasia.

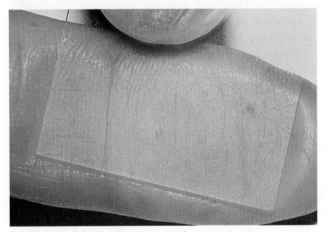
Fig. 72.4. Hereditary telangiectasia: diascopy positive.

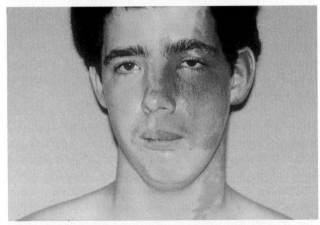
Fig. 72.5. Sturge-Weber angiomatosis.‡ port-wine stain.

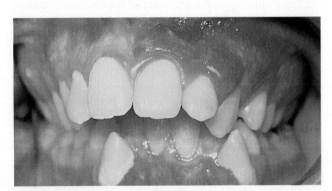
Fig. 72.6. Sturge-Weber angiomatosis.‡ oral involvement.

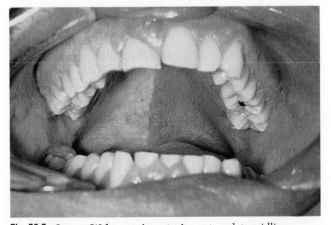
Fig. 72.7. Sturge-Weber angiomatosis:** up to palate midline.

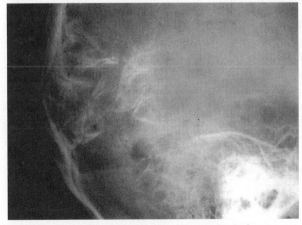
Fig. 72.8. Sturge-Weber angiomatosis:** cranial calcifications.

Erythroplakia (Figs. 73.1–73.4) is defined as a persistent red patch that cannot be characterized clinically as any other condition. Like leukoplakia, the term has no histologic connotation. However, unlike leukoplakia, most **erythroplakias** are histologically diagnosed as epithelial dysplasia or worse and have a much higher propensity for progression to carcinoma. Erythroplakias are most prevalent in the mandibular mucobuccal fold, oropharynx, tongue, and floor of the mouth and are often associated with tobacco or alcohol use. They are usually painless and appear as flat and velvety patches but can be speckled with white areas. The redness of the lesion is a result of atrophic mucosa overlying a highly vascular (reddish) and inflamed submucosa. The border is often well demarcated. There is no sex predilection, and patients older than 55 years are most commonly affected.

Three clinical variants of erythroplakia are recognized: (1) the **homogeneous** form, which is completely red; (2) **erythroleukoplakia**, which mainly has red patches interspersed with occasional white areas; and (3) **speckled erythroplakia**, which contains white specks or granules scattered throughout the red lesion. Biopsy is mandatory for all types of erythroplakia because 91% represent severe dysplasia, carcinoma in situ, or invasive squamous cell carcinoma. Inspection of the entire oral cavity is required because 10% to 20% of these patients have several erythroplakic areas, a phenomenon known as **field cancerization**.

Erythroleukoplakia and Speckled Erythroplakia (Fig. 73.5) are precancerous red and white lesions. Both are usually asymptomatic. Erythroleukoplakia and speckled erythroplakia (also called speckled leukoplakia) have a male predilection, and most are detected in patients older than 50 years. They may occur at any intraoral site but frequently affect the lateral border of the tongue, buccal mucosa, and soft palate. Lesions are often associated with heavy smoking, alcoholism, and poor oral hygiene.

Fungal infections are common in speckled erythroplakias. *Candida albicans*, the predominant organism, has been isolated in most cases. Thus, management of these lesions should include analysis for candida. The cause-and-effect relationship between candidiasis and speckled leukoplakia is unknown, but erythroplakia with leukoplakic regions confers a high risk for atypical cytologic changes and progression to carcinoma.

Squamous Cell Carcinoma (Figs. 73.6–73.8) is an invasive malignancy of oral epithelium. It is the most common type of oral cancer, accounting for more than 90% of all malignant neoplasms of the oral cavity. Oral cancer may occur at any age, but it is primarily a disease of the elderly. Recent studies demonstrate that 90% of oral cancers occur in persons older than 45 years and the prevalence is higher in men than women (2.6:1).

The exact cause of oral squamous cell carcinoma is unknown but appears to involve mutations of genes on chromosomes 3 and 9 (*p53*, *ras*) that regulate cell proliferation and death (apoptosis). Cytological changes occur with excessive use of tobacco, areca nut, and alcohol and can be influenced by infection with human papillomavirus, *Treponema pallidum*, or *C. albicans*. Other contributory factors are those associated with aging, immune compromise, poor nutrition, iron deficiency, oral neglect, chronic trauma, and ultraviolet radiation.

In the United States, the most common site of intraoral squamous cell carcinoma is the lateral border and ventral surface of the tongue, followed by the oropharynx, floor of the mouth, gingiva, buccal mucosa, lip, and palate. The buccal mucosa is a common site in persons of developing countries who chronically use quid (areca/betel nut) tobacco. The occurrence of carcinoma of the lip has decreased dramatically in the past decade because of the increased use of protective sunscreen agents. The dorsal surface of the tongue is almost never affected.

The appearance of squamous cell carcinoma is variable; more than 90% of cases are erythroplakic, and about 60% have a leukoplakic component. A combination of colors and surface patterns—such as a red and white lesion that is exophytic, infiltrative, or ulcerated—indicates instability of the oral epithelium and is highly suggestive of carcinoma. Early lesions are often asymptomatic and slow growing. As the lesion develops, the borders become diffuse and ragged, and induration and fixation ensue. If the mucosal surface becomes ulcerated, the most frequent oral symptom is that of a persistent sore or irritation that fails to heal. Advancing disease can cause numbness, mobile teeth, swelling, or difficulty in speaking or swallowing. Lesions can extend to several centimeters in diameter if treatment is delayed. This delay permits lesions to invade and destroy vital tissues.

Squamous cell carcinoma spreads by local extension or by way of lymphatic vessels. Affected patients may have palpable regional (submandibular or anterior cervical) lymph nodes. These nodes can be large, firm, rubbery, and possibly fixed to underlying tissue. Staging of the tumor according to the TNM system—**size (T)**, **regional lymph nodes (N)**, and **distant metastases (M)**—allows assessment of the extent of disease. Surgery and radiation therapy are the principal forms of treatment. In advance disease, cetuximab plus chemotherapy can help to improve overall survival. The prognosis for oral cancer depends, in large measure, on the site involved (posterior tumors having worse prognosis), the clinical stage at the time of diagnosis and treatment, tumor diameter, the patient's access to adequate health care, treatment provided, and the patient's ability to cope and mount an immunologic response. Because early treatment is paramount, biopsy should be done if neoplasia is suspected. Unfortunately, the majority of tumors are not localized at the time of diagnosis. Use of vital stains and new imaging devices can help in early recognition and speed the diagnostic process.

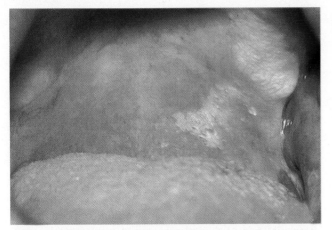

Fig. 73.1. **Erythroplakia:** seen after tongue was depressed.*

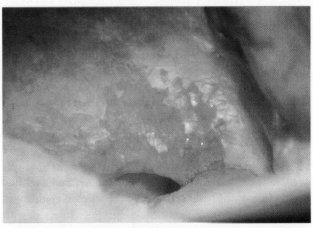

Fig. 73.2. **Erythroplakia:** on soft palate; tongue depressed.*

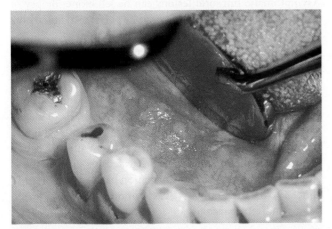

Fig. 73.3. **Erythroplakia:** of floor of the mouth.

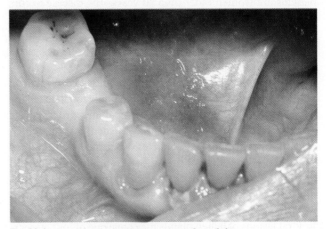

Fig. 73.4. **Carcinoma appearing as erythroplakia.**

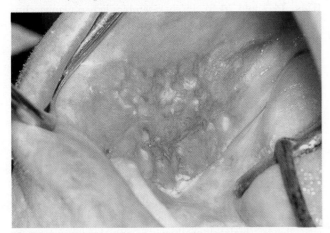

Fig. 73.5. **Erythroleukoplakia:** squamous cell carcinoma.‡

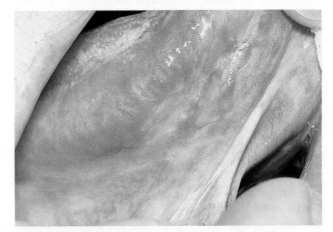

Fig. 73.6. **Squamous cell carcinoma:** ulcer ventral tongue.‡

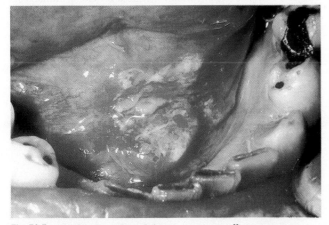

Fig. 73.7. **Speckled erythroplakia:** squamous cell carcinoma.

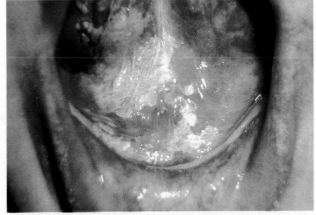

Fig. 73.8. **Squamous cell carcinoma:** floor of the mouth.

9

163

Lichen Planus (Figs. 74.1–74.6) is a common skin disease that can appear at mucosal sites. The cause and pathogenesis are unknown, but evidence suggests that it is an autoimmune disorder in which T lymphocytes are attracted to an antigen within the epithelium. Both CD4 and CD8 T-cell subsets are found heavily dispersed at the epithelial-connective tissue interface of the diseased tissue. This chronic inflammatory state leads to epithelial changes, excessive amounts of fibrinogen deposited at the basement membrane, and eventual destruction of the basal cell layer of the affected epithelium. Anxious, high-strung persons and persons infected with hepatitis C virus are predisposed to lichen planus. Most patients are women older than 40 years. The disease occurs in 1% of adults and exhibits a protracted course with periods of remission and exacerbation.

The skin lesions of **lichen planus** are classically described as *purple, polygonal, pruritic papules.* Initially, they consist of small, flat-topped, red papules with a depressed central area. The lesions may enlarge and become polygonal in shape or coalesce into larger plaques. The papules progressively acquire a violaceous hue and surface lichenification, which consists of fine white striae. Skin lesions usually itch and may change color to yellow or brown before resolution. Bilateral distribution on the flexor surfaces of the extremities is common, occasionally involving the fingernails, causing dystrophic changes. The vulva or glans penis is sometimes affected.

Oral lesions of lichen planus may have one of four appearances: **atrophic, erosive, striated (reticular),** or **plaquelike**. More than one form may affect a single patient. The most frequently affected site is the buccal mucosa. The tongue, lips, palate, gingiva, and floor of the mouth may also be affected. Bilateral and relatively symmetric lesions are common. Patients with reticular oral lichen planus characteristically have several delicate white lines and tiny papules arranged in a lacy, weblike network known as **Wickham striae**. The glistening white areas are often asymptomatic but may be of cosmetic concern. They may involve large areas.

Atrophic lichen planus results from atrophy of the epithelium and predominantly appears as a red, nonulcerated mucosal patch. Wickham striae are often present at the border of the lesion. When the attached gingiva is affected, the term **desquamative gingivitis** has been used (see Figs. 87.5 –87.7).

Erosive lichen planus occurs if the surface epithelium is completely lost and erosion results. The buccal mucosa and tongue are commonly affected sites. A vesicle or bulla may initially appear. This eventually breaks down and produces an erosion or ulcer. Mature lesions are red, raw looking, and painful, with irregular borders. Often, there is a yellowish necrotic central pseudomembrane and an annular white patch at the periphery. The condition can be intermittently painful and may develop rapidly. All of these features are helpful in differentiating oral lichen planus from other lesions with a similar clinical appearance, such as leukoplakia, erythroplakia, candidiasis, lupus erythematosus, pemphigoid, and erythema multiforme.

The least common type of lichen planus is the asymptomatic **plaque form**. This lesion is a solid white plaque or patch that has a smooth to slightly irregular surface and an asymmetric configuration. Lesions are commonly found on the buccal mucosa or tongue. Patients may be unaware of the lesions.

In many cases, clinical appearance alone can confirm the diagnosis of oral lichen planus, and biopsy is not necessary. Asymptomatic intraoral lesions can be left alone. Biopsy of the atrophic or erosive form should be performed at the border of the lesion, away from areas of ulceration.

Oral lesions of lichen planus tend to be more persistent than those of the skin. A vacation, change in routine, or discharge of psychologically burdensome problems can bring about abrupt and dramatic resolution of the lesions. Chronic, symptomatic, erosive lichen planus lesions are best managed with topical steroids or short courses of systemic steroids and immunosuppressant agents. A few patients with oral lichen planus are diabetic and should be tested for glucose intolerance. Carcinomatous transformation has been reported in about 1% of cases and has an association with erosive lichen planus and/or tobacco use.

Lichenoid Mucositis (Lichenoid Drug Reaction/Eruption) (Figs. 74.7 and 74.8) closely resembles lichen planus, clinically and histologically. This disorder is more apparent after 30 years of age and frequently occurs on the buccal mucosa, immediately adjacent to a metallic material (usually an older or corroding restoration). Mild cases are asymptomatic, whereas erosive cases can cause a burning type of pain. The histologic features of this lesion mimic those of lichen planus. Current evidence suggests that **lichenoid mucositis** results from a delayed hypersensitivity reaction to antigens in various substances (such as metals, particularly mercury). Interestingly, a **lichenoid drug reaction** can be caused by the systemic administration or application of the same metals (mercury and gold) found in dental restorations. Other drugs shown to induce lichenoid eruptions include antihypertensive drugs (hydrochlorothiazide, angiotensin-converting enzyme inhibitors), antimalarials, beta blockers, nonsteroidal anti-inflammatory drugs, sulfasalazine, and sulfonylurea compounds (Figs. 75.5–75.8). Also, cinnamon (in chewing gum or food) can induce lichenoid mucositis at the site of contact. Patch testing, to confirm contact allergens, aids in the diagnosis. Treatment consists of removing the causative agent. If a restoration is to be replaced, a different restorative material, preferably porcelain, or composite materials should be used. The prognosis is excellent, and healing occurs within weeks of removing the offending agent.

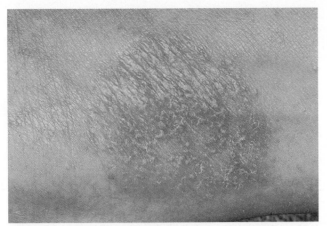

Fig. 74.1. Lichen planus: violaceous skin plaque of the wrist.

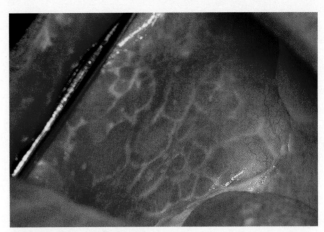

Fig. 74.2. Reticular lichen planus: striae on buccal mucosa.

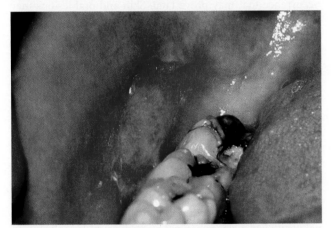

Fig. 74.3. Erosive lichen planus: of buccal mucosa.*

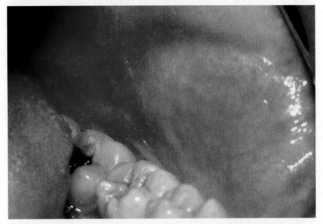

Fig. 74.4. Erosive lichen planus: opposite buccal mucosa.*

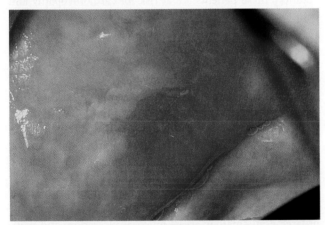

Fig. 74.5. Atrophic (erythematous) lichen planus: of buccal mucosa.

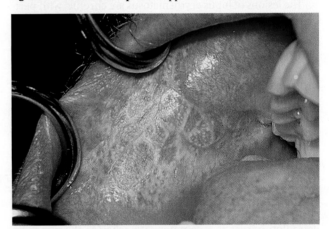

Fig. 74.6. Plaque form of lichen planus.

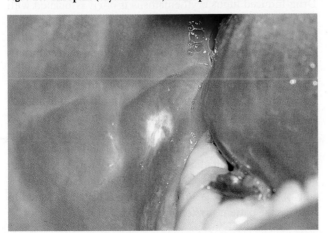

Fig. 74.7. Lichenoid mucositis: adjacent to facial alloy.‡

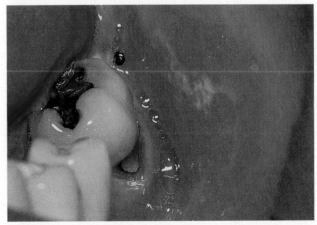

Fig. 74.8. Lichenoid mucositis: opposite buccal mucosa.‡

9

RED AND RED-WHITE LESIONS

Lupus Erythematosus (Figs. 75.1–75.4) Systemic lupus erythematosus (SLE) is an autoimmune disorder that develops when the body's immune system mistakenly attacks the body's own cells and tissue, resulting in inflammation and tissue damage. Affected patients produce antinuclear antibodies (ANA), anti-DNA, and antihistone antibodies against components in the cell nucleus. They also have antibodies directed against the basement membrane of epithelium. All of these antibodies participate in immunologically mediated attack of self-antigens, resulting in tissue injury. Three forms exist: (1) **chronic discoid lupus erythematosus**, also known as **chronic cutaneous lupus erythematosus**, which only involves the skin; (2) **systemic lupus erythematosus**, in which multiple organ systems are involved; and (3) **subacute cutaneous lupus erythematosus**, an intermediate form that produces nonscarring skin lesions, mild musculoskeletal (arthritis) symptoms, and limited or no organ disease. The cause of all three types is unknown; however, sensitivity to sunlight is a feature of all three forms.

Chronic cutaneous or **discoid lupus erythematosus**, the benign form of the disease, is a purely mucocutaneous disorder. It may appear at any age but predominates in women older than 40 years. The condition classically produces a red butterfly rash distributed symmetrically on the cheeks across the bridge of the nose. Other prominent sun-exposed areas of the face—including the malar areas, forehead, scalp, and ears—may be involved.

The lesions of lupus erythematosus are chronic, with periods of exacerbation and remission. Mature lesions exhibit three zones: an atrophic center lined by a hyperkeratotic margin, which is surrounded by an erythematous periphery. As the center heals, hypopigmentation (or in some cases hyperpigmentation) results from melanocyte damage at the epidermal-dermal junction. Telangiectasias, blackheads, a fine scale, and hair loss at sites of involvement are common findings. The lesions are usually limited to the upper portion of the body, particularly the head and neck.

Oral lesions are found in 20% to 40% of patients with lupus erythematosus. These lesions may develop before or after skin lesions develop. Lip lesions are red with a white to silvery, scaly margin. A sun-exposed lower lip at the vermilion border is a common site, whereas the upper lip is usually involved as a result of direct extension of dermal lesions. Intraoral lesions are frequently diffuse erythematosus plaques, with erosive, ulcerative, and white components.

Chronic discoid lupus erythematosus sometimes appears as isolated red-white plaques. The buccal mucosa is the most frequent intraoral site, followed by the tongue, palate, and gingiva. Oral lesions are characterized by a central, red atrophic area sometimes covered by a fine stippling of white dots. The peripheral margins are irregular and are composed of alternating red and keratotic white lines extending for a short length up to about 1 cm in a radial pattern. These lesions may mimic lichen planus, but concurrent ear involvement helps to exclude the diagnosis of lichen planus. Ulcerative lesions are painful and require treatment. Avoidance of emotional stress, cold, sunlight, and hot spicy foods is necessary. The use of sunscreens, topical steroids, systemic steroids, and antimalarial and immunosuppressive agents has proven effective. Patients using antimalarial agents require close ophthalmologic follow-up.

Systemic manifestations of the disease often begin with reports of fatigue, fever, and joint pain. Generalized nontender lymphadenopathy is often present. Hepatomegaly, splenomegaly, peripheral neuropathy, and hematologic abnormalities may be seen. Strict avoidance of sun exposure is necessary because sunlight can trigger acute exacerbations. Involvement of the kidneys and heart is a common occurrence that may prove fatal. Skin and oral lesions may accompany the condition, but there is little chance of conversion from discoid to systemic lupus. Patients with systemic lupus erythematosus often have other concurrent autoimmune collagen-vascular diseases, such as Sjögren syndrome and rheumatoid arthritis. Allergic mucositis, candidiasis, leukoplakia, erythroleukoplakia, and lichen planus must be considered in the differential diagnosis of oral lupus erythematosus lesions. Biopsy and histologic examination with immunofluorescence confirm the diagnosis. Precautions are advised in the dental treatment of patients with lupus erythematosus, who may be taking high doses of systemic steroids, because of their predisposition to delayed wound healing, risk for infection, and the possibility of stress-induced adrenal insufficiency characterized by cardiovascular collapse. In addition, these patients are at risk for cardiomyopathy and defective heart valves.

Lichenoid and Lupuslike Drug Eruption (Figs. 75.5– 75.8) **Stomatitis medicamentosa** is a general term used to describe an oral hypersensitivity reaction to a drug that results in oral lesions. Two subcategories of oral hypersensitivity, called **lichenoid drug eruption** and **lupuslike drug eruption**, have been described. They produce reticular or erosive lesions similar in appearance to lichen planus and lupus erythematosus. Although the appearance may vary, white linear plaques with red margins are common. The lesions may erupt immediately or after prolonged use of a drug. Persistent inflammatory changes may result in large erythematous areas, mucosal ulceration, and pain. Drug-induced lupus erythematosus is often associated with arthritis, fever, and renal disease. Hydralazine and procainamide are the most common instigators of lupuslike drug eruptions. Other drugs known to cause lupuslike eruptions include gold, griseofulvin, isoniazid, methyldopa, penicillin, phenytoin, procainamide, streptomycin, and trimethadione. Drugs known to induce lichenoid eruptions include allopurinol, carbamazepine, chloroquine, dapsone, furosemide, methyldopa, penicillamine, phenothiazines, quinidine, sulfasalazine, thiazides, certain antibiotics, and heavy metals (gold, mercury, palladium). Consultation with a physician and withdrawal of the offending medication leads to regression of the lesion(s). A substitute drug is usually selected to manage the patient's systemic problem.

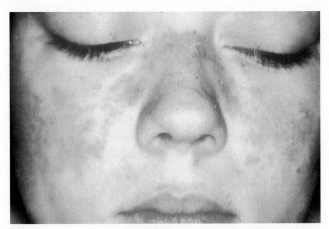

Fig. 75.1. **Discoid lupus erythematosus:** butterfly rash.

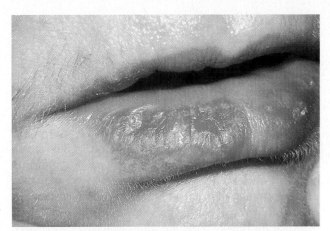

Fig. 75.2. **Discoid lupus erythematosus:** sun-exposed area.

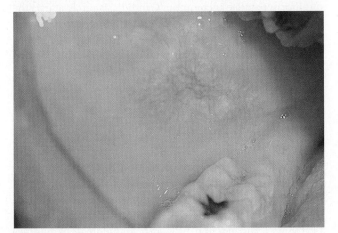

Fig. 75.3. **Alternating red-white lines of lupus erythematosus.**

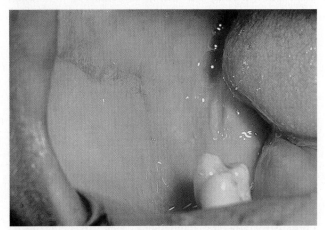

Fig. 75.4. **Atrophic lesion of lupus erythematosus.**

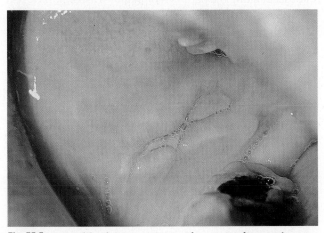

Fig. 75.5. **Lupuslike drug eruption:** with amitriptyline use.[*]

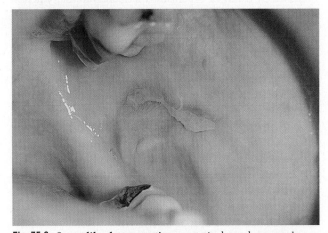

Fig. 75.6. **Lupuslike drug eruption:** opposite buccal mucosa.[*]

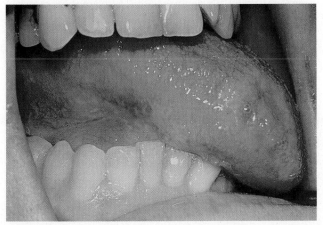

Fig. 75.7. **Lichenoid drug eruption:** lateral tongue.[‡]

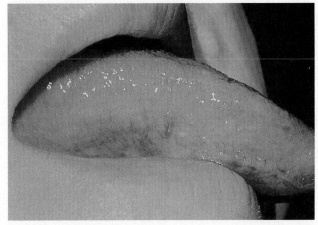

Fig. 75.8. **Lichenoid drug eruption:** after drug withdrawal.[‡]

9

RED AND RED-WHITE LESIONS

Candidiasis is the most common fungal infection of the oral cavity. Several different types of candidiasis exist and are discussed here.

Pseudomembranous Candidiasis (Thrush) (Figs. 76.1 and 76.2) is an opportunistic infection caused by overgrowth of the superficial fungus *C. albicans*. It appears as diffuse, velvety, white mucosal plaques that are nonpainful until they are wiped off, leaving a red, raw, or bleeding surface. *C. albicans* is a common inhabitant of the oral cavity, gastrointestinal tract, and vagina. Infants whose mothers have vaginal thrush at the time of birth and adults who have experienced a change in normal oral microflora because of antibiotics, steroids, or systemic alterations such as diabetes, immunodeficiency, or chemotherapy are frequently affected. There is no racial or sex predilection. **Pseudomembranous candidiasis** is usually found on the buccal mucosa, tongue, and soft palate. In patients with asthma who use a steroid inhaler, the pattern appears as a circular or oval reddish-white patch at the site of aerosol contact on the palate. Diagnosis is made by clinical examination, fungal culture, or direct microscopic examination of tissue scrapings. A cytologic smear treated with potassium hydroxide, Gram, or periodic acid–Schiff (PAS) stain will reveal budding organisms with branching pseudohyphae. Topical or systemic antifungal medication for 2 weeks usually produces resolution.

Chronic Hyperplastic Candidiasis (Figs. 76.3 and 76.4) is caused by candidal organisms that penetrate the mucosal surface and stimulate a hyperplastic response. Chronic irritation, poor oral hygiene, and xerostomia are predisposing factors. Thus, smokers, denture wearers, and diabetics are commonly affected. Immunosuppression, such as HIV infection, can be contributory. Sites most affected are the dorsum of the tongue, palate, buccal mucosa, and labial commissures. The lesion invariably has a distinctive raised border, a white or grayish pebbly surface, and red zones caused by destruction of the mucosa. Thus, the condition may resemble leukoplakia, erythroleukoplakia, or verrucoid growths.

Chronic hyperplastic candidiasis cannot be peeled off. Thus, the diagnosis must be made by biopsy. On microscopy, the organisms may be identified by routine hematoxylin and eosin stain or, more appropriately, by PAS stain. With adequate topical application of an antifungal agent, the condition usually resolves. In some instances, surgical stripping may be required. All patients with hyperplastic candidiasis should be followed closely because this form may be related to speckled erythroplakia, a lesion that is often premalignant or worse.

Erythematous Candidiasis There are several "red"-appearing forms of candidiasis. Three are discussed here; median rhomboid glossitis (a fourth form) is discussed elsewhere (Figs. 58.2 and 58.3).

Acute Atrophic Candidiasis (Antibiotic Sore Mouth) (Fig. 76.5) The use of broad-spectrum antibiotics, particularly tetracyclines, or topical steroids can result in a form of erythematous candidiasis known as **acute atrophic candidiasis**. This fungal infection is the result of an imbalance in the oral ecosystem between *Lactobacillus acidophilus* and *C. albicans*. Antibiotics taken by the patient can reduce the *Lactobacillus* population and permit candidal organisms to flourish. The infection produces desquamated areas of surface mucosa that appear as diffuse, atrophic red patches that cause burning pain. The location of the patches can indicate the cause. Lesions affecting the buccal mucosa, lips, and oropharynx often suggest the systemic use of antibiotics, whereas redness of the tongue and palate are more common after use of antibiotic troches. When the tongue is affected, a surface devoid of filiform papillae is common. Candidiasis rarely affects the attached gingiva. If this is the clinical finding, severe immunosuppression is a distinct possibility. The diagnosis is confirmed by demonstration of budding organisms or hyphal forms on a stained cytologic smear. Treatment should be the withdrawal of offending antibiotics followed by use of antifungal drugs.

Angular Cheilitis (Fig. 76.6) Angular cheilitis, or *perlèche* ("*per lecher*" meaning "thoroughly + to lick" in French), is a chronic painful erosive condition involving the labial commissures caused by *C. albicans*, *Staphylococcus aureus*, lip licking, and pooling saliva. It appears at the corners of the lips as red erosions with central fissures that may ulcer. Erythema, crusting, and brownish granulomatous nodules may occur along the peripheral margins. Discomfort caused by opening the mouth may limit normal oral function. Predisposing factors include poor nutrition, loss of vertical dimension, and high sucrose intake. Treatment involves antifungal-antibacterial agents, correction of predisposing factors, and habit cessation.

Chronic Atrophic Candidiasis (Denture Stomatitis) (Figs. 76.7 and 76.8) is the most common form of chronic candidiasis. It presents as an asymptomatic red lesion on the palate of complete and partial denture wearers, particularly elderly women who wear their dentures at night. Only rarely are dentate patients and the mandible affected. Misnomers for this disease are denture sore mouth and denture base allergy.

Chronic atrophic candidiasis is caused by candidal organisms under the denture base. There are three stages of denture stomatitis. The earliest lesions are red pinpoint areas of hyperemia limited to the orifices of the palatal minor salivary glands. The second stage produces a diffuse erythema that is sometimes accompanied by epithelial desquamation. **Papillary hyperplasia**, consisting of multiple fibroma-like papules, is the third stage. With time, the papules may enlarge to form red nodules. Effective therapy requires antifungal treatment of the mucosa and denture base. Traumatic influences, such as the rocking action of an ill-fitting denture, should be eliminated to speed healing. Occasionally, surgical stripping is required.

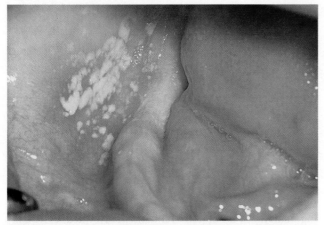

Fig. 76.1. **Acute pseudomembranous candidiasis:** in a patient with diabetes.

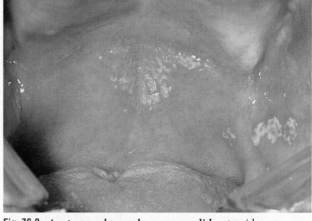

Fig. 76.2. **Acute pseudomembranous candida:** steroid user.

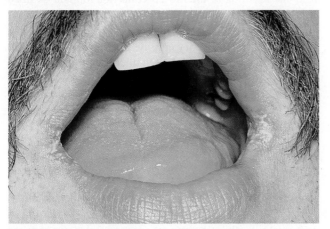

Fig. 76.3. **Chronic hyperplastic candidiasis:** at commissures.

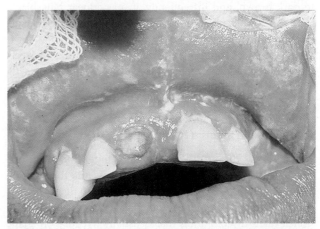

Fig. 76.4. **Chronic hyperplastic candidiasis:** of labial mucosa.

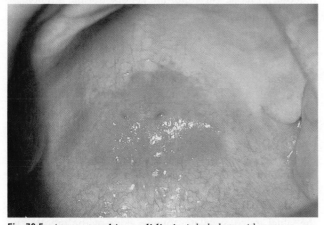

Fig. 76.5. **Acute atrophic candidiasis:** inhaled steroid use.

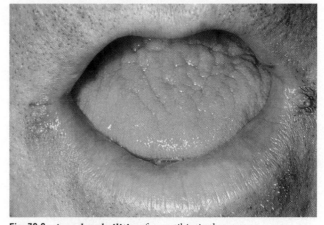

Fig. 76.6. **Angular cheilitis:** after antibiotic therapy.

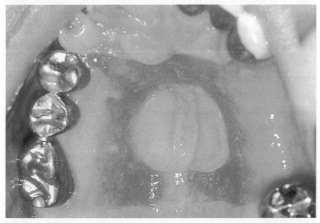

Fig. 76.7. **Chronic atrophic candidiasis:** denture-bearing area.

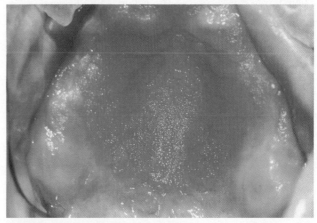

Fig. 76.8. **Papillary hyperplasia:** third stage.

9

169

Melanoplakia (Physiologic Pigmentation) (Fig. 77.1) is a generalized and constant dark pigmentation of the oral mucosa, commonly seen in dark-skinned persons. The condition is physiologic, not pathologic. It results from increased amounts of melanin (an endogenous pigment) that are deposited in the basal layer of the mucosa and lamina propria. The most common site for observing melanoplakia is the attached gingiva. It often appears as a diffuse, ribbonlike, dark band with a well-demarcated and curvilinear border that separates it from the alveolar mucosa. Melanoplakia is characteristically symmetric and asymptomatic. Infrequently, it can be patchy or asymmetric. The degree of pigmentation varies from light brown (Fig. 7.10) to dark brown, and infrequently, it may appear blue-black. Other sites of occurrence are the buccal mucosa, hard palate, lips, and tongue. At these sites, the deposition of pigment is often multifocal and diffuse. Melanoplakia requires no treatment, but should be differentiated from similar-appearing conditions that produce oral pigmentations, such as Addison disease, Albright syndrome, Peutz-Jeghers syndrome, heavy metal pigmentation, and antimalarial drugs and other conditions discussed in this section.

Tattoo (Figs. 77.2–77.5) is caused by intentional or accidental implantation of exogenous pigments into the mucosa. The most common intraoral type is the amalgam tattoo. The amalgam tattoo appears as a slate-gray to blue-black, nonelevated discoloration that is usually irregular in shape and variable in size. It results from the entrapment of amalgam in a soft tissue wound, such as an extraction socket or a gingival abrasion from a rotating bur. Deterioration of the metallic compounds of the amalgam imparts the characteristic blue-gray color. Focal discolorations may occasionally appear green to dark gray because of the deposition of high copper alloys.

Amalgam tattoos are usually seen in the gingiva in posterior areas adjacent to a large amalgam restoration or gold casting. These lesions are not limited to the gingiva and may also be seen on the edentulous ridge, vestibular mucosa, palate, buccal mucosa, and floor of the mouth. The clinical diagnosis of an amalgam tattoo can be confirmed by finding radiographic evidence of the foreign metal in the paradental tissue (Fig. 77.4). The radiographic appearance may vary from the absence of demonstrable particles to pinpoint or globular radiopacities several millimeters in diameter. If radiographs fail to demonstrate suspected metallic particles or there are no restorations in the vicinity, a biopsy is required to rule out more serious pigmented lesions.

Other types of tattoos seen in the oral cavity are the graphite pencil wound (graphite implantation) and India ink tattoos. Graphite implantation appears as a focal, slate-gray macule after trauma embeds the pencil tip into the mucosa.

Sites frequently affected are the lip and the palate. The nature of the lesion can be easily ascertained by questioning the patient. Ordinary India ink tattoos are occasional findings on the labial mucosa of the lower lip, sometimes conveying a message. In general, tattoos are harmless and of no clinical significance. However, they may be indistinguishable from more potentially ominous lesions.

Ephelis (Freckle) (Fig. 77.6) is a small, light- to dark-brown macule that appears on the lip or skin after active deposition of melanin triggered by exposure to sunlight. Unlike some pigmentations, an ephelis remains nonelevated, essentially unchanged in size (less than 3 mm) with time, darkens in response to sunlight, and has a predilection for light-skinned or red-headed persons. A single freckle is clinically distinguished from an oral melanotic macule by the history of a traumatic or inflammatory episode that precedes the development of the latter condition. On microscopic examination, an ephelis shows an increase in melanin pigment without an increase in the number of melanocytes. Multiple freckles on the lip can be a feature of Peutz-Jeghers syndrome (Figs. 79.1 and 79.2). This syndrome is associated with lip ephelides, intraoral and palmar pigmentations, and intestinal polyposis. In general, ephelides may be of cosmetic concern, but most only require clinical observation.

Smoker's Melanosis (Tobacco-Associated Pigmentation) (Figs. 77.7 and 77.8) Smoking tobacco imparts smoker's melanosis, a characteristic change in color to exposed mucosal surfaces. The condition is not a normal physiologic process but instead results primarily from the deposition of melanin in the basal cell layer of the mucosa. It arises as a result of inflammatory changes that are caused by chronic exposure to heat, smoke inhalation, and the absorption of exogenous pigments. It has been suggested that the deposition of melanocytes is a protective response against the toxic substances in tobacco smoke.

Smoker's melanosis affects older persons who are heavy smokers. It appears as a diffuse smoky-gray-brown patch up to several centimeters in size. Dark-brown foci or zones are often distributed asymmetrically throughout the patch. The mandibular anterior gingiva and buccal mucosa are the most frequently affected sites. Other susceptible sites include the labial mucosa, palate, tongue, floor of the mouth, and lips. The degree of pigmentation ranges from light to dark brown and appears to be directly related to the amount of tobacco smoked. Brown-stained teeth and halitosis usually accompany the condition. Smoker's melanosis itself is not premalignant. However, the clinician should closely inspect the adjacent tissues for other tobacco-induced lesions, which may be more significant. Smoking cessation programs should be offered to these patients.

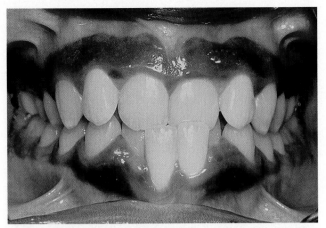

Fig. 77.1. Melanoplakia: along the attached gingiva.

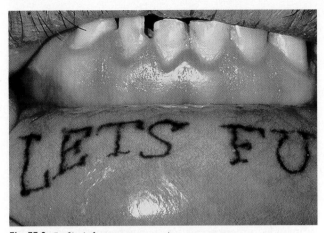

Fig. 77.2. India ink tattoo: conveying a message.

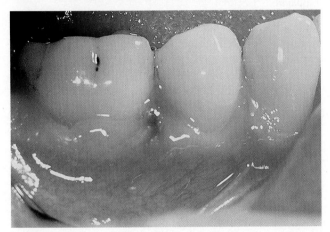

Fig. 77.3. Amalgam tattoo: in attached gingiva.*

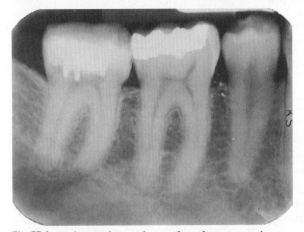

Fig. 77.4. Radiographic evidence of amalgam tattoo.*

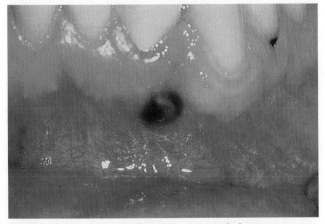

Fig. 77.5. Focal argyrosis: after silver-point endodontics.

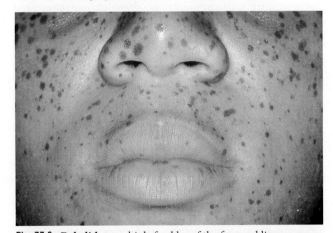

Fig. 77.6. Ephelides: multiple freckles of the face and lips.

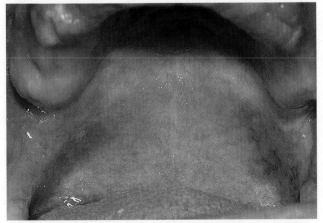

Fig. 77.7. Smoker's melanosis: of lateral soft palate.

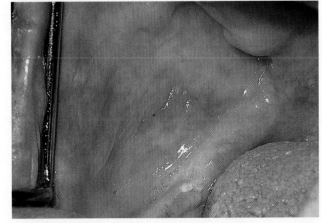

Fig. 77.8. Smoker's melanosis: of the buccal mucosa.

PIGMENTED LESIONS

Oral Melanotic Macule (Focal Melanosis) (Figs. 78.1 and 78.2) is a small, flat circumscribed pigmentation of the lip or mouth. It results from focal deposition of melanin along the basal layer of the epithelium and superficial layer of connective tissue. These asymptomatic pigmentations are usually single, less than 1 cm, and common in light-skinned persons between 25 and 45 years of age. They represent reactions to trauma, inflammation, or sun damage. The most common site is the lower lip, close to the midline. Other sites include the gingiva, buccal mucosa, and palate. The color is uniform and may be blue, gray, brown, or black. Biopsy is recommended unless no visible change has occurred in many years. Periodic observation should be provided.

Nevus (Figs. 78.3–78.6) is a flat or sometimes raised growth comprised of a collection of nevus (melanin-producing) cells, called *thèques*, in the epithelium or dermis. A **nevus** is commonly dark and seen on the skin, and occasionally it occurs in the oral mucosa. There are many types of nevi, which are broadly classified as either congenital or acquired. **Congenital nevi** are present at birth and are also known as birthmarks or garment trunk nevi. They are usually larger than acquired nevi and have a higher incidence of malignant transformation.

Acquired nevi, or **moles**, occur later in life and usually appear as dark, slightly raised, papules. They are often symmetrical and uniform in color, but can be pink (amelanotic), brown, grayish, or black. Oral nevi are rare. Most are asymptomatic, small, well-circumscribed, dome-shaped pigmented papules or macules on the palate and buccal mucosa mainly in women. Their size tends to remain constant after puberty.

Benign nevi are classified into four types according to histologic appearance and location of the thèques, which extend deeper as the lesion matures. Least to most common are the junctional nevus, compound nevus, blue nevus, and intramucosal nevus.

The **junctional nevus** is an early-stage nevus in which the nevus cells are located at the junctional layer of the epithelium and lamina propria. These lesions are the rarest of oral nevi and usually appear flat and brown and have a diameter of less than 1 cm. The palate and buccal mucosa are common locations.

The **compound nevus**, as the name implies, is composed of nevus cells located in the epithelium and the lamina propria. The compound nevus rarely undergoes malignant transformation.

The **intramucosal nevus** has ovoid nevus cells located in the connective tissue only. This entity is analogous to the intradermal nevus, which appears as a dark, raised papule on the skin, often seen with a hair growing from it. It is rare, however, to find a hair associated with the intramucosal nevus of the mouth. The intramucosal nevus is usually brown, raised, and less than 0.8 cm in diameter.

The term **blue nevus** originates from the typical blue or blue-black color imparted by the spindle-shaped nevus cells located deep in the connective tissue. It appears as a persistent small, focal blue macule, most commonly on the palate of young adults. Malignant transformation of intraoral blue nevi is very rare.

On rare occasions **Hutchinson freckle** (lentigo maligna) is found in the mouth. The melanotic freckle is usually seen on sun-exposed skin (face) or dorsum of the hands of persons older than 50 years. This lesion is flat and irregularly shaped, with zones of varying brown color. It tends to spread superficially (laterally) and undergo malignant transformation.

Nevi may be difficult to distinguish from their malignant counterparts. Thus, all intraoral pigmented lesions should be biopsied.

Melanoma (Figs. 78.7 and 78.8) is a malignant tumor that begins in the cells (melanocytes) that produce skin-coloring pigment. **Melanomas** occur primarily in sun-exposed skin surfaces and infrequently in the oral cavity. They occur about twice as frequently in men as women and often in light-skinned persons between 20 and 50 years of age. However, the majority of melanomas appear after age 50. There is no sex predilection. About 30% of melanomas arise from previously existing pigmented lesions, such as moles, particularly ones with a history of chronic trauma. They may appear flat or raised, nonpigmented or pigmented. Pigmented lesions are usually deep brown, gray, blue, or jet black. Eighty percent of oral melanomas occur on the palate or maxillary alveolar ridge. Less commonly, the anterior gingivae and labial mucosa are affected. Malignant changes are the result of DNA damage of genes critical for cell cycle control often induced by ultraviolet light.

Melanoma begins as a small superficial or slightly raised patch that grows slowly and laterally over several months. Early recognizable signs are *A,* **asymmetrical lesion;** *B,* **border irregularity;** *C,* **color variation within the lesion;** and *D,* **diameter enlarging.** Eventually, a prominent, nonmovable, dark lesion develops. The clinician should be alert to features that include multiple colors (the combination of red together with blue-black is particularly ominous), change in size, satellite lesions arising at the periphery of the lesion, and signs of inflammation, such as a peripheral zone of erythema. Late signs include bleeding and ulceration, firmness, and firm regional lymph nodes. Intraoral melanomas are extremely dangerous and more serious than their cutaneous counterpart because of early and wide metastasis, which results in poor prognosis. Early diagnosis when tumors are less than 1.5 mm in size and complete resection are critical to long-term survival. The 5-year survival rate of oral melanoma is only about 40% compared to 91% for skin melanoma. Spread to regional lymph nodes reduces the 5-year survival rate; however, targeted immunotherapies have improved treatment outcomes. About 11% of melanomas recur by 25 years, dictating long-term follow-up care.

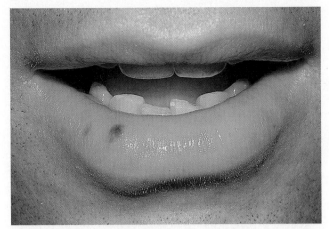

Fig. 78.1. **Oral melanotic macule:** in the lower lip.

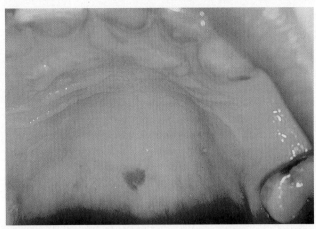

Fig. 78.2. **Oral melanotic macule:** of the hard palate.

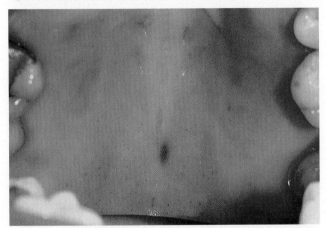

Fig. 78.3. **Compound nevus:** uniform color, on palate.

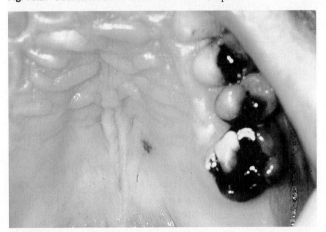

Fig. 78.4. **Intramucosal nevus:** amelanotic, next to molar.

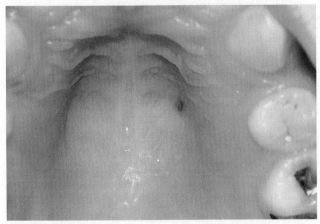

Fig. 78.5. **Blue nevus:** uniform slate-blue color, hard palate.

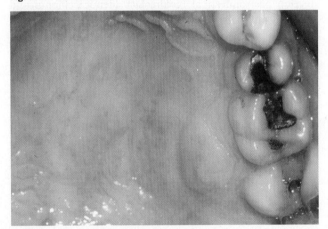

Fig. 78.6. **Blue nevus:** of the lateral palatal vault.

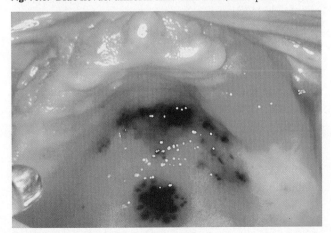

Fig. 78.7. **Melanoma:** satellite lesions of palate.

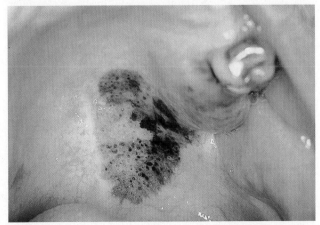

Fig. 78.8. **Melanoma:** color variation, in soft palate and tuberosity.

9

173

PIGMENTED LESIONS

Peutz-Jeghers Syndrome (Hereditary Intestinal Polyposis) (Figs. 79.1 and 79.2) is an autosomal dominant condition characterized by multiple pigmented macules and benign polyps, primarily in the intestines. It is caused by a germline mutation in the *LKB1* gene of chromosome 19 that encodes a multifunctional serine-threonine kinase. The multiple benign intestinal polyps are hamartomatous tissue growths that usually occur in the ileum but also are found in the stomach and colon. Symptoms such as intermittent colicky pain and reports of obstruction may be concurrent. Signs of **Peutz-Jeghers Syndrome** are pigmented macules distributed on the skin around the eyes, nose, mouth, lips, perineum, oral mucosa, gingiva, and palmar and plantar surfaces of the hands and feet. The perioral pigmentations must be distinguished from multiple ephelides and lentigines of the LEOPARD syndrome.

The most common intraoral locations for the macules are the lips and buccal mucosa. Characteristically, the density of macules is higher on the vermilion than the adjacent skin. The macules are asymptomatic, small, flat brown ovals that do not darken with exposure to the sun, as freckles do. In contrast to their cutaneous counterparts, the intraoral spots tend to persist into adulthood, whereas the dermal macules may fade with age. No treatment is necessary for the macules, which on microscopic examination contain elongated melanocytes along the basal cell layer and lamina propria. Although the macules are benign, they are of considerable clinical significance because affected patients are prone to develop gastrointestinal (colorectal) adenocarcinoma and are at an increased risk for tumors of the reproductive system. The diagnosis of Peutz-Jeghers syndrome therefore necessitates prompt medical evaluation.

Addison Disease (Adrenal Cortical Insufficiency) (Figs. 79.3 and 79.4) is an endocrine disorder in which the adrenal gland produces insufficient amounts of steroid hormones. It commonly results from autoimmune-induced destruction of the adrenal gland. Other causes include pituitary insufficiency, tumor invasion, adrenalectomy, infectious diseases, and gram-negative sepsis. Progression of the disease results in anemia, anorexia, diarrhea, hypotension, nausea, salt craving, weakness, and weight loss.

As serum cortisol levels drop, a feedback loop from the adrenal gland to the pituitary gland triggers the production of melanocyte-stimulating hormone by the pituitary gland. This leads to the deposition of melanin in the skin, especially in sun-exposed areas. Classically, the skin acquires a bronze tan that persists after sun exposure. Darkening may be initially noted on the knuckles, elbows, palmar creases, and intraoral mucosa.

In the mouth, **Addison disease** is characterized by hypermelanosis that is similar in appearance to physiologic pigmentation. The pattern is not unique and may consist of multiple focal brown-bronze to blue-black spots or generalized, diffuse streaks of dark-brown pigmentation. The pigmented areas are usually macular, nonraised, brown, and varied in shape. The buccal mucosa and gingiva are most commonly affected, but pigmentation may also extend onto the tongue and lips. Biopsy is not diagnostic, and serum cortisol tests are recommended. Replacement therapy with corticosteroids produces a gradual diminution of the hyperpigmentation. Thus, the degree of oral pigmentation is a sensitive indicator of therapeutic effectiveness. Transient changes in pigmentation in a treated patient may indicate inadequate therapy.

Heavy Metal Pigmentation (Figs. 79.5–79.8) Excessive ingestion of heavy metals (bismuth, lead, mercury, silver) and certain drugs (cis-platinum, antimalarial agents, antipsychotic agents, birth control pills) can produce mucocutaneous pigmentations. Bismuth is commonly found in diarrhea medications, which if used for a long term results in diffuse deposition of the metal in the gingiva. The discoloration is confined to the marginal gingiva, particularly in areas where inflammation is present. The **bismuth line** usually appears blue to black in a linear distribution along the gingival sulcus. A metallic taste and burning mucosa are common symptoms.

Lead poisoning, or **plumbism**, is usually a result of occupational exposure to excessive doses of lead used in paints, batteries, or plumbing. The most prominent intraoral change and early diagnostic sign is a gray-black lead line that occurs from the deposition of lead sulfide in the marginal gingiva. Spotty gray macules on the buccal mucosa, a coated tongue, neurologic deficits (tremor of the extended tongue), and hypersalivation are other intraoral findings. The condition is reversible if exposure to lead is eliminated.

Mercury poisoning, or **acrodynia**, can be acquired by absorption, inhalation, or ingestion. Although uncommon today, acrodynia was the result of treatment for syphilis earlier in the century. Inadequate mercury hygiene measures, such as handling mercury, breathing mercury vapors, and spilling mercury, place dental personnel at risk for acrodynia. Like bismuth and lead intoxication, mercury poisoning produces a dark mercury gingival line. In addition, the disease is often accompanied by many signs and symptoms, including abdominal pain, anorexia, headaches, insomnia, psychological symptoms, vertigo, oral ulcerations, hemorrhage, a metallic taste, sialorrhea, burning mouth, and periodontal destruction.

Silver pigmentation, or **argyria**, is a rare occurrence that most often results from prolonged exposure to silver-containing ocular, nasal, or oral medications. Asymptomatic pigmentations accumulate in the sun-exposed areas of the skin, along with the hair, fingernails, and oral mucosa. A blue-gray pigmentation is characteristic. Once evident, the pigmentation is irreversible. Nasal inhalation of solutions containing silver salts has a propensity to deposit in the palatal mucosa, imparting a color similar to that seen on the skin. Treatment is immediate withdrawal of the medication.

174

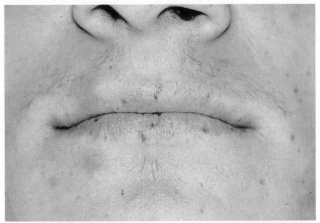

Fig. 79.1. Peutz-Jeghers syndrome: of the lips and perioral skin.

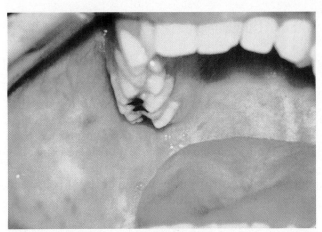

Fig. 79.2. Peutz-Jeghers syndrome: of the buccal mucosa.

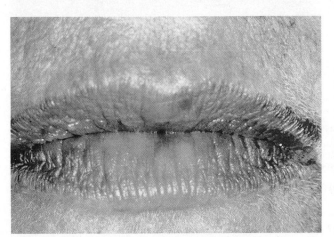

Fig. 79.3. Addison disease: pigmentation of the lips.˙

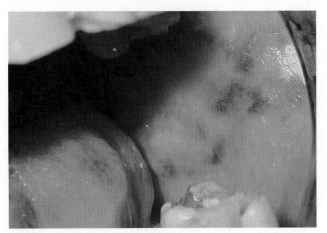

Fig. 79.4. Addison disease: of the buccal mucosa.˙

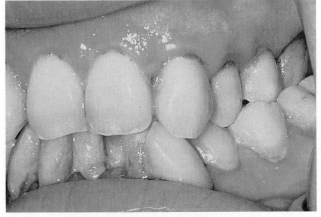

Fig. 79.5. Lead line: along marginal gingiva.

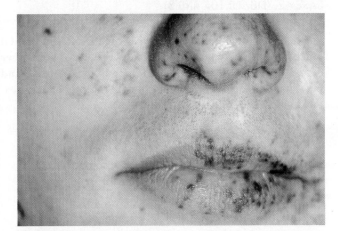

Fig. 79.6. Pigmentation: from silver acetaldehyde detonation.

9

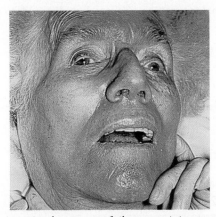

Fig. 79.7. Argyria: chronic use of silver-containing nose drops.‡

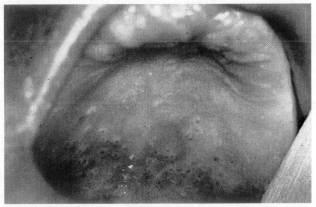

Fig. 79.8. Heavy silver pigmentation (argyria): of palate.‡

CASE STUDIES

CASE 41. (FIG. 79.9)

This 28-year-old Hispanic woman presents to your office for a recall visit. She has good daily oral self-care and has nice restorations with no visible decay but has not been in for a while. She claims to smoke four cigarettes per day and has done this for about 11 years. She is not married and is socially active. You saw her about 2½ years ago, and the lesion was much smaller then.

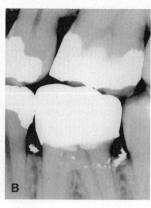

1. What is the pink, raised, midline, linear soft tissue structure?

2. Describe the clinical findings (appearance and location).

3. Which term best describes the lesion?
   A. Leukoplakia
   B. Erythroplakia
   C. Speckled erythroplakia
   D. Morsicatio buccarum

4. What term more specifically describes this lesion?

5. Is this lesion a normal finding, a variant of normal, or disease? What clinical features are suggestive that this condition is benign or malignant?

6. Is this condition associated with smoking? Is there any clinical evidence that she smokes?

7. If this lesion is removed, do you expect it to resolve or recur?

8. Do you expect this condition to be symptomatic?

9. What should a dental hygienist communicate to the dentist?

CASE 42. (FIG. 79.10A AND B)

You take this photograph of a 50-year-old man in your dental office. He has many restorations that were placed at another dental office and is asymptomatic. He is hypertensive and takes medication for this condition. He recently had a prostate biopsy. The results are pending.

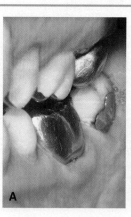

1. Based on the clinical photograph only, with what materials are the molars restored?

2. What part of the tooth is the yellowish component seen at the gingival margin of lower premolar in the clinical photograph? Why is this apparent?

3. Describe the soft tissue changes affecting the gingiva.

4. In a similar case, you take a bitewing radiograph (Fig. 79.10B). Describe the radiographic findings.

5. Is this condition shown in the clinical photograph and radiograph normal, a variation of normal, or disease? Do you expect this condition to be symptomatic?

6. After reviewing the radiograph, does it appear that the alveolar bone is affected by this condition?

7. Which of the following is the most likely diagnosis?
   A. Amalgam tattoo
   B. Blue nevus
   C. Intramucosal nevus
   D. Melanoma

8. Why is taking a radiograph and interpretation of the film important in this case?

Additional cases to enhance your learning and understanding of this section are available Online through the book's Navigate 2 Advantage Access site.

Intraoral Findings by Surface Change

Objectives:

- Define clinical entities that appear as nodules, papulonodules, vesicles, bullae, and ulcerative lesions of the oral cavity.
- Recognize the causes of these conditions.
- In the clinical setting, document the clinical features of oral conditions discussed in this section in terms of anatomic location, color, border, and configuration.
- Use the diagnostic process to distinguish similar-appearing nodules, papulonodules, and vesiculobullous and ulcerative lesions of the oral cavity.
- Recommend appropriate treatment options for these conditions.
- Identify conditions discussed in this section that would (1) require the attention of the dentist, (2) affect the delivery of noninvasive and invasive dental procedures, or (3) need to be further evaluated by a specialist.

In the figure legends, *‡ denotes the same patient.

NODULES

Retrocuspid Papilla (Figs. 80.1 and 80.2) Not all persons have a **retrocuspid papilla**. This particular growth appears as a firm, round, fibroepithelial papule about 1 to 4 mm in diameter. It is located on the lingual surface of the attached gingiva of the mandibular cuspids just below or a few millimeters below the marginal gingiva. The surface mucosa is pink, soft, and smooth. Rarely, the structure may be pedunculated, and the stalk can be lifted off the gingiva by a periodontal probe. The retrocuspid papilla is a variation of normal and is frequently found bilaterally. Some authorities state that it is a developmental anomaly that represents a variant form of fibroma. It is seen in children but regresses with maturity; thus, the incidence and size decrease with increasing age. The retrocuspid papilla has no sex predilection, and no treatment is necessary unless interference with a removable prosthesis is anticipated.

Oral Lymphoepithelial Cyst (Figs. 80.3 and 80.4) The **oral lymphoepithelial cyst** usually presents as a small, movable, painless swelling that is characterized by a well-circumscribed, soft, doughy mass. It is an encapsulated dermal or submucosal papule that arises from epithelium entrapped in lymphoid tissue that has undergone cystic transformation. The cyst is benign and asymptomatic but may enlarge and spontaneously drain. Most appear in children and young adults. No sex predilection has been demonstrated.

Common sites for the oral **lymphoepithelial cyst** are the floor of the mouth, lingual frenum, ventral tongue, posterior lateral border of the tongue, and, rarely, the soft palate. These small swellings rarely exceed 1 cm in diameter and are characteristically yellow when superficial and pink when deeper. Palpation yields a slightly moveable nodule. When located in the anterior floor, the lesion may resemble a mucus retention cyst. Infrequently, multiple lymphoepithelial cysts can be found, and HIV-infected persons are predisposed to occurrences in major salivary glands.

When the lymphoepithelial cyst is derived from degenerative tissue of the second branchial arch, it is referred to as a **cervical lymphoepithelial cyst** or a **branchial (cleft) cyst**. This developmental cyst appears in children on the lateral aspect of the neck just anterior and deep to the superior third of the sternocleidomastoid muscle near the angle of the mandible. The cyst may occur in the proximity of the parotid gland. It is a well-circumscribed, soft, fluctuant mass that is rubbery to the touch. It may enlarge to 1 or 2 cm and can drain externally.

Histologic examination shows that lymphoepithelial cysts are usually lined with stratified squamous epithelium; occasionally, pseudostratified, columnar, or cuboidal epithelium is found. Surrounding the cystic epithelial lining is a fibrous connective tissue wall that contains dark-staining lymphoid aggregates with prominent germinal centers. The luminal fluid may contain yellow, viscous, keratinaceous content. Excisional biopsy should be performed to provide histologic confirmation. Lymphoepithelial cysts rarely recur.

Torus, Exostosis, and Osteoma (Figs. 80.5–80.8; Figs. 34.1–34.4) Tori, exostoses, and peripheral osteomas are readily recognizable, bony hard nodules that appear histologically identical. The term used depends on location, appearance, and systemic associations.

Tori are bony protuberances of the jaws, localized to the palatal midline or lingual surface of the mandible in the canine-premolar-molar area. They are the most common intraoral lesion. Women are more frequently affected. Tori are hard growths with smooth, rounded contours, normal-appearing or slightly pale mucosa, and a sessile base. They often have a lobulated surface. Internally, they are composed of dense cortical bone with an occasional central core of spongy bone. Hereditary factors contribute to the development of tori.

Exostoses are bony outgrowths in alternate locations of tori. The facial aspects of the maxillary and mandibular alveolar ridge are common sites. Infrequently, the palatal alveolar ridge adjacent to maxillary molars is affected. Most exostoses are multiple hard lobulated nodules. The surface mucosa is firm, taut, and white to pale pink.

Tori and exostoses tend to increase slowly in size with advancing age but remain asymptomatic unless traumatized. After a traumatic incident, patients may be concerned about neoplasia and state that the bony mass is enlarging or that it was not present before the injury. Removal is generally unnecessary unless prompted by cosmetic, prosthodontic, psychological, or traumatic considerations.

Osteomas are benign neoplastic growths that are distinct from the developmental lesions (tori and exostoses) because osteomas have more growth potential, tend to be larger, and may rarely be confined to soft tissue. Almost all osteomas occur in the bones limited to the face and head. Two types are described based on surface of bone from which they arise. Those that arise on the outer surface of the bone are known as **periosteal osteomas** (Figs. 34.3 and 34.4), whereas those arising within medullary bone are **endosteal osteomas**. Both types appear as radiodense structures with well-defined, smooth, and rounded borders. The presence of more than one osteoma dictates that a radiographic examination be performed to see if the patient has multiple impacted supernumerary teeth and odontomas, which is suggestive of **Gardner syndrome** (Figs. 20.7 and 20.8). This inherited condition, associated with a gene abnormality on chromosome 5, is characterized by osteomas, dermal cysts, multiple impacted and supernumerary teeth, odontomas, abnormal retinal pigmentation, and intestinal polyposis. The bowel polyps have a high propensity for malignant transformation. Most patients with Gardner syndrome demonstrate malignant polyposis by age 40; thus, all patients with this condition require close medical management and genetic counseling. In addition, there is an increased risk of thyroid carcinoma in these patients.

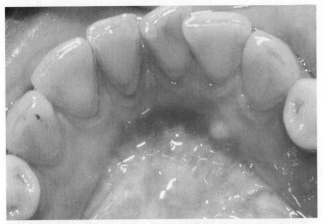

Fig. 80.1. Retrocuspid papilla. Usual pink nodule appearance.

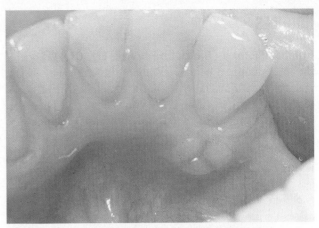

Fig. 80.2. Retrocuspid papilla: with unusual clefting.

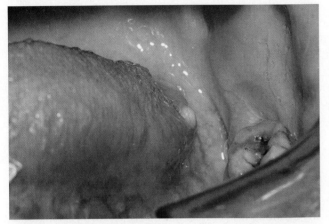

Fig. 80.3. Oral lymphoepithelial cyst: yellow, lateral tongue.

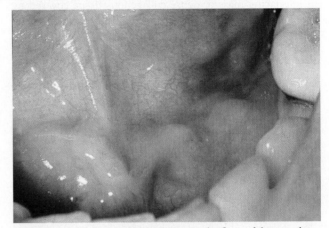

Fig. 80.4. Oral lymphoepithelial cyst: in the floor of the mouth.

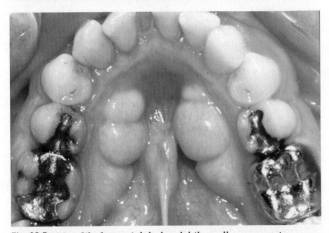

Fig. 80.5. Mandibular tori: lobulated, bilaterally symmetric.

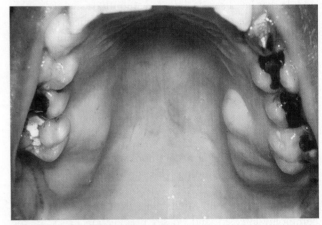

Fig. 80.6. Exostoses: palatal location.

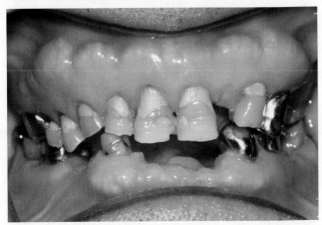

Fig. 80.7. Exostoses: maxilla and mandible.

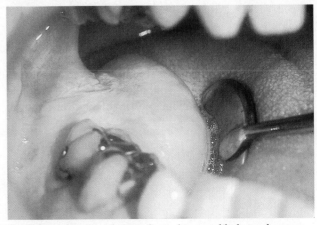

Fig. 80.8. Osteoma: enlarging, lingual to mandibular molars.

NODULES

Irritation Fibroma (Traumatic Fibroma; Fig. 81.1) is one of the most common benign lesions of the oral cavity. It is a reactive **focal fibrous hyperplasia** that arises in response to a chronic irritant; thus, this lesion is not a true neoplasm as the term implies. True intraoral neoplastic fibromas are rare (see below). The **irritation fibroma** appears as a well-defined, pale pink papule that slowly enlarges to form a nodule. It is smooth, symmetrically round, firm, and painless. Infrequently, a white, roughened, or ulcerated surface is present because of repeated trauma. Most occur in adults as sessile growths that arise on the buccal mucosa, labial mucosa, gingiva, or tongue. Histologic examination shows an interlacing mass of dense collagenous tissue covered by thinned epithelium. Fibromas are treated by removing the source of the irritation together with surgical excision. They recur infrequently if treated properly. Multiple intraoral (angio)fibromas, which resemble fibromas, are associated with **tuberous sclerosis**, an autosomal dominant disorder characterized by seizures, mental deficiency, and angiofibromas of the face.

Peripheral odontogenic fibroma is clinically similar to the irritation fibroma but characterized by its unique location and tissue of origin—arising from cells of the periodontal ligament. Accordingly, it is generally found in the region of the interdental papilla. An example is shown in Figure 49.7.

Giant Cell Fibroma (Fig. 81.2) is a painless, pink papule or nodule that has a sessile base and smooth or slightly pebbly surface. Unlike the irritation fibroma, evidence of chronic irritation is generally lacking. The giant cell fibroma has many large, polynucleated stellate-shaped fibroblasts scattered among a loosely arranged vascular connective tissue; the irritation fibroma does not. Most giant cell fibromas occur before 35 years of age on the mandibular gingiva, tongue, or palate. Excision is recommended, and recurrence is rare.

Lipoma (Fig. 81.3) is a common benign dermal tumor, but a rare intraoral finding. This slow-growing neoplasm is composed of mature fat cells surrounded by a thin, fibrous, connective tissue wall. Adults older than 30 years of age are commonly affected, and no sex predilection exists. In the mouth, the **lipoma** presents as a painless, smooth dome-shaped, slightly lobulated, or diffusely elevated nodule that is yellow to pale pink. Sometimes, they are polypoid, pedunculated, or lobulated. Most occur on the buccal mucosa or vestibule. Less common sites include the tongue, floor of the mouth, and lip. The palate is rarely involved (Fig. 63.2). Palpation reveals a doughy soft, movable, and compressible submucosal mass. Treatment consists of surgical removal; recurrence is rare.

Fibrolipoma (Fig. 81.4) is a rare benign intraoral neoplasm of mixed connective tissue origin. It is a well-demarcated submucosal mass consisting of mature lobules of fat cells intermixed with a significant fibrous connective tissue component. Clinical examination shows a blend of a fibroma and lipoma. It is generally found on labial and buccal mucosa as a nonindurated, movable, painless, and soft or firm lesion, depending on the fat-to-collagen content. **Fibrolipomas** grow slowly but can obtain several centimeters in diameter.

Traumatic Neuroma (Figs. 81.5 and 81.6) A **neuroma** is a benign tumor of neural tissue. It arises de novo or as a result of trauma (amputation or traumatic neuroma). The **traumatic neuroma** results from a hyperplastic response to nerve damage after severance of a large nerve fiber. In the mouth, the traumatic neuroma is frequently encountered in the mandibular mucobuccal fold in the region adjacent to the mental foramen. It also arises facial to the mandibular incisors, lingual to the retromolar pad, and in ventral tongue. The size of the lesion depends on the degree of insult and hyperplastic response.

Traumatic neuromas are usually small nodules, measuring less than 0.5 cm in diameter. Visualization may be difficult if the lesion is located deep below the normal oral mucosa. Neuromas are painful when palpated. Pressure applied to the neuroma elicits a response often described as an electric shock. Multiple neuromas discovered on the lips, tongue, or palate may indicate **multiple endocrine neoplasia type 2b**—an autosomal dominant condition characterized by numerous mucosal neuromas, marfanoid body type (thin elongated limbs), and multiple endocrine tumors, especially thyroid cancer. Treatment of the traumatic neuroma is surgical excision or intralesional injection with corticosteroids. Excision may further damage the nerve and lead to recurrence.

Neurofibroma (Figs. 81.7 and 81.8) are benign tumors resulting from proliferation of peripheral nerve components: the Schwann cells and perineural fibroblasts. They commonly appear as sessile, firm, pink nodules. They may be solitary or multiple. Solitary nodules are rare. More commonly, multiple, slowly enlarging neurofibromas are encountered with **neurofibromatosis** (von Recklinghausen disease; see "Swellings of the Face" [Fig. 66.6]).

Intraoral **neurofibromas** usually appear on buccal mucosa, tongue, and lips, and less commonly within bone. Most soft tissue neurofibromas are asymptomatic, but those within deeper tissues or bone may produce pain and paresthesia. Large neurofibromas can be soft and baggy or firm and physically deforming. Within bone, they can expand the inferior alveolar canal (Fig. 39.8A). Solitary neurofibromas have no tendency for malignant transformation, but neurofibromatosis does.

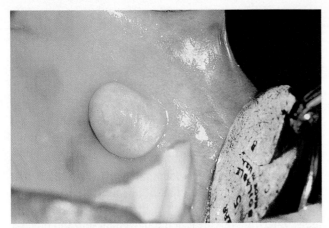

Fig. 81.1. Irritation fibroma: on buccal mucosa.

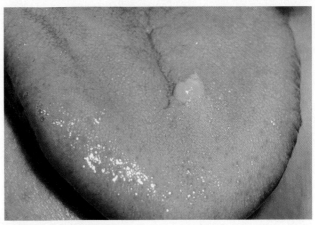

Fig. 81.2. Giant cell fibroma: on dorsum of the tongue.

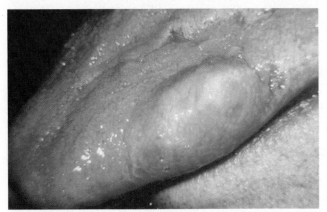

Fig. 81.3. Lipoma: on lateral margin of the tongue.

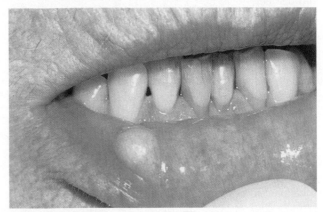

Fig. 81.4. Fibrolipoma: on labial mucosa.

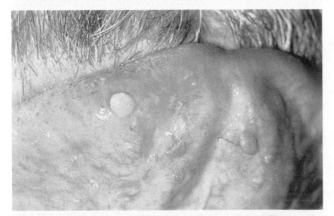

Fig. 81.5. Traumatic neuroma: near midline and a papilloma.

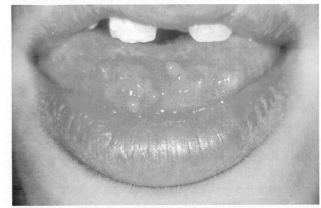

Fig. 81.6. Neuromas of multiple endocrine neoplasia.

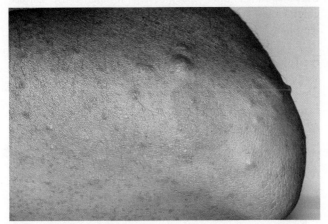

Fig. 81.7. Neurofibromatosis: multiple tumors, café au lait spot.

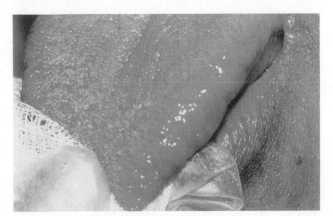

Fig. 81.8. Neurofibroma: nodule on lateral tongue.

10

PAPULONODULES

Oral Squamous Papilloma (Papilloma) (Figs. 82.1 and 82.2)

is the most common benign epithelial neoplasm of the oral cavity. They appear as small, pink-white, painless, exophytic masses that are usually less than 1 cm in diameter. The surface of the **papilloma** may be smooth, pink, and pebbly (vegetative) or have numerous small fingerlike projections. The base is pedunculated and well delineated. Intraoral lesions are typically soft, whereas keratin-producing lesions are rough or scaly. Lesions are generally solitary, but multiple lesions are occasionally seen. Human papillomavirus (HPV) types 6 and 11 have been detected in more than 50% of papillomas examined and are generally accepted as the cause of this disease.

The mean age of occurrence of papilloma is 35 years; both sexes are affected equally. Most occur on the palate, uvula, tongue, frenum, lips, buccal mucosa, and gingiva. Other HPV-induced lesions, such as the condyloma acuminatum, focal epithelial hyperplasia (Heck disease), and verruca vulgaris, share similar clinical features but are microscopically distinct. Histologic features of the squamous papilloma include fingerlike epithelial projections and a fibrovascular core. Treatment is complete excision, including the base. Recurrence is rare. If left untreated, they can enlarge, spread to other sites, and serve to transmit HPV to other persons. Malignant transformation does not occur.

Verruca Vulgaris (Fig. 82.3)

is the common skin *wart* that seldom occurs intraorally. When present, it is most frequently seen in children or young adults. The etiologic agents of **verruca vulgaris** are HPV types 2, 4, 6, 11, and 40. Virally induced cellular changes result in the characteristic clinical findings. The lesional surface is typically rough and raised, with white fingerlike projections. The whiteness of intraoral verrucae varies, depending on the amount of surface keratinization. Pink areas are not unusual at the lesional base. Verrucae are contagious and commonly located on the skin, lip, labial/buccal mucosa, tongue, and attached gingiva. The base of the lesion is broad, but the size is usually less than 1 cm. On clinical examination, it may appear identical to a papilloma, although the clefts are more shallow and the mass more sessile. Viral inclusion bodies and elongated rete ridges that converge toward the center of the lesion are frequently seen on histologic examination. Patients with skin verrucae are more likely to have oral lesions as a result of autoinoculation. A lesion may sometimes regress spontaneously. If not, treatment is effective by excision, laser removal, cryosurgery, or chemical applications. Recurrence is possible.

Focal Epithelial Hyperplasia (Heck Disease) (Fig 82.4)

is a virus-induced disease associated with multiple asymptomatic, papulonodular growths of the oral mucosa, particularly the tongue and labial and buccal mucosa. It was first described in Native Americans and Eskimos but now has been reported in many populations. The etiologic agents are HPV types 13 and 32. The virus is transmitted during kissing. Virus replication in epithelial cells produces soft papular growths in children and teenagers. Lesions are initially small, discrete, flat papules that are pink or whitish pink. Later lesions enlarge, become papillary or cobblestoned, and can coalesce. Some lesions undergo spontaneous regression; surgical excision can be performed for those that do not regress.

Condyloma Acuminatum (Venereal Wart) (Figs. 82.5 and 82.6)

is a venereal disease that occurs much less frequently in and around the mouth than the papilloma. The warm, moist, intertriginous areas of the anogenital skin and mucosa are frequent sites of this transmissible papillomatous growth. In more than 85% of cases, HPV types 6 and 11 DNA are present in the epithelium. The virus is transmitted by sexual and oral contact.

Condyloma acuminata is usually small, pink to dirty gray, solitary or multiple growths. The surface is often pebbly, resembling a cauliflower, but may be flat. The base is sessile, and the borders are raised and rounded. When multiple lesions are present, proliferation of adjacent condylomas can form extensive clusters that may appear as a single mass. Any oral mucosal surface may be affected, but the labial mucosa is the most common site. Other sites include the tongue, lingual frenum, gingiva, and soft palate. Histologic examination shows parakeratosis, cryptic invagination of cornified cells, and koilocytosis. Wide excision or antiviral agents are used in treatment, as condylomata have a high rate of recurrence. Occasional oncogenic transformation of long-standing anogenital growths has been reported, but this is not the case with oral lesions.

Lymphangioma (Figs. 82.7 and 82.8)

is a collection of lymph vessels (benign hamartomas) that are overgrown and clumped together. **Lymphangiomas** develop early in life with no sex predilection. They may occur on the skin or mucous membrane. In the oral cavity, they occur commonly in the dorsal and lateral surface of the anterior portion of the tongue, lips, and labial mucosa.

Small superficial lymphangiomas have irregular papillary projections that resemble a papilloma. They are soft and compressible and vary from normal pink to whitish, slightly translucent, or blue. Deep-seated lesions cause diffuse enlargement and stretching of the surface mucosa. A diffuse lymphangioma in the tongue can cause **macroglossia**; in the lips, it can cause **macrocheilia**; and in the neck, it is called a **cystic hygroma**. Aspiration or diascopy is mandatory before surgical excision of a lymphangioma to prevent complications associated with the similar-appearing hemangioma. Patients with a large, diffuse lesion often require hospitalization to monitor postoperative edema and possible airway obstruction. Lymphangiomas do not undergo malignant change. Some lymphangiomas, especially congenital types, regress spontaneously during childhood.

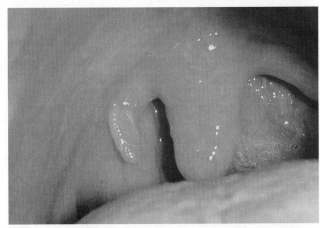

Fig. 82.1. Oral squamous papilloma: on soft palate.

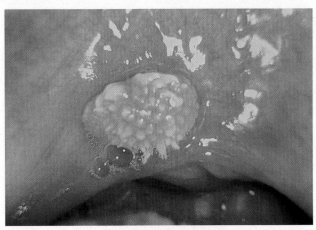

Fig. 82.2. Papilloma: with fingerlike projections.

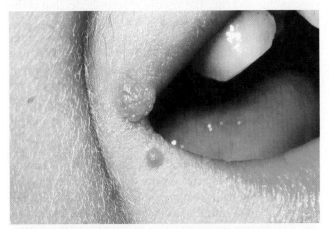

Fig. 82.3. Verruca vulgaris: autoinoculation from fingers.

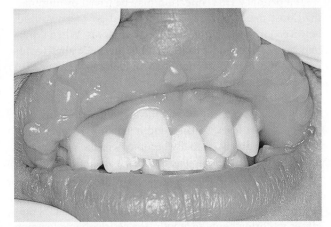

Fig. 82.4. Focal epithelial hyperplasia: multiple on labial mucosa.

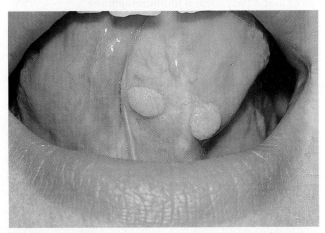

Fig. 82.5. Condyloma acuminata: on ventral tongue.

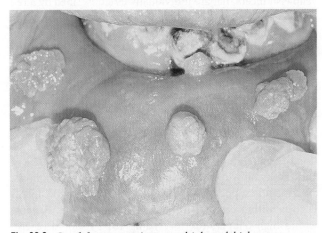

Fig. 82.6. Condyloma acuminata: multiple on labial mucosa.

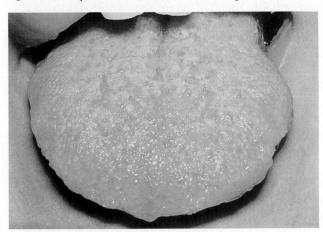

Fig. 82.7. Lymphangioma: causing macroglossia.*

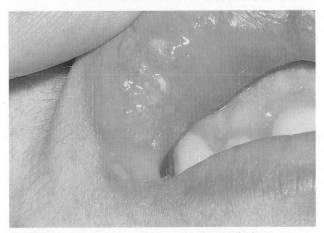

Fig. 82.8. Lymphangioma: pebbly, pink-white in the lip.*

183

VESICULOBULLOUS LESIONS

Primary Herpetic Gingivostomatitis (Figs. 83.1–83.3)

Herpes simplex virus (HSV) types 1 and 2 belong to the family Herpesviridae, which includes eight DNA viruses (cytomegalovirus, varicella-zoster virus, Epstein-Barr, and human herpesvirus types 6, 7, and 8). Approximately 75% to 90% of the adult human population has been infected with HSV. Transmission occurs by contact of infected oral secretions with the mucosa or skin of a susceptible person. In most cases of primary infection, HSV-1 is the causative organism; however, HSV-2, which has a propensity to infect the skin below the waist, can cause herpetic gingivostomatitis by oral-genital or oral-oral contact.

The primary HSV infection may be trivial or fulminating. Most infections are subclinical and go unrecognized, however a minority produce flulike symptoms. When symptomatic, the infection is called primary herpetic gingivostomatitis. It occurs most commonly in children younger than 10 years and second most commonly in young adults. The acute inflammatory response of the primary HSV infection usually follows a 2- to 10-day incubation period. Infected patients report fever, malaise, and irritability. Focal areas of the marginal gingiva initially become fiery red and edematous. The interdental papillae abruptly swell and bleed after minute trauma because of capillary fragility and increased permeability. Widespread inflammation of the marginal and attached gingiva develops, and small clusters of vesicles rapidly erupt throughout the mouth. The vesicles burst, forming yellowish ulcers that are individually circumscribed by a red halo. Coalescence of adjacent lesions forms large ulcers of the buccal mucosa, labial mucosa, gingiva, palate, tongue, and lips. Shallow erosions of the perioral skin and hemorrhagic crusts of the lips are characteristics. Headache, lymphadenopathy, and pharyngitis are common, especially in persons infected with HSV-2.

Pain is a significant problem in patients with primary herpetic gingivostomatitis. Mastication and swallowing may be impaired, resulting in dehydration and subsequent elevation of temperature. Viral culturing, serum antibody levels, and results of cytologic testing are helpful in the diagnosis. Treatment is supportive and should include antiviral agents if given within the first few days of disease onset. Patients with a high temperature (exceeding 101°F) should receive nonaspirin antipyretic drugs and antibiotics.

Primary herpetic gingivostomatitis is a contagious disease that usually regresses spontaneously within 12 to 20 days without scarring. Complications associated with the primary infection include autoinoculation of other epidermal sites, producing keratoconjunctivitis (eye) and herpetic whitlow (finger); extensive epidermal infection in the atopic patient, which is called Kaposi varicelliform eruption; and disseminated infections in immunosuppressed patients. Immunity to HSV is relative, and patients previously infected with the virus may be reinfected with a different strain of HSV.

Recurrent Herpes Simplex Infection (Figs. 83.4–83.7)

After the acute infection, HSV infects sensory nerve endings, migrates to regional sensory ganglia, and enters latency within infected neurons. Reactivation of virus and clinical recurrences develop in about 40% of persons who harbor latent virus. Recurrences are often precipitated by sunlight, heat, stress, trauma (dental procedures), or immunosuppression. Normal immune mechanisms are required to eliminate reactivated HSV. Asymptomatic shedding of virus into saliva in the absence of oral lesions occurs in 10% of the population on any given day.

Recurrent herpes simplex infection produces clusters of vesicles that ulcerate. The vesicles repeatedly develop at the same site, following the distribution of the infected nerve. Recurrences on the vermilion border of the lip (recurrent herpes labialis) are clinically more apparent than intraoral recurrences (recurrent herpetic stomatitis). The lesions of recurrent herpes labialis appear as a small cluster of vesicles that erupt, coalesce, ulcerate, form a scab, and heal without scarring. Spread to perioral skin is common, especially with the use of greasy lip ointments that permit horizontal weeping of vesicular fluid. Contact of vesicular fluid at other epidermal sites can result in spread of the infection. In relatively healthy persons, recurrent herpetic stomatitis produces small ulcers with red halos that are limited to periosteal-bound, keratinized mucosa (i.e., the attached gingiva and hard palate). Recurrences on the buccal mucosa and tongue are infrequent unless the patient is immunosuppressed.

Most patients with recurrent herpes simplex report pain and tenderness of affected tissues. Prodromal neurogenic symptoms, such as tingling, throbbing, and burning, often precede the eruption of lesions by 6 to 24 hours. Sunscreens are effective in the prevention of lip and skin recurrences. Management also includes lysine, desiccating agents, and antiviral drugs (acyclovir, famciclovir, penciclovir, and valacyclovir). Patients should be informed that lesions are contagious and that their saliva is contaminated with virus.

Herpangina (Fig. 83.8)

is a highly contagious but self-limiting infection involving the oral cavity that is caused by group A and sometimes group B coxsackieviruses and echovirus. The disease is spread by infected saliva. Herpangina is seen mainly in children during the warmer months of summer and early fall. Young adults are occasionally affected. It produces a small number of light-gray papillary vesicles that rupture to form discrete, shallow ulcers. The ulcers have an erythematous border and are limited to the posterior oral cavity (tonsillar pillars, soft palate, uvula). Diffuse pharyngeal erythema, dysphagia, and sore throat are common features, as are fever, malaise, headache, lymphadenitis, abdominal pain, and vomiting. Convulsions rarely occur. Treatment is palliative, and spontaneous healing occurs within 7 to 10 days.

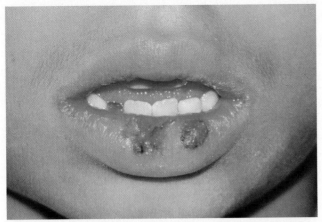

Fig. 83.1. **Primary herpetic gingivostomatitis:** in a 7-year-old.*

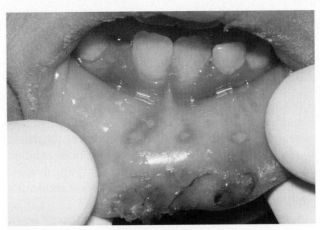

Fig. 83.2. **Primary herpetic gingivostomatitis.***

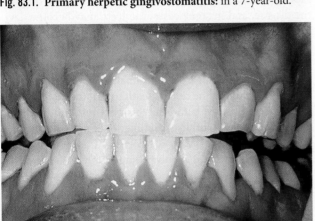

Fig. 83.3. **Primary herpetic gingivitis:** a 27-year-old man.

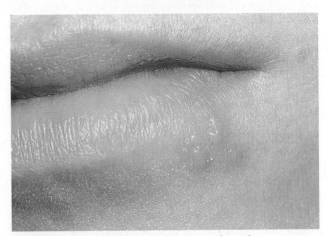

Fig. 83.4. **Recurrent herpes labialis:** clustered vesicles.

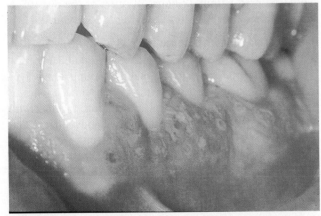

Fig. 83.5. **Recurrent herpes simplex:** multiple gingival ulcers.

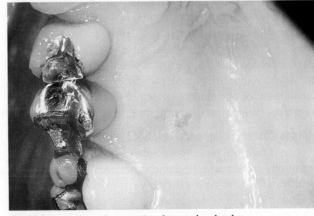

Fig. 83.6. **Recurrent herpes simplex:** on hard palate.

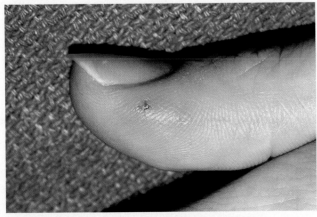

Fig. 83.7. **Herpetic whitlow:** caused by autoinoculation.

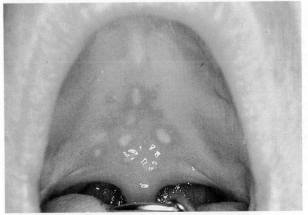

Fig. 83.8. **Herpangina:** multiple, soft palate ulcers and redness.

10

185

Varicella (Chickenpox) (Figs. 84.1 and 84.2) Varicella and herpes zoster are caused by the same virus, varicella-zoster virus (VZV)—a type of human herpesvirus. **Varicella** (chickenpox) is the highly contagious primary infection transmitted by aerosolized nasopharyngeal droplets; **herpes zoster (shingles)** is the recurrent neurodermal infection. Unvaccinated persons are susceptible. Typically, children become infected during the late winter and spring months. After exposure to the virus and a 2- to 3-week incubation period, mild prodromal features appear.

Chickenpox is usually a mild childhood illness. Fever, malaise, and a distinctive red and very itchy rash on the face and trunk are the first recognizable signs of the disease. The pruritic rash spreads quickly to the neck and extremities and is followed shortly by the eruption of papules that form vesicles and pustules. On bursting, the pus-laden vesicles have the appearance of a dewdrop on a rose petal. The first and largest skin lesion is called the *herald spot*. It is often located on the face and, if scratched, may heal with scarring. Infected persons are contagious from 2 days before the rash appears until all lesions crust over.

Intraoral lesions of varicella are few and often go unnoticed. They appear as vesicular lesions that break down and form ulcers with an erythematous halo. The soft palate is the predominant site, followed by the buccal mucosa and mucobuccal fold. Anorexia, fever, chills, headache, nasopharyngitis, and muscle aches may accompany the condition. Complications such as pneumonitis and encephalitis are infrequent. Infections are worse in adults and immunosuppressed persons. In the United States, about 100 people die each year as a result of complications. In the majority, vesicles typically crust over and resolve spontaneously within 7 to 10 days. Infection during pregnancy poses a significant risk to the fetus. A live-attenuated two-dose vaccine (Varivax) is recommended for infants between 12 and 18 months to prevent the development of chickenpox.

Herpes Zoster (Shingles) (Figs. 84.3 and 84.4) is the recurrent infection of chickenpox. Suppression of cell-mediated immunity associated with aging, cancer, and stress results in reactivation of dormant varicella virus from sensory ganglia and migration of virus along the affected sensory nerves. The prevalence of **shingles** increases with age, with up to 30% of the population being affected, usually after age 50. Rarely, young adults or children are affected. Before eruption, prodromal signs of itching, tingling, burning, pain, or paresthesia occur. Lesions are characterized by acutely painful vesicular eruptions of the skin and mucosa that are unilaterally distributed along one dermatome and stop abruptly at the midline. The skin lesions begin as itchy erythematous macules that become vesicular and pustular eruptions. Crust formation occurs within 7 to 10 days and persists for several weeks. The pain is intense but usually dissipates after crusts

fall off. Two areas most affected are (1) the trunk between vertebrae T3 and L2 and (2) the face along the ophthalmic division of the trigeminal nerve.

Intraoral lesions (also see Fig. 93.3) appear as clusters of vesicles that ulcerate with an intense red border. Within several days, a yellowish surface slough forms, and zones of bleeding occur. Involvement of the mandibular branch of the trigeminal nerve results in ulcers of the lips, tongue, and buccal mucosa that extend to the midline. Involvement of the maxillary nerve branch typically produces unilateral palatal ulcerations that extend up to but not beyond the palatal raphe. Considerable malaise, fever, and distress accompany the disease, and in some cases, the teeth may become devitalized or bone necrosis can result.

Herpes zoster usually heals without scar formation in about 3 weeks. However, scarring can occur, and many patients may experience persistent pain after the lesions have faded. This condition, called **postherpetic neuralgia**, may continue for months before regressing. Immunosuppressed patients are particularly susceptible to shingles and have a high morbidity rate. Varicella-zoster virus infection that causes unilateral facial paralysis and involves the auditory nerves (ear eruptions) is known as **Ramsay Hunt syndrome**. The disease can be associated with **Reye syndrome** (high fever, cerebral edema, liver degeneration, high mortality) if salicylates are used to manage the disease in children. Antiviral agents, such as famciclovir (Famvir) and valacyclovir (Valtrex), block varicella-zoster virus replication and should be used within 72 hours of onset of the disease. A vaccine is recommended for those over age 50 years.

Hand-Foot-and-Mouth Disease (Figs. 84.5–84.8) is a mildly contagious disease caused by many Coxsackie A and B viruses. It usually affects children and sometimes young adults, typically during spring and summer. As the name implies, it produces small ulcerative lesions in the mouth together with an erythematous rash on the skin of the hands, fingers, and soles of the feet. Rarely, the legs and lower trunk are involved. Multiple pinpoint vesicles that ulcerate and crust are characteristic. Patients may have several to more than 100 pinpoint lesions with distinctive erythematous halos.

Oral lesions of **hand-foot-and-mouth** disease are scattered mainly on the tongue, hard palate, and buccal and labial mucosa. In time, they coalesce to form large eroded areas. Unlike herpangina, the oropharynx is usually unaffected, and the total number of intraoral lesions ranges up to 30. Pain and flulike symptoms (fever, malaise, and lymphadenopathy) are common, along with cough, anorexia, vomiting, and diarrhea. The diagnosis can be made by viral culture and serum antibody studies. However, the classic distribution of lesions on the palms of hands, soles of feet, and oral mucosa is diagnostic in most instances. Healing occurs regardless of treatment in about 10 days.

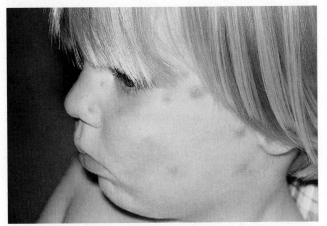

Fig. 84.1. **Varicella (chickenpox):** herald spot lateral to eye.

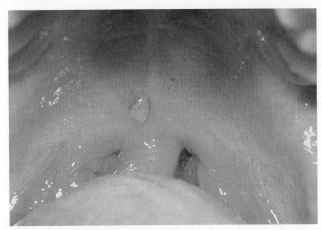

Fig. 84.2. **Varicella (chickenpox):** vesicle near midline.

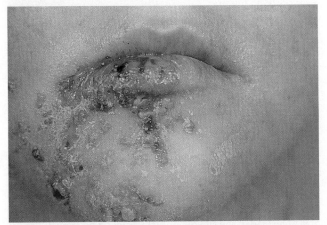

Fig. 84.3. **Herpes zoster (shingles):** mandibular eruption.*

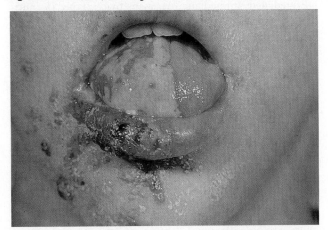

Fig. 84.4. **Herpes zoster (shingles):** painful oral lesions.*

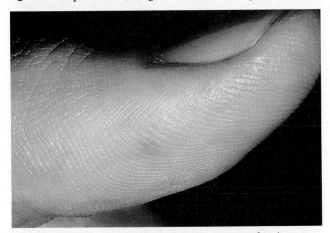

Fig. 84.5. **Hand-foot-and-mouth disease:** pinpoint ulcer.‡

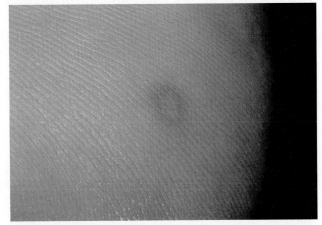

Fig. 84.6. **Hand-foot-and-mouth disease:** foot ulcer.‡

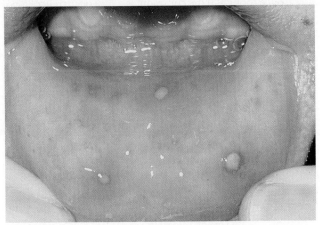

Fig. 84.7. **Hand-foot-and-mouth disease:** labial ulcers.

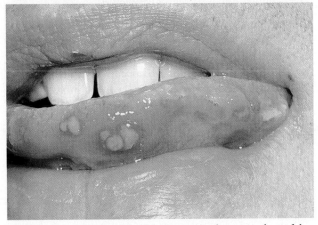

Fig. 84.8. **Hand-foot-and-mouth disease:** coalescing and painful.

10

187

VESICULOBULLOUS LESIONS

Allergic Reactions (Figs. 85.1–85.8)

Allergy is an abnormal or hypersensitive response of the immune system to a usually harmless substance in the environment, such as mold or pollen. These reactions are acquired by repeated exposure to an allergen, which results in inappropriate tissue damage from antigen-antibody reactions. Manifestations may be generalized or localized and occur at any age. A genetic predisposition is common.

Hypersensitivity reactions are classified into several types according to the following factors: the speed with which the symptoms occur (immediate or delayed), clinical appearance, and cellular and tissue response (**type I**, IgE-mediated immediate hypersensitivity; **type II**, antibody-dependent cytotoxic hypersensitivity; **type III**, complex-mediated hypersensitivity; and **type IV**, cell-mediated, or delayed, hypersensitivity). Reactions of dental significance include immediate type I reactions (anaphylactic shock, urticaria, angioneurotic edema, allergic stomatitis) and delayed type IV reactions (contact allergy).

Localized Anaphylaxis (Figs. 85.1 and 85.2)

is an immediate allergic response mediated by IgE and histamine that occurs within minutes of exposure to an antigen. **Localized anaphylaxis** produces vasodilation and increased permeability of superficial blood vessels, tissue swelling, and pruritus. The localized form manifests as wheals, urticaria, or hives that arise after the ingestion of such foods as shellfish, citrus fruits, peanuts, chocolate, or systemically administered drugs.

Generalized Anaphylaxis is a rapid and potentially life-threatening allergic (type I hypersensitivity) reaction. This sudden systemic reaction causes constriction of the airways, resulting in difficulty breathing or even unconsciousness and death. It results from an antigen-antibody (IgE) interaction that results in mast cell degranulation and the release of vasoactive amines and mediators such as histamine. In severe cases, a generalized increase in vascular permeability and smooth muscle contraction causes urticaria, dyspnea, hypotension, airway edema, and vascular collapse. Mild localized immediate hypersensitivity reactions are treated with antihistamines. Epinephrine 1:1,000 (0.3 to 0.5 mL, subcutaneously) and airway management is required to effectively manage severe reactions. Treatment should always target elimination of the causative allergen.

Allergic Stomatitis (Fig. 85.3)

also called **allergic mucositis**, is an oral type I hypersensitivity reaction to a systemically administered drug or food. The oral manifestations (eruptions) of **allergic stomatitis** occur rapidly but are varied in appearance. Some resemble erythema multiforme or lichen planus. In the mouth, a dry, glistening, red area is usually apparent. Focal white areas may be adjacent. Multiple vesicles form that break down and produce fibrin-covered ulcers. The ulcers have red, inflammatory borders and are painful or burn. The reaction may be limited to the buccal/labial mucosa, gingiva, lips, or tongue or may involve the entire oral cavity. Concurrent dermal lesions are possible. Treatment requires withdrawal of the allergen and administration of antihistamines.

Angioedema (see Figs. 61.1, 61.2, and 67.1)

is a swelling within the tissues usually occurring around the eyes and lips. Angioedema results from a hypersensitivity reaction brought about by histamine-induced vascular leakage. Hereditary and acquired forms exist. The hereditary form, caused by activation of complement, is more serious. Both forms are characterized by swelling that rapidly appears and lasts for 24 to 36 hours. Sensations of warmth, tenseness, and itchiness are concurrent. See "Swellings of the Lip" (Fig. 61.1) and "Swellings and Nerve Weakness of the Face" (Fig. 67.1) for a full discussion.

Delayed Hypersensitivity (Figs. 85.4 and 85.5)

or type IV hypersensitivity is a response of the immune system to a locally or systemically introduced allergen that usually develops slowly and reaches its maximum 24 to 48 hours after antigenic exposure. Topically applied allergens, such as latex gloves or chemical disinfectants, may produce a delayed hypersensitivity response evident as itchy, erythematous skin lesions (contact dermatitis) that eventually become inflamed and ulcerated at the site of contact. **Delayed hypersensitivity** is treated with corticosteroids and avoidance of the allergen.

Contact Stomatitis (Figs. 85.6 and 85.7)

is a form of type IV delayed hypersensitivity that is due to T-cell attack. It produces erythema at the site of contact with the allergen. Reactions to lipstick or sunscreens may cause the lips to burn and appear red, swollen, fissured, or dry. Toothpastes, mouthwashes, antibiotic lozenges, topical anesthetics, and eugenol preparations can cause diffuse reactions. Intraoral lesions typically appear on the alveolar mucosa, dorsum of the tongue, or palate as erythematous ulcers that are covered by a gray-white pseudomembrane. Cast alloy restorations and partial denture frameworks that contain heavy metals (cobalt, mercury, nickel, or silver) can induce **contact stomatitis** reactions of the mucosa adjacent to the restored area. The area is usually red and ulcerated and often burns. Allergy to the free monomer in dentures, once thought to be common, is a rare occurrence.

Plasma Cell Gingivitis (Fig. 85.8)

affects the gingiva, producing diffusely edematous and fiery red gingiva because of the flavoring ingredients (such as cinnamon) in some toothpastes and chewing gums. The lips and commissures are frequently involved, resulting in cheilitis. Microscopy shows tissue infiltrated with plasma cells, a type of differentiated B cell that produces antibodies. Withdrawal of the causative agent is curative.

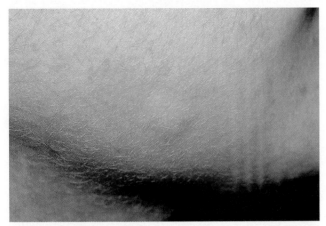

Fig. 85.1. **Immediate (type 1) hypersensitivity:** facial wheal.

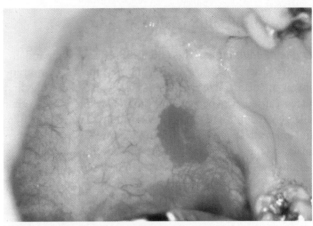

Fig. 85.2. **Immediate (type 1) hypersensitivity:** bee sting.

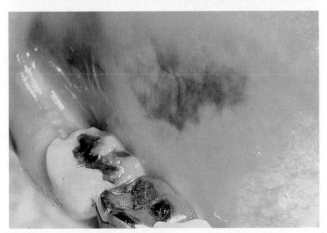

Fig. 85.3. **Immediate (type 1) hypersensitivity:** penicillin.

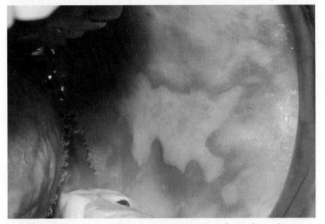

Fig. 85.4. **Delayed (type IV) hypersensitivity:** from thiazide.

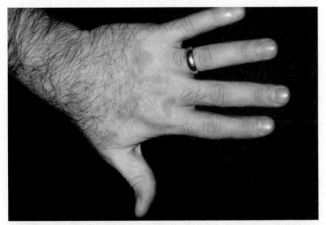

Fig. 85.5. **Delayed (type IV) hypersensitivity:** latex allergy.

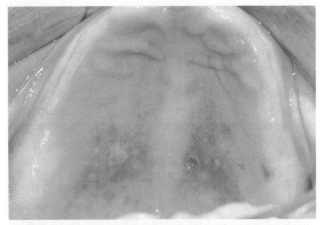

Fig. 85.6. **Delayed (type IV) hypersensitivity:** benzocaine.

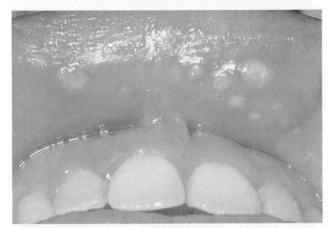

Fig. 85.7. **Delayed (type IV) hypersensitivity:** alloy contact.

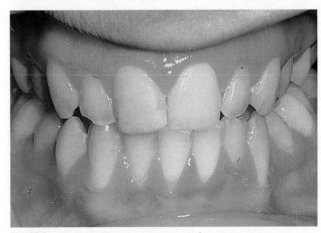

Fig. 85.8. **Plasma cell gingivitis:** type IV hypersensitivity.

10

VESICULOBULLOUS LESIONS

Erythema Multiforme (Figs. 86.1–86.4) is an acute inflammatory disease of varied skin and/or mucous membrane involvement characterized by red target-shaped macules and ulcers caused by hypersensitivity to a drug, microbe, or other allergen. It commonly affects young adults, particularly men, but may affect children and the elderly. Low-grade fever, malaise, and headache typically precede the emergence of lesions by 3 to 7 days. Most cases of erythema multiforme are the result of an immunological response to drug administration, especially drugs containing sulfa (antibiotics or hypoglycemic agents) or barbiturates. Other cases are precipitated by radiation, infections with herpes simplex virus or *Mycoplasma pneumoniae*, or an unidentified allergen. Immune complexes form that settle in small blood vessels, resulting in perivascular inflammation and necrosis of the epithelium.

Erythema multiforme can be classified into four types according to its spectrum of clinical presentations. These are discussed below.

Oral Erythema Multiforme (Fig. 86.1) is the minimal manifestation of erythema multiforme. It is usually limited to the gingiva, but eruptions may also affect the tongue, lips, or palate. A history of infection or drug therapy is common. Constitutional symptoms such as anorexia, malaise, and low-grade fever may or may not be present. As the name multiforme (*many forms*) suggests, the lesions have a *varied appearance*. Affected gingiva appears fiery red, similar to the appearance of desquamative gingivitis; mucosal surfaces of the tongue and lips often show diffuse red patches with zones of ulceration. The borders of lesions are irregular (wavy) and red but seldom hemorrhagic, as is seen in pemphigoid and pemphigus.

Erythema Multiforme (Figs. 86.2–86.4) The hallmarks of classic erythema multiforme are the red-white, concentric, ringlike macules termed *target, bull's-eye,* or *iris lesions* that rapidly appear on the extremities (arms, legs, knees, and palms of the hands). The trunk of the body is classically exempt from lesions, except in the most severe cases. The skin lesions are initially small, dusky red, circular macules that vary in size from 0.5 to 2.0 cm in diameter. The macules then enlarge and develop a pale white or central clear area. Shortly thereafter, the lesions slightly elevate and become urticarial plaques that form vesicles and bullae. The vesicles may go unnoticed until they rupture and become confluent, forming large, raw, and shallow ulcers with erythematous borders. A necrotic slough and a yellowish fibrin pseudomembrane typically cover the ulcers.

In the mouth, red macular areas, multiple ulcerations, and erosions with a gray-white fibrinous surface may be seen. These are generally limited to the buccal mucosa, labial mucosa, or tongue or involve all of those areas. The gingiva and palate are sometimes involved. Dark red-brown, hemorrhagic (bloody) crusts are characteristically present on the lips, which helps establish the diagnosis. Lesions are usually short-lived and last about 2 weeks. Erythema multiforme rarely persists for more than 1 month. About 20% of patients experience recurrent episodes and chronic disease.

Pain is the most common symptom. Oral hygiene may be neglected, resulting in secondary bacterial infection. Treatment consists of topical palliative rinses and, in some instances, systemic corticosteroids. If a viral infection precedes the episode, antiviral therapy is provided. Evidence of a drug trigger dictates that drug administration be stopped. Complications resulting from erythema multiforme are uncommon unless the disease progresses to its major form, Stevens-Johnson syndrome.

Stevens-Johnson Syndrome (Erythema Multiforme Major) (Figs. 86.5–86.7) A severe form of erythema multiforme is termed erythema multiforme major or Stevens-Johnson syndrome, named for the two investigators who first described the appearance of the disease in the early 1920s. It frequently affects children and young adults, predominantly men. Stevens-Johnson syndrome is typically triggered by a drug and is characterized by skin detachment of up to 10% of body surface area. Both cutaneous and oral structures are involved, and constitutional signs such as fever, malaise, headache, chest pain, diarrhea, vomiting, and arthralgia are concurrent.

The classic clinical triad of Stevens-Johnson syndrome consists of *ocular (conjunctivitis), oral (stomatitis), and genital lesions (balanitis, vulvovaginitis).* Other features include characteristic target skin lesions on the face, chest, and abdomen that later develop into painful weeping bullae. Like erythema multiforme, the gingiva is less commonly affected by desquamating bullae than is the nonkeratinized mucosa. Extensive ulcerative and hemorrhagic lesions of the lips and denuded areas of oral mucosa are intensely painful and usually prevent affected patients from eating and swallowing. Inadequate nutritional intake, dehydration, and debilitation are common sequelae that necessitate rehydration and hospitalization. Healing takes about 6 weeks.

Toxic Epidermal Necrolysis (Fig. 86.8) is the most severe form of erythema multiforme. By definition, toxic epidermal necrolysis involves skin detachment of greater than 30% of the body surface area. Its occurrence is rare, and most cases are associated with drug therapy. Unlike other forms of erythema multiforme, older persons are most commonly affected, especially women. The condition primarily affects the skin, eyes, and oral mucosa. Large areas of the skin are severely affected with coalescing bullae that slough, leaving huge areas of denuded skin. Management is similar to that of a burn patient. Significant morbidity will occur if supportive therapy is not promptly initiated. Treatment consists of intravenous fluid, nutritional therapy, corticosteroids, anesthetic and antiseptic rinses, and prevention of secondary infection with antibiotics. Affected areas take weeks to heal, and permanent eye damage is a frequent outcome. Both Stevens-Johnson syndrome and toxic epidermal necrolysis have been fatal.

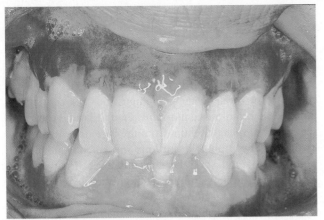

Fig. 86.1. **Oral erythema multiforme:** gingival involvement.

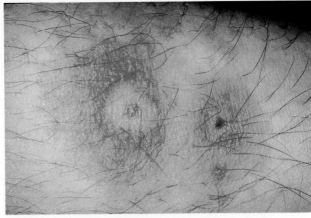

Fig. 86.2. **Erythema multiforme:** classic target skin lesions.

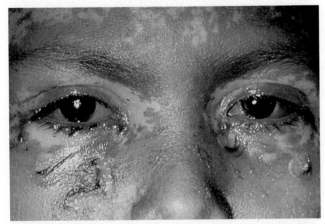

Fig. 86.3. **Erythema multiforme:** hemorrhagic lip crusts.

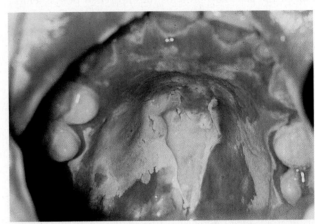

Fig. 86.4. **Erythema multiforme:** erythema and ulceration.

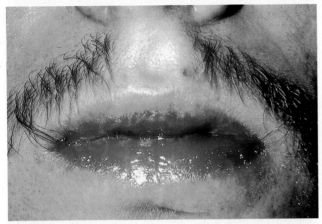

Fig. 86.5. **Stevens-Johnson syndrome:** eye, skin involvement.

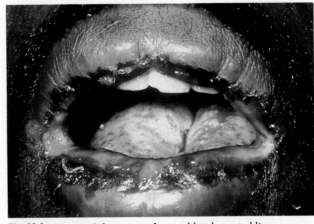

Fig. 86.6. **Stevens-Johnson syndrome:** blood-crusted lips.

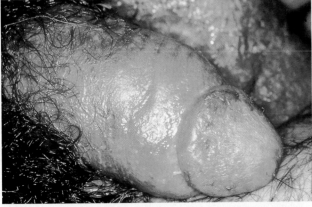

Fig. 86.7. **Stevens-Johnson syndrome:** genital involvement.*

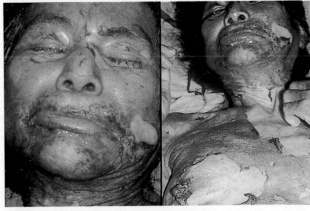

Fig. 86.8. **Toxic epidermal necrolysis:** life threatening.

191

Pemphigus Vulgaris (Figs. 87.1–87.4) is a potentially fatal, autoimmune skin disease that often causes large bullae (blisters) and erosions of the skin and mucous membranes. Four types have been described: *vulgaris* and *vegetans*, which have intraoral manifestations, and *foliaceous* and *erythematosus*, which generally do not. **Pemphigus vulgaris**, the most common intraoral type, develops more often in women between 40 and 60 years of age and in light-pigmented patients of Jewish or Mediterranean origin. It is infrequent in children and the elderly. Acute and chronic forms exist; the slow chronic form is more common.

Pemphigus vulgaris is caused by autoantibody destruction of the adhesion proteins (desmogleins) of epithelium that compose the desmosome. Desmosomes are the intercellular gluelike substance that holds epithelial cells together. Autoantibody destruction of desmogleins (types 3 and 1) causes cell-to-cell separation (*acantholysis*), particularly the basal cell layer from the overlying stratum spinosum. Events that induce autoantibody production (antidesmoglein 3 IgG) are unknown, but occasionally are induced by drugs (e.g., penicillamine, ACE inhibitors). Destruction of the attachment proteins produces *intraepithelial splitting* or blisters (bullae) that rupture, quickly leaving painful erosions of skin and oral mucosa. Lesions develop rapidly and form weeping bullae or clear gelatinous plaques (a collapsed bulla). The bullae are extremely fragile and rapidly disintegrate, bleed, and crust. They tend to recur and spread. Light lateral pressure applied to a bulla causes the blister to enlarge by extension (the **Nikolsky sign**). A characteristic mucosal finding is the appearance of a whitish superficial covering, which is the roof of a collapsed bulla that can be easily stripped away.

Pemphigus may appear as sloughing or folded epithelium, a flaccid blister, an ulcer, or multiple, large irregular ulcers. Most often, the buccal mucosa, gingiva, palate, floor of the mouth, and lips are involved. Less frequently, the tongue and oropharynx are affected. Individual lesions have circular or serpiginous borders, whereas extensive erosions of the buccal mucosa appear red and raw and have diffuse irregular borders. New eruptions may superimpose over healing lesions so periods of remission are absent. Fetor oris (bad odor), hemorrhagic lip crusts, and severe pain are characteristic.

The diagnosis of pemphigus is made by positive Nikolsky sign, biopsy, and immunofluorescent staining. Early recognition of oral lesions, which precede skin involvement by several months in more than half the cases, is important because early diagnosis greatly enhances the initiation of treatment and the prognosis. Remission and control are gained with the use of corticosteroid and immunosuppressive agents. Dehydration and septicemia are potentially fatal complications. A small percentage of cases are associated with an underlying neoplasm such as a lymphoma or leukemia, which induce autoantibodies and **paraneoplastic pemphigus**.

Pemphigoid (Figs. 87.5–87.8) is a chronic, self-limiting, autoimmune subepithelial blistering disease of older adults that involves the oral cavity in about 90% of cases. It is more common intraorally than pemphigus, but associated with much less morbidity and mortality. **Pemphigoid** is caused by separation of the epithelium from the basement membrane. Two types of pemphigoid (**bullous and mucous membrane pemphigoid**) and several subgroups exist. They produce identical oral lesions and are distinguished by clinical and immunohistologic features.

In **bullous pemphigoid**, the less common of the two, skin lesions predominate over oral lesions. Skin folds of the axilla, inguinal, and abdominal regions are commonly affected. **Mucous membrane pemphigoid**, also historically called **cicatricial pemphigoid**, is more common and is characterized by lesions predominantly of mucous membranes, particularly the ocular and oral mucosa. It occurs twice as frequently in women as men and usually develops after 50 years of age. There is no racial predilection.

Pemphigoid occurs when autoantibodies (IgG, IgG4, IgM, IgA, or IgE) bind and destroy the anchoring filament complex of the basement membrane (i.e., the hemidesmosome) at the dermal-epidermal junction. Basement proteins BP180 and BP230, which comprise the hemidesmosome, are the main targets of autoantibody destruction. Additional antigenic targets are laminin 332 and a subunit of $\alpha6\beta4$ integrin. This leads to detached epithelium at the level of the lamina lucida (*subepithelial clefting*), thus exposing the underlying connective tissue. Immunofluorescence staining reveals linear deposits of immunoglobulin (Ig)G and IgA and/or C3 along the basement membrane.

Pemphigoid skin lesions usually precede oral lesions, tend to be desquamative and localized, and heal spontaneously. The lips are rarely affected. Intraoral bullae are usually small, yellow, or hemorrhagic blebs. They form slowly and favor the palate, gingiva, and buccal mucosa. Because pemphigoid bullae result from subepithelial separation (Nikolsky positive), they are thicker walled, less fragile, and longer lasting than those of pemphigus. Rupture leads to patchy ulcers that coalesce. The ulcers are symmetric, curvilinear, and surrounded by a red border. When limited to the gingiva, the clinical term **desquamative gingivitis** has been used to describe the bright red, burning, and denuded tissue. Desquamative gingivitis is a descriptive term and may represent several clinically similar vesiculobullous conditions.

Mucous membrane pemphigoid may affect the nasal mucosa, skin, anal, vaginal, and pharyngeal mucosa, but the most severe complication is ocular involvement, producing conjunctivitis, occasional bullae, clouding of the cornea, and healing marked by scarring and possibly blindness. Although the condition is rarely fatal, close follow-up by a physician is suggested because rare reports of carcinoma of the rectum and uterus have been associated with pemphigoid. Topical corticosteroids alone or in conjunction with immunosuppressive agents such as azathioprine, dapsone, mycophenolate mofetil, or tacrolimus have provided effective management. Tetracycline with niacinamide serves as an alternative therapy.

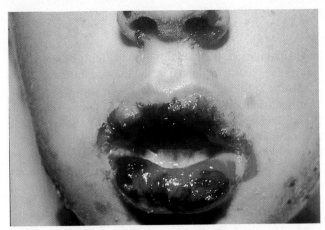

Fig. 87.1. Pemphigus vulgaris: lip and nose crusts.

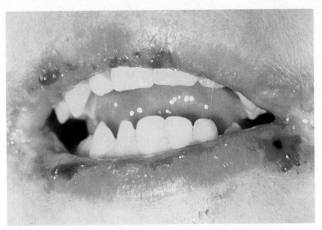

Fig. 87.2. Pemphigus vulgaris: hemorrhagic lip crusts.

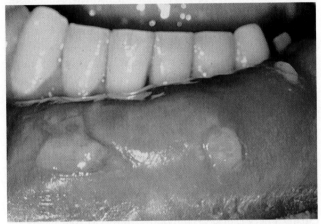

Fig. 87.3. Pemphigus vulgaris: rare, intact bullae on mucosa.*

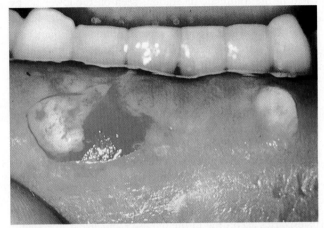

Fig. 87.4. Pemphigus vulgaris: erythema below ruptured bullae.*

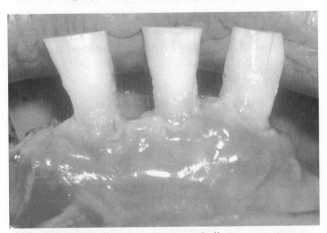

Fig. 87.5. Cicatricial pemphigoid: intact bulla.

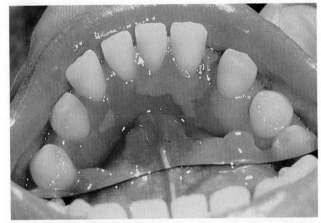

Fig. 87.6. Cicatricial pemphigoid: sloughing gingiva.

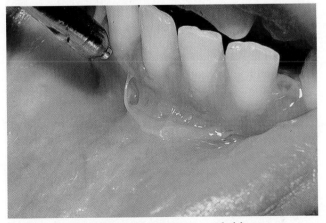

Fig. 87.7. Cicatricial pemphigoid: positive Nikolsky sign.

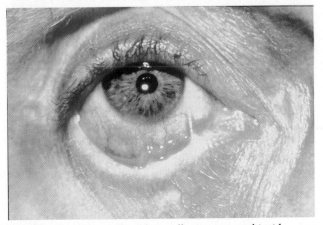

Fig. 87.8. Symblepharon: a lid-eye adhesion in pemphigoid.

10

193

Traumatic Ulcer (Figs. 88.1–88.3) Recurrent oral ulceration is a common condition caused by several factors, primarily trauma. Ulcers may occur at any age and in either sex. Likely locations for traumatic ulcers are the labial/buccal mucosa, palate, and borders of the tongue.

Traumatic ulcers may result from chemicals, heat, or mechanical force and are often classified according to the exact nature of the insult. Pressure from an ill-fitting denture base or flange or from a partial denture framework is a source of a **decubitus** or **pressure ulcer**. **Trophic**—or **ischemic**—**ulcers** occur particularly on the palate at the site of a previous injection. Dental injections have also been implicated in the traumatic ulcerations seen on the lower lip by children who chew their numb lip after dental appointments. In addition to factitial injury, young children and infants are prone to traumatic ulcers of the soft palate from thumb sucking, called **Bednar aphthae**.

Ulcers may be precipitated by contact with a fractured tooth or restoration, a partial denture clasp, or inadvertent biting of the mucosa. Ulcers on the palate appear after the mucosa is burned by hot food or drink. Other traumatic ulcers are caused by factitial injury from inappropriate use of fingernails or other objects on the oral mucosa. The diagnosis is simple and often established from a careful history and examination of the physical findings.

The appearance of a mechanically induced traumatic ulcer varies according to the intensity and size of the agent. The ulcer usually appears slightly depressed and oval. An erythematous zone is initially found at the periphery; this zone progressively lightens as the ulcer heals. The center of the ulcer is usually yellow-gray. Chemically damaged mucosa, such as that seen with an aspirin burn, is less well defined and contains a loosely adherent, coagulated, white surface slough. After removal of the traumatic influence, the ulcer should heal within 2 weeks. If healing does not occur, other causes should be suspected and a biopsy should be performed.

Recurrent Aphthous Stomatitis (Minor Aphthae, Aphthous Ulcer) (Figs. 88.4–88.6) is characterized by recurrent, painful ulcers of the oral mucosa. The disorder is classified into three categories according to size: **minor aphthae, major aphthae**, and **herpetiform ulcers**. Approximately 20% of the population is afflicted with minor aphthae, or *canker sores,* as they are commonly called. They may be seen in anyone, but women and young adults are slightly more susceptible. Familial patterns have been demonstrated, and persons who smoke are less frequently affected than nonsmokers. Although the cause is unknown, studies suggest an immunologic process involving T-cell–mediated cytolytic activity and tumor necrosis factor in response to human leukocyte antigen or foreign antigens. Factors that promote thinned mucosa (trauma, endocrinopathies, menstruation, nutritional deficiencies), immune dysfunction (atopy, stress), or exposure to antigens (food allergies) contribute to this condition, because the presentation of antigens to Langerhans cells is facilitated by the thinned mucosa.

Minor aphthae have a propensity for movable mucosa that is situated over minor salivary gland tissue. The labial, buccal, and vestibular mucosa are frequently affected, as are the tonsillar fauces, tongue, and soft palate. Ulcers are rarely seen on keratinized mucosa, such as the gingiva and hard palate. Prodromal symptoms of paresthesia or hyperesthesia are sometimes reported. The ulcers are shallow, yellow-gray, oval, well demarcated, and small (less than 1 cm; usually about 3 to 5 mm in diameter). A prominent erythematous border surrounds the fibrinous pseudomembrane. No vesicle formation is seen in this disease—a distinctive diagnostic feature. Ulcers that occur along the mucobuccal fold often appear more elongated. Burning is a preliminary symptom that is followed by intense pain lasting a few days. Tender submandibular, anterior cervical, and parotid lymph nodes are sometimes present, particularly when the ulcer becomes secondarily infected.

Aphthae are recurrent, and the pattern of occurrence varies. Most persons exhibit single ulcers once or twice a year, beginning during childhood or adolescence. The ulcers occasionally appear in crops, but usually, fewer than five occur at one time.

Minor aphthae usually heal spontaneously without scar formation within 14 days. Some patients have multiple ulcers during a period of several months. In these cases, ulcers are in various stages of erupting and healing and produce constant pain. Although no medication has been totally successful for treating aphthous stomatitis, patients have responded to 5% amlexanox (Aphthasol), topical corticosteroids, and coagulating and cauterizing agents, as well as specific food and toothpaste avoidance.

Pseudoaphthous (Figs. 88.7 and 88.8), a term coined by Dr. Bill Binney, refers to recurrent, aphthouslike mucosal ulcers of the mouth that are associated with nutritional deficiency states. Studies indicate that 20% of patients with recurrent aphthous stomatitis are deficient in folic acid, iron, or vitamin B_{12}. Pseudoaphthae are frequently seen with inflammatory bowel disease, Crohn disease, gluten intolerance (celiac disease), and pernicious anemia.

Pseudoaphthae resemble both minor and major aphthous stomatitises but are characteristically more persistent. There is a slight predilection for women between 25 and 50 years of age. The ulcers are depressed, rounded, painful, and sometimes multiple. The borders may be raised, firm, and irregular. Occasionally, lesions are accompanied by mucosal fissures and nodules. Alterations of the tongue papillae may suggest an underlying nutritional deficiency state. Healing is slow, and patients may report that they are rarely free of ulceration. Chronic and persistent presence of aphthae necessitates evaluation for nutritional deficiencies, including hematologic studies. If the laboratory results are abnormal, a medical referral is required.

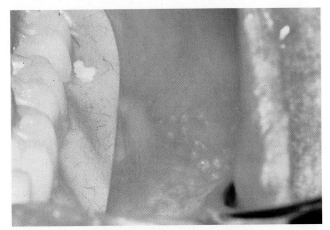

Fig. 88.1. **Traumatic ulcer:** denture flange induced.*

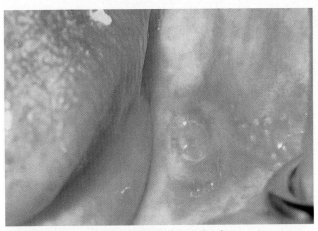

Fig. 88.2. **Traumatic ulcer:** molar area, under denture.*

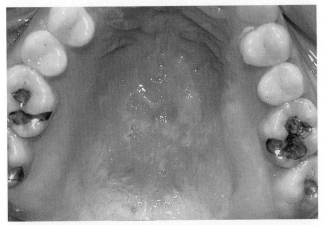

Fig. 88.3. **Traumatic ulcer:** irregular, caused by hot food.

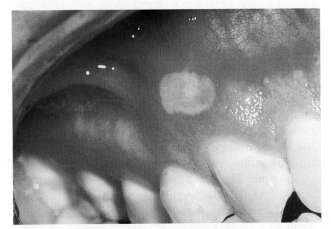

Fig. 88.4. **Aphthous:** oval ulcer on alveolar mucosa.

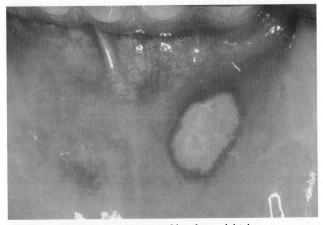

Fig. 88.5. **Aphthous:** prominent red border on labial mucosa.

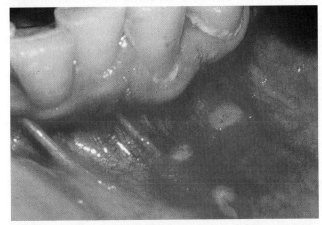

Fig. 88.6. **Aphthae:** a cluster of ulcers with typical shapes.

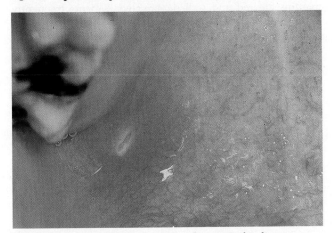

Fig. 88.7. **Pseudoaphthous:** irregular ulcer in Crohn disease.

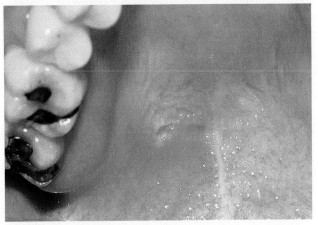

Fig. 88.8. **Pseudoaphthae:** corrugated ulcers, Crohn disease.

10

Major Aphthous (Figs. 89.1–89.4) is a severe form of aphthous stomatitis that produces larger (≥1 cm), more destructive, and deeper ulcers that last longer and recur more frequently than minor aphthae. The cause is the same as for minor aphthae, namely, an immune defect in T-lymphocyte function. Young women with anxious personality traits and HIV-seropositive persons are commonly affected. Historically, this condition was also known as **Sutton disease** or **periadenitis mucosa necrotica recurrens (PMNR)**.

Major aphthae are usually multiple. They involve the soft palate, tonsillar fauces, labial mucosa, and tongue and occasionally extend onto the attached gingiva. Characteristically, the ulcers are crateriform, asymmetric, and unilateral. Prominent features include the large size, an irregular border, and a depressed necrotic center. A red raised inflammatory border is common. Depending on size, traumatic influences, and secondary infection, ulcers may last from several weeks to months. Because the ulcers erode deep into the connective tissue, they may heal with scar formation after repeated recurrences. Muscle destruction can result in tissue fenestration. If the periodontium is involved, tissue attachment may be damaged. Extreme pain and lymphadenopathy are common symptoms.

Use of steroids (topical, intralesional, or systemic) can accelerate healing and reduce scarring. Ulcers similar to those of major aphthae are seen with some frequency in association with cyclic neutropenia, agranulocytosis, and gluten intolerance. Ulcers located on the tongue may strongly resemble carcinoma. The presence of scarring is of diagnostic importance to rule out a malignant condition.

Herpetiform Ulceration (Figs. 89.5 and 89.6) is the least common variant of aphthous stomatitis. Clinically, the ulcers resemble those seen in primary herpes (hence the name *herpetiform*). The most prominent feature of the disease is the numerous, pinhead-sized, gray-white erosions that enlarge and coalesce into ulcers. Initially, the ulcers are 1 to 2 mm in diameter and occur in clusters of 10 to 100. The mucosa adjacent to the ulcer is erythematous, and pain is a predictable symptom.

Any part of the oral mucosa may be affected by **herpetiform ulcerations**, but the tip and margins of the tongue and labial mucosa are particularly affected. The smaller size of these ulcerations distinguishes them from minor aphthae, and the absence of vesicles and gingivitis together with their frequent and recurrent nature distinguishes them from primary herpes and other oral viral infections. Virus cannot be cultured from these lesions, and the ulcers are not contagious.

The first episode of herpetiform ulceration usually occurs in patients in their late 20s and 30s, 10 years after the peak incidence of minor aphthae. The duration of recurrent attacks is variable and unpredictable. Most patients experience healing within 2 weeks; however, some patients have constant lesions for months. The trigger of this disease has yet to be determined. Recurrent herpetiform ulcerations respond especially well to tetracycline suspensions, both topically and systemically, and the condition often regresses spontaneously after several years.

Behçet Syndrome (Oculo-Oral-Genital Syndrome) (Figs. 89.7 and 89.8), named for the Turkish physician who described the ulcerative disorder, principally involves the oral cavity, eye, and genitals. Although the condition primarily occurs at these three sites, it is now considered a multisystem disorder. In its fully developed state, cutaneous rashes, arthritis of the major joints, gastrointestinal ulcerations, cardiovascular disease, thrombophlebitis, and neurologic manifestations (headaches) are seen, although rarely are all components present in the same patient. The syndrome appears to be the result of a delayed hypersensitivity reaction, immune complexes, and *vasculitis* triggered by the presentation of human leukocyte antigens (HLA-B51) or environmental antigens, such as viruses, bacteria, chemicals, heavy metals, or pesticides. Behçet syndrome is two times more prevalent in men than in women and typically develops between 20 and 30 years of age. Persons from Asia, Eastern Mediterranean countries (along the ancient Silk Route), and Great Britain are most commonly affected.

Eye manifestations of Behçet syndrome include photophobia, conjunctivitis, and posterior uveitis. Rarely, pus in the anterior eye chamber (hypopyon) occurs that can lead to blindness. Eye lesions may be concurrent or occur years after oral and genital ulcers. Skin changes are characterized by subcutaneous nodules and macular and papular eruptions that vesiculate, ulcerate, and encrustate. Genital ulcers may involve the mucosa or skin and tend to be smaller and less common than the oral lesions.

Oral ulcers, the most prevalent manifestation of Behçet syndrome, are the initial sign of disease in about 50% of patients. Although they may manifest as any of the three forms of aphthous stomatitis, they most often occur in crops of six or more on the soft palate and oropharynx (infrequent sites and numbers for routine aphthae). Characteristically, the ulcers are recurrent, shallow, oval, and variable in size. Small lesions tend to occur more frequently than larger lesions. A serofibrinous exudate covers the surface, and the margins are red and well demarcated. Patients frequently report pain, and recurrent periods of exacerbation and remissions are characteristic. Topical and systemic steroids are used to treat the symptoms of patients with limited mucocutaneous involvement. Protracted disease involving the neuro-ocular structures requires the care of a physician. Azathioprine, cyclophosphamide, thalidomide, and colchicine have been used successfully in select cases. All of these agents have potentially serious side effects; they are best prescribed by experts.

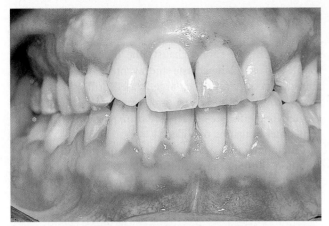

Fig. 89.1. Major aphthous: persistent ulcers on gingiva.*

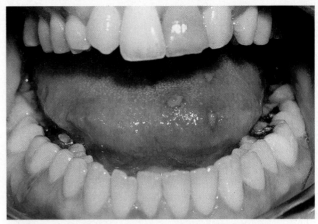

Fig. 89.2. Major aphthous: multiple, irregular tongue ulcers.*

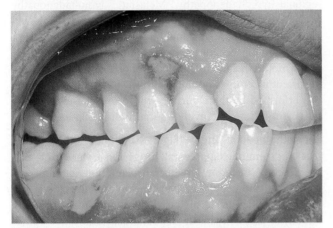

Fig. 89.3. Major aphthous: deep, painful gingival ulcers.*

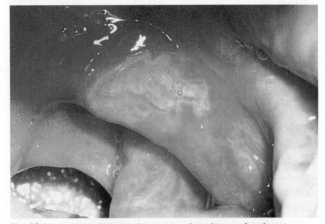

Fig. 89.4. Major aphthous: large irregular ulcer, soft palate.*

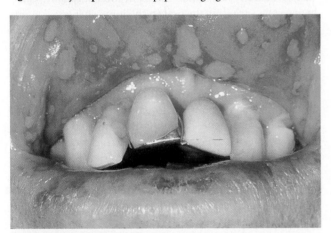

Fig. 89.5. Herpetiform ulceration: many ulcers of mucosa.‡

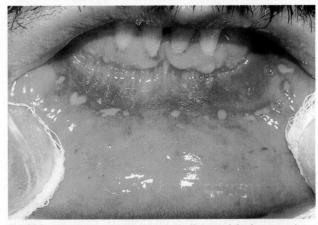

Fig. 89.6. Herpetiform ulceration: small crops, labial mucosa.‡

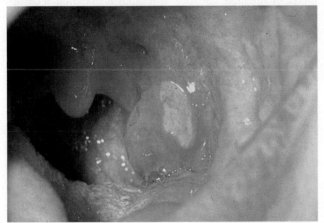

Fig. 89.7. Behçet syndrome: a 27-year-old man, tonsillar ulcer.

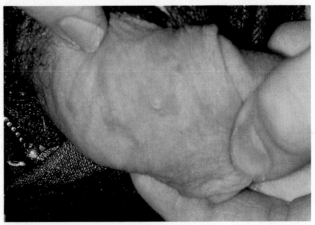

Fig. 89.8. Behçet syndrome: genital ulcers.

10

Granulomatous Ulcer (Figs. 90.1 and 90.2)

Granulomatous infections may produce oral ulcers. Two of the more common oral granulomatous infections are **tuberculosis** and **histoplasmosis**. These two infections exhibit primary, latent, and reactivated states. Although the oral lesions are relatively uncommon, they occur with frequency when infected respiratory secretions are implanted into oral mucosa following trauma. Adults with advanced pulmonary disease and persons with acquired immune deficiency syndrome (AIDS) are more often affected. Pulmonary lesions usually precede oral lesions. Thus, symptoms of persistent cough, fever, night sweats, weight loss, and chest pain are important historic findings.

Dissemination of organisms (*Mycobacterium tuberculosis* or *Histoplasmosis capsulatum*) from the lungs via infected sputum is the primary mode of oral infection. The classic oral manifestation of tuberculosis and histoplasmosis infection is a chronic nonhealing ulcer. Most oral tuberculous ulcers occur on the dorsum of the tongue, labial mucosa at the commissure, gingiva, and palate. Oral ulcers of histoplasmosis most often occur on the tongue, palate, and buccal mucosa. The clinical picture varies. The ulcer may resemble a traumatic ulcer or epidermoid carcinoma, particularly when the location is on the lateral tongue border. Lesions on the alveolar ridge often resemble a granulating extraction site. The center of the ulcer is necrotic, yellow-gray, and depressed. The periphery of the ulcer is undulating or lumpy and cobblestoned. The margin of the lesion is irregular, well demarcated, and undermined. Nodular and vegetative components are often seen in conjunction with the ulcers of histoplasmosis. Cervical lymphadenopathy is a common finding. Some patients report pain; in these patients, the discovery may be an incidental finding. Other patients experience severe, unremitting discomfort or bony involvement. Tuberculous and histoplasmosis lesions are contagious; the organisms can be transmitted by coughing and aerosols.

A biopsy or culturing is required to confirm the diagnosis. Histologic features and special stains (Ziehl-Neelsen for tuberculosis) demonstrate the presence of the causative organisms and groups of macrophages organized into granulomas. Treatment of the primary lung problem is with specific long-term antibiotics. For tuberculosis, isoniazid, rifampin, ethambutol, and pyrazinamide are administered for 2 months followed by drug combinations for 4 to 7 months. Specific drug combinations are selected based on drug resistance exhibited by the infecting organism. For symptomatic histoplasmosis, itraconazole, fluconazole, and amphotericin B are administered. Clinicians should be aware that the lung disease should be effectively treated before initiating dental treatment.

Squamous Cell Carcinoma (Figs. 90.3–90.6)

often appears as a chronic, nonhealing ulcer. In early stages, the lesion is usually small, nonpainful, and nonulcerative. However, the persistent nature of the disease results in neoplastic proliferation that soon exhausts the blood supply, resulting in surface telangiectasia and eventual ulcer formation. Chronic ulcers tend to be large, crateriform, granular, and covered by a central yellow-gray necrotic slough. Red, raw foci are frequent. The borders are firm, raised, irregular, and sometimes fungating or rolled.

Carcinomas may occur anywhere in the mouth. The most common sites are the posterior third of the lateral margin of the tongue and the floor of the mouth. The retromolar trigone, soft palate, and tonsillar fauces are also frequently affected. Associated features may include pain, numbness, leukoplakia, erythroplakia, induration, fixation, and regional lymphadenopathy. Metastatic lymphadenopathy is characterized by nonpainful rubbery or hard nodes that are fixed at the base and matted together. Excessive use of alcohol and tobacco, or the detection of HPV-16 or HPV-18 in the mouth, heightens suspicion of oral carcinoma when a persistent ulcer does not heal within 14 days. Biopsy should be performed by the clinician, who provides the definitive treatment. Treatment involves surgery and radiation therapy.

Chemotherapeutic Ulcer (Figs. 90.7 and 90.8)

Patients receiving immunosuppressant drugs for a variety of serious illnesses, including organ transplantation, autoimmune conditions, and neoplasia, may develop oral ulcerations and mucositis. Side effects of the chemotherapeutic drug may directly or indirectly harm the oral mucosa. Antimetabolites such as methotrexate inhibit the replication of rapidly reproducing cells, including the oral epithelium, whereas alkaloids such as cyclophosphamide induce leukopenia and secondary ulcer formation.

A **chemotherapeutic ulcer**, an early sign of drug toxicity, appears during the 2nd week of therapy and usually persists for 2 weeks. These ulcers may occur on any oral mucosal site, but more commonly affect nonkeratinized mucosa (lips, buccal mucosa, tongue, floor of the mouth, and soft palate) before keratinized mucosa (gingival, hard palate, and dorsal tongue). The affected area initially turns red and burns. The surface epithelium is lost (mucositis), then a large, deep, necrotic, and painful ulcer forms. The margins of the ulcer are irregular, and the characteristic red inflammatory border is often not present because of the lack of an inflammatory response by the host. If the pain becomes severe and the intake of adequate nutrition and fluids is impaired, a reduction in chemotherapy drug dose may be necessary.

Culturing is highly recommended for all oral lesions in patients on chemotherapy because of the propensity for infection with gram-negative organisms, fungi, or recurrent herpes simplex virus. Topical anesthetics and Benadryl mouth rinses are used to minimize symptoms, whereas oral hygiene measures, including antimicrobial agents such as chlorhexidine, are critical to prevent secondary infection, soft tissue necrosis, and osseous necrosis. Consultation and open communication between the physician and the dentist can help reduce complications and promote oral comfort.

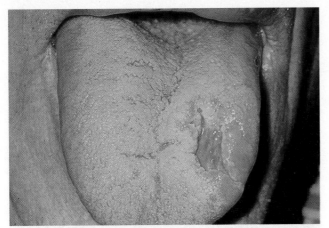

Fig. 90.1. Granulomatous ulcer: caused by *M. tuberculosis*.

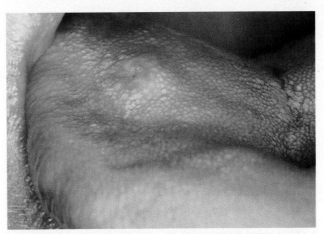

Fig. 90.2. Granulomatous ulcer: caused by histoplasmosis.

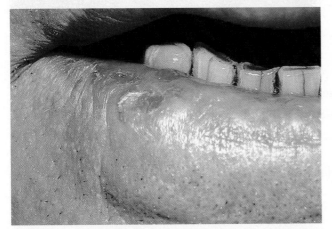

Fig. 90.3. Squamous cell carcinoma: indurated and raised.

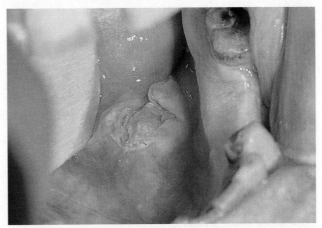

Fig. 90.4. Squamous cell carcinoma: ulcer on the floor of the mouth.

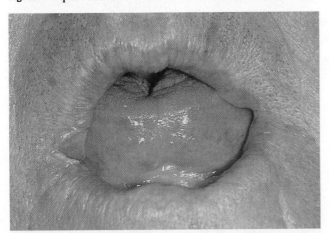

Fig. 90.5. Squamous cell carcinoma: at labial commissure.*

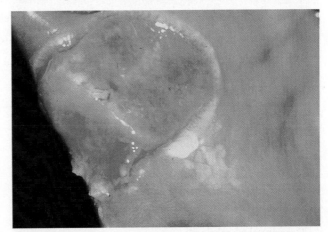

Fig. 90.6. Squamous cell carcinoma: spreading, buccal mucosa.*

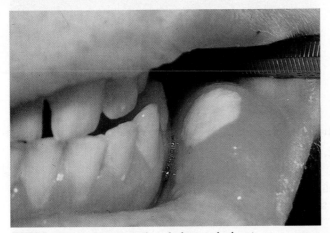

Fig. 90.7. Chemotherapy-induced ulcer: in leukemia.

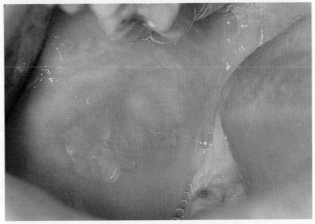

Fig. 90.8. Chemotherapy-induced ulcer: by methotrexate.

10

199

CASE STUDIES

CASE 46. (FIG. 90.9)

This 67-year-old Caucasian woman presents to your office for the first time. She is edentulous and wants new dentures. Her current dentures are about 11 years old, and she has not been to a dentist in a while. She does not smoke tobacco, although she did for about 35 years. She quit 4 years ago. She drinks a glass of wine once a week. She is widowed and has dated a couple of men during the last 4 years. She is asymptomatic and feels fine.

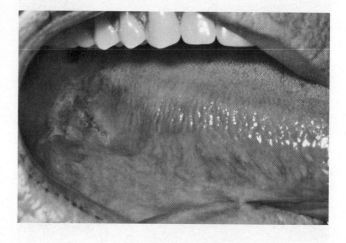

1. Describe the features in the clinical photograph.

2. Which term best describes the lesion?
   A. Leukoplakia
   B. Erythroplakia
   C. Speckled erythroplakia
   D. Ulcer

3. Why is it important to pull the tongue out during the examination?

4. Is this lesion a normal finding, a variant of normal, or disease? What clinical features are suggestive that this condition is benign or malignant?

5. What is the most likely diagnosis of this condition?

6. Which of the following would *not* be expected to occur with this condition?
   A. Induration
   B. Rapid appearance
   C. Lymphadenopathy
   D. History of smoking

7. What factors place this patient at risk for this condition being neoplasia?

8. Should the dental hygienist proceed with treatment prior to informing the dentist of the lesion?

9. What should the dentist communicate to the patient about this lesion?

CASE 47. (FIG. 90.10)

This 57-year-old women presents with pain near the back of her maxillary denture. The pain has been present for about 5 days and makes it difficult for her to swallow. She works at a local factory in the accounting department. She had a cold last week, but feels like she is recovered. No other significant medical findings were noted on her medical history form.

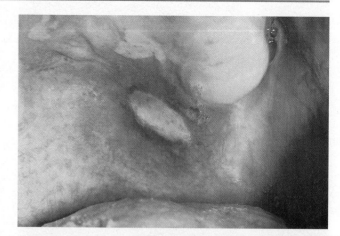

1. Describe the oral findings.

2. What is the significance of the location of the lesion?

3. What questions should you ask the patient that might provide diagnostic clues of what this condition is?

4. What is the significance of the lesion's red border?

5. What is the most likely diagnosis of this condition?

6. What is the cause of this condition?

7. What other conditions should be considered in the differential diagnosis?

8. Should the dentist suggest a biopsy of this lesion to the patient?

Additional cases to enhance your learning and understanding of this section are available Online through the book's Navigate 2 Advantage Access site.

Oral Manifestations of Sexual Conditions and Systemic Drug Therapies

Objectives:

- Define oral entities that appear as a result of sexual activity, sexually transmitted infections, or drug therapy.
- Recognize the causes of these conditions.
- In the clinical setting, document the clinical features of these conditions in terms of anatomic site, border, color, and configuration.
- Use the diagnostic process to distinguish similar-appearing oral conditions that result from sexual activity, sexually transmitted infections, or drug therapy.
- Recommend appropriate treatments for oral conditions that result from sexual activity, sexually transmitted infections, or drug therapy.
- Identify conditions discussed in this section that would (1) require the attention of the dentist, (2) affect the delivery of noninvasive and invasive dental procedures, or (3) need to be further evaluated by a specialist.

In the figure legends, *‡ denotes the same patient.

Traumatic Conditions (Figs. 91.1 and 91.2) Injury to the lingual frenum and soft palate are common oral conditions associated with sexual activity. Ulceration of the lingual frenum may occur when the tongue is rubbed against the incisal edge of the mandibular incisors during orogenital sexual activity. The ulcer has a gray-white fibrinous coating and an erythematous border. A history of cunnilingus confirms the diagnosis, and abstinence is recommended to permit healing. Chronic irritation may lead to secondary bacterial infection, development of leukoplakia or a traumatic fibroma, or it may permit ingress of the human papillomavirus. Fellatio can traumatize oral soft tissues and produce erythema and submucosal hemorrhage of the soft palate. Isolated bright red petechiae initially appear (see Figs. 71.1 and 91.5). They eventually become a confluent patch (ecchymosis) that bridges the palatal midline. The purpuric patch is painless and does not blanch on diascopy. It clinically resembles the petechial patch produced by infectious mononucleosis. However, swollen lymph nodes and fever are characteristically absent. Petechiae darken and fade away in about a week.

Sexually Transmitted Pharyngitis (Figs. 91.3 and 91.4) Pharyngitis is inflammation of the back of the throat that is often due to infection. Venereal organisms, such as herpes simplex virus (HSV) type 2, *Neisseria gonorrhoeae*, and *Chlamydia trachomatis*, may cause pharyngitis by transmission from direct contact with infected genital or oral secretions or lesions. These infections occur most often in sexually active persons between 15 and 35 years of age. When primary HSV-2 infection manifests in the oral cavity, it produces inflammation of the pharynx and tonsils, fever, and generally less gingival inflammation than that caused by primary HSV-1 infection. Multiple small vesicles are usually apparent in the early stages; the vesicles collapse to form ulcers that resolve in 10 to 21 days. Antiviral agents initiated the first few days of clinical presentation provide effective treatment.

N. *gonorrhoeae*, a gram-negative bacterium, infects nonkeratinized mucosal epithelium, producing a diffuse erythematosus pharyngitis, small tonsillar pustules, or an erythematous and edematous patch involving the throat, tonsillar area, and uvula. Burning is the initial symptom, followed by increased salivary viscosity and halitosis. Other oral manifestations include painful, discrete ulcerations of the oral mucosa; fiery red and tender gingiva with or without necrosis of the interdental papilla; tongue ulcerations; and glossodynia. A single injected dose of ceftriaxone with either azithromycin or doxycycline is effective in managing this condition. C. *trachomatis*, a gram-negative bacterium, may also cause a sore throat, mild pharyngitis, and tonsillar inflammation with pustule formation. Treatment is with azithromycin or doxycycline.

Infectious Mononucleosis (Figs. 91.5 and 91.6) is an acute viral infection characterized by fatigue, fever, sore throat, swollen lymph nodes, stomatitis, and occasional hepatosplenomegaly. It is most commonly caused by the Epstein-Barr virus and occurs chiefly in adolescents and young adults. The disease is of low contagiousness, and transmission is through exchange of virus-contaminated saliva during deep kissing or sharing of straws. Oral lesions are often the earliest manifestations of infectious mononucleosis. Multiple red petechiae located at the junction of the hard and soft palate occur during the first few weeks of infection. These lesions turn brown and fade after several days. As the condition progresses, fatigue, exudative tonsillitis, and bilateral, posterior, painful cervical lymphadenopathy become prominent findings. Less frequently, patients develop a rash, cough, necrotizing ulcerative gingivitis (NUG), or pharyngeal ulcers. Blood analysis reveals modest lymphocytosis, atypical lymphocytes, heterophile antibodies, and mildly elevated transaminase levels. Treatment mainly involves bed rest, soft diet, analgesics, and antipyretic agents. Recovery usually occurs within 1 to 2 months.

Syphilis (Figs. 91.7 and 91.8) is a venereal disease caused by *Treponema pallidum*, an anaerobic spirochete. The hallmark of primary oral syphilis is the nonpainful chancre, which represents a granulomatous reaction to vascular obliteration. Chancres may affect any oral soft tissue. However, the lips are the most common site of involvement, followed by the tongue, palate, gingiva, and tonsils. Oral syphilis is more often observed in sexually active young men.

The syphilitic chancre initially appears as a small solitary papule that elevates, enlarges, erodes, and ulcerates. The lesion is usually punched out, indurated, and 2 or 3 cm in diameter and lacks a red inflammatory border. The surface is covered by a yellowish, highly infectious serous discharge. Palatal erythema or an asymptomatic, reddish ulcer may be the initial lesion, along with swollen, nontender, firm, anterior cervical lymph nodes. Chancres typically persist for 2 to 4 weeks and heal spontaneously, causing patients to erroneously believe that treatment is not necessary. After a latent period of 4 weeks to 6 months, the secondary stage of syphilis appears. During this stage, the patient may report headaches, tearing of the eyes, nasal discharge, sore throat, generalized joint pain, enlarged lymph nodes, elevated temperature, and weight loss. A painless, symmetric maculopapular skin rash on the palms of the hands and bottoms of the feet soon follows. Concurrent oral lesions of secondary syphilis appear as oval red macules, pharyngitis, or isolated or multiple mucous patches (painless, shallow, highly infectious ulcers surrounded by an erythematous halo). The borders are often irregular and resemble snail tracks. Tertiary syphilis occurs in infected persons many years after nontreatment of secondary syphilis. It is primarily characterized by palatal perforation and neurologic symptoms. Parenteral penicillin G remains the drug of choice for treating all stages of syphilis.

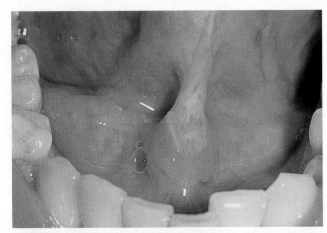
Fig. 91.1. **Traumatic ulcer:** of lingual frenum.

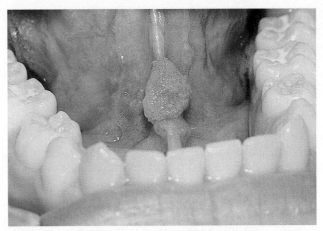
Fig. 91.2. **Condyloma acuminatum:** of lingual frenum.

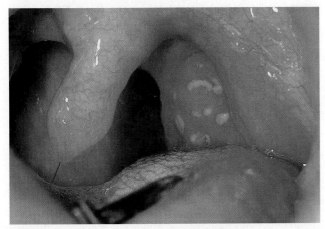
Fig. 91.3. **Sexually transmitted HSV-2 pharyngitis.***

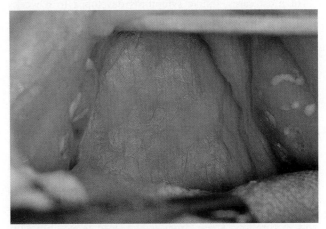
Fig. 91.4. **Primary HSV-2 infection.***

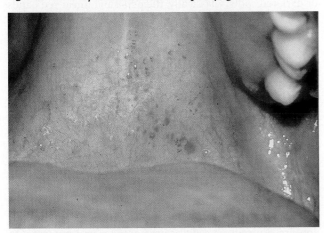
Fig. 91.5. **Infectious mononucleosis:** palatal petechiae.

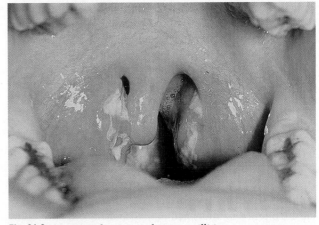
Fig. 91.6. **Mononucleosis:** exudative tonsillitis.

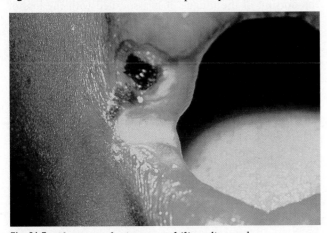
Fig. 91.7. **Chancres of primary syphilis:** split papule.

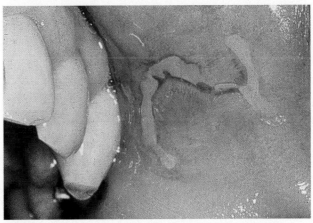
Fig. 91.8. **Mucous patch secondary syphilis:** snail track.

11

203

HIV INFECTION AND AIDS

Acquired Immunodeficiency Syndrome (AIDS) is a communicable disease caused by the human immunodeficiency virus (HIV), first reported by the Centers for Disease Control in 1981. HIV is an RNA retrovirus that infects CD4$^+$ T lymphocytes, brain glial cells, and macrophages. The virus is harbored in blood, tears, saliva, breast milk, and other bodily fluids and tissues of infected persons. It is predominantly spread by sexual contact, blood or blood products, or perinatally. Infection results by exposure to the virus through sharing of injected needles during drug use, having unprotected sex, receiving infected blood or blood products, or being accidentally exposed to infected materials.

In most cases, flulike symptoms develop 2 to 6 weeks after infection; then *persistent, generalized lymphadenopathy* occurs, followed by a latent phase. Initially, the latent phase is asymptomatic. Later, lymphadenopathy, respiratory infections, weight loss, fever, chronic diarrhea, fatigue, skin anergy, oral candidiasis, hairy leukoplakia, parotid enlargement, and recurrent herpesvirus infections develop. **AIDS** is defined as an immune deficiency caused by HIV infection when CD4$^+$ T-cell counts decrease to <200 cells/mm^3 or when 1 of 30 opportunistic infections or certain forms of cancer develop. Treatment involves the use of antiretroviral drugs (ARVs), such as reverse transcriptase inhibitors, protease inhibitors, entry inhibitors, fusion inhibitors, and integrase inhibitors in combination to block virus replication and maturation. These drugs, when used in combination called highly active antiretroviral therapy (HAART), have extended the lives of infected patients for more than 20 years. Oral manifestations of HIV infection are often numerous, concurrent, and recurrent. Recognition of the oral features warrants patient referral to a physician.

HIV-Associated Oral Bacterial Infections (Figs. 92.1–92.3)

Oral bacterial infections in HIV-infected patients often involve periodontal tissues. These include the two **necrotizing periodontal diseases** discussed below.

Necrotizing Ulcerative Gingivitis (Figs. 92.1 and 92.2) or

NUG is common in HIV-infected patients. It is characterized by sudden onset of fiery red, swollen, painful, bleeding gingiva and a fetor oris (bad breath). The interdental papillae are blunted or "punched out," ulcerated, and covered by a grayish necrotic slough, without loss of bone. Fusiform and spirochetal organisms and immunosuppression are contributing causes. The affected gingiva responds quickly to debridement. Metronidazole is used when constitutional signs (fever, malaise, and lymphadenopathy) are present.

Necrotizing Ulcerative Periodontitis (Fig. 92.3) or NUP

is a rapidly progressive and destructive loss of periodontal attachment and bone. It initially manifests in the anterior periodontal tissues, then radiates to the posterior areas and has a distinct propensity for the incisor and molar teeth. This bacterial infection (caused by typical and atypical pathogens) is associated with pronounced immunosuppression.

It is characterized by pain and spontaneous gingival bleeding, gingival edema, ulceration and necrosis, rapid gingival recession (often interdentally), extremely rapid and *irregular bone loss*, delayed wound healing, and spread to adjacent mucosa. Aggressive periodontal measures and antibiotics are required for control.

HIV-infected patients with waning immune responses are also prone to infections with bacterial flora uncommon to the oral cavity. The most commonly isolated bacteria are respiratory and coliform flora, *Klebsiella* species, and *Escherichia coli*. Infections by these organisms often produce diffuse, erythematous, and ulcerated changes of the tongue.

HIV-Associated Oral Fungal Infections (Figs. 92.4–92.8)

Candidiasis is a mild fungal infection of the skin or mucous membranes caused by an overgrowth of *C. albicans*. Candidiasis is the most common oral mucosal infection of patients with AIDS and is often the first oral manifestation. Candidal infections are usually chronic and may appear red, white, flat, raised, or nodular. Any oral mucosal surface may be infected, but the palate, tongue, and buccal mucosa are the most frequent sites. The different types of candidiasis are discussed below and in Figures 76.1–76.8.

Linear Gingival Erythema (Fig. 92.4) is a candidal infection

in immunosuppressed persons characterized by a distinct red linear band along the marginal gingiva. It can also appear on attached and nonattached gingiva as patches of tiny red or dark red spots. Classically, the persistent linear red bands appear in the absence of apparent local factors such as plaque. The maxilla and mandible are equally affected. Spontaneous gingival bleeding and lack of response to conventional therapy are common unless antifungal agents are used in combination with plaque removal.

Pseudomembranous Candidiasis (Figs. 92.5 and 92.6)

is characterized by creamy white plaques that on scraping reveal a red, raw, or bleeding mucosal surface. The organisms when smeared and stained with potassium hydroxide or cultured reveal hyphal forms typical of *Candida albicans*.

Erythematous (atrophic) Candidiasis (Figs. 92.7 and 92.8)

appears clinically as a diffuse red area on oral mucosa. On the dorsum of the tongue, it is associated with the loss of filiform papillae and is called **median rhomboid glossitis**. A diffuse, erythematous contact lesion corresponding in size and shape to the tongue lesion may be apparent on the palate. Although usually asymptomatic, patients may report mild discomfort, burning, or altered taste. **Chronic hyperplastic candidiasis**, a late stage of candidal infection, appears as nonpainful, diffuse, white keratotic plaques on the buccal mucosa (Fig. 76.4). The plaques cannot be wiped off. Affected patients require systemic antifungal drugs. This disease is often chronic and recurrent and may predict esophageal candidiasis in immunosuppressed persons.

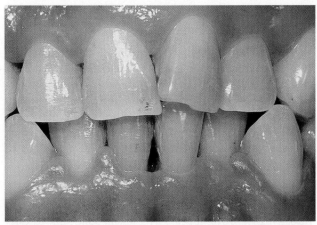

Fig. 92.1. HIV-associated necrotizing ulcerative gingivitis (NUG).

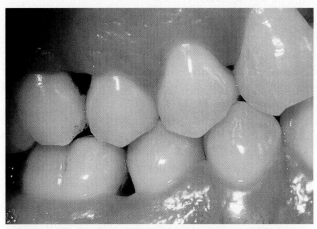

Fig. 92.2. HIV-associated necrotizing ulcerative gingivitis (NUG).

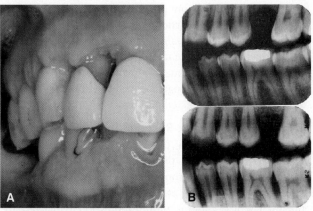

Fig. 92.3. NUP: anterior (**A**) and posterior (**B**) bone loss in 6 months.

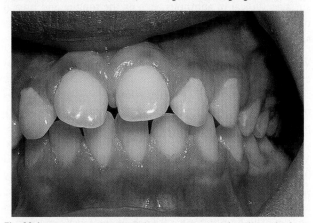

Fig. 92.4. Linear gingival erythema: on marginal and attached gingiva.

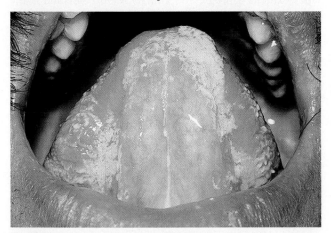

Fig. 92.5. Pseudomembranous candidiasis: in AIDS.‡

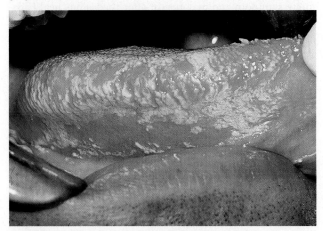

Fig. 92.6. Pseudomembranous candidiasis: in AIDS.‡

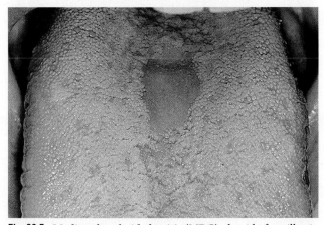

Fig. 92.7. Median rhomboid glossitis (MRG): devoid of papillae.*

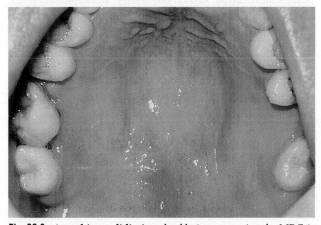

Fig. 92.8. Atrophic candidiasis: palatal lesion contacting the MRG.*

11

205

HIV-Associated Oral Viral Infections (Figs. 93.1–93.8)

There are eight human herpesviruses (HHVs), including HSV-1 and HSV-2, varicella-zoster, cytomegalovirus, Epstein-Barr virus, HHV-6, HHV-7, and HHV-8. All but HHV-6 and HHV-7 figure prominently in acute and chronic oral disease in AIDS. **HSV infections** (Figs. 93.1 and 93.2) usually appear on the lips or in the mouth on keratinized epithelium. Recurrent infection forms small vesicles that rapidly erupt, leaving shallow yellow ulcers bordered by a red halo. Coalescence of adjacent vesicles into large ulcers is common. Unlike patients with normal immune function, patients with AIDS may have herpetic infections on mucosal surfaces typical of aphthous such as the tongue and buccal mucosa. Recurrent HSV infections are more frequent, persistent, and severe (larger) in immunosuppressed patients.

Varicella-Zoster Virus (VZV; Fig. 93.3)

is a herpesvirus that causes chickenpox and—in immunosuppressed adults—may reactivate to cause herpes zoster (shingles). VZV recrudesces more frequently in HIV-positive patients than the ordinary population. The clinical appearance is similar in both groups, but the prognosis is worse for immunosuppressed patients. VZV produces multiple vesicles that are commonly located on the trunk or face, extend to the midline, and are usually self-limiting and unilateral. The vesicles erupt, coalesce, and then form pustules and ulcers before scabbing. Vesicles are typically found along a branch of the trigeminal nerve, inside or outside the mouth. Deep, searing pain is the premiere symptom and may persist after the lesions heal (**postherpetic neuralgia**). Antiviral agents are used to accelerate healing and alleviate symptoms.

Cytomegalovirus (CMV; Fig. 93.4)

infection occurs in nearly 100% of untreated HIV-positive men who have sex with men and approximately 10% of children with AIDS. The virus has a predilection for secretory tissue (salivary glands) and is prevalent in the saliva of HIV-seropositive persons. Inflammatory changes associated with CMV in HIV-infected persons include unilateral and bilateral parotid gland swelling and xerostomia. CMV-induced oral ulcerations are nonspecific, often resemble aphthae, and can occur on any mucosal surface. They are more frequent when the CD4 count is <100 cells/mm³.

Epstein-Barr Virus (EBV) and Hairy Leukoplakia (Figs. 93.5, 56.7, and 56.8)

Hairy leukoplakia is a raised, corrugated white lesion on the lateral border of the tongue that is associated with EBV and immunosuppression. Early lesions appear as discrete, white, vertically oriented plaques on the lateral borders of both sides of the tongue. Mature lesions may cover the entire lateral and dorsal surface of the tongue and extend onto the buccal mucosa and palate. The lesions are asymptomatic, cannot be rubbed off and may pose an esthetic problem to the patient. Histologic features are hyperkeratotic hairlike projections, koilocytosis (swollen epithelial cells), minimal inflammation, and, frequently, candidal coinfection. Electron microscopic examination shows EBV particles. Treatment is with antiviral agents.

Human Papillomavirus (HPV) Oral manifestations of HPV occur frequently in persons infected with HIV, even in spite of ART. So far, more than 100 genotypes of HPV have been identified. A variety of benign mucocutaneous lesions are induced by the virus, including squamous papilloma, verruca vulgaris, focal epithelial hyperplasia (Heck disease), and condyloma acuminatum. These entities are discussed below and in Section 10.

Condyloma Acuminatum (Fig. 93.6)

is a slow-growing HPV-induced venereal wart often seen in HIV-positive patients. This benign growth appears as a small, soft, pink to dirty gray papule that has a cauliflowerlike surface. **Condyloma acuminata** are often multiple, recurrent, and coalescent to form large, sessile, pebbly growths. They can be found on any mucosal surface, particularly the ventral tongue, gingiva, labial mucosa, and palate. Transmission is by (1) direct contact that results in contagious spread from anal or genital sites or (2) self-inoculation. Treatment consists of local excision or antiviral therapy together with simultaneous eradication of all lesions of infected partners.

Oral Malignancies (Figs. 93.7 and 93.8)

Kaposi sarcoma (Fig. 93.7) is a vascular tumor that exhibits endothelial proliferation that affects the skin and mucosa. HHV-8, a herpesvirus capable of promoting angiogenesis, is the causative agent. Three types are recognized: indolent (classic), endemic (African), and immunosuppression associated; the latter exhibits a progressive course. Kaposi sarcoma is the most common cancer associated with HIV infection, with at least 20% of all AIDS patients affected.

Kaposi sarcoma is characterized by three clinical stages. Initially, it appears an asymptomatic red macule or patch. In the second stage, the tumor enlarges into a red-blue plaque. Advanced lesions (third stage) appear as lobulated, violet nodules that ulcerate and cause pain. Oral lesions are limited to the immunosuppression-associated form. The hard palate is the most common location, followed by the gingiva and buccal mucosa. Lesions are frequently multiple, uncomfortable, and esthetically displeasing. Similar-appearing lesions, such as erythroplakia, purpura, hemangiomas, pyogenic granuloma, and bacillary angiomatosis, should be ruled out by biopsy. Localized radiation therapy, direct injection of chemotherapeutic drugs (vinblastine) or sclerosing agents, and use of HAART have proven beneficial.

Non-Hodgkin Lymphoma (NHL, Fig. 93.8) and Squamous Cell Carcinoma

are both associated with HIV infection, probably as a result of abnormal immune surveillance and dysregulation of apoptosis. **NHL** is linked with EBV infection and often appears as a rapidly proliferating, purplish, nodular mass of the palatal-retromolar complex. **Squamous cell carcinoma** is most frequently found as a reddish white or ulcerated lesion on the posterolateral border of the tongue, floor of the mouth (Fig. 90.4), or, less frequently, the gingiva. These neoplasms occur at a younger age when associated with HIV infection and when the usual cofactors—such as alcohol abuse, advanced age, and poor oral hygiene—are absent. Treatment involves chemotherapy and radiation.

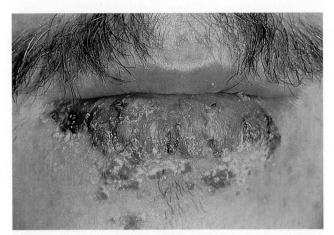

Fig. 93.1. Recurrent herpes labialis: in AIDS.

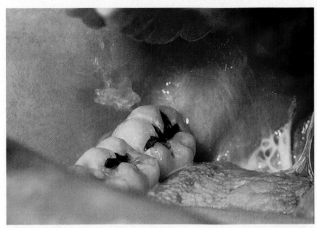

Fig. 93.2. HIV-associated recurrent herpes simplex: ulcer.

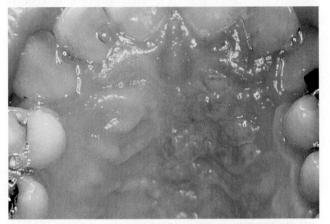

Fig. 93.3. HIV-associated herpes zoster: up to midline.

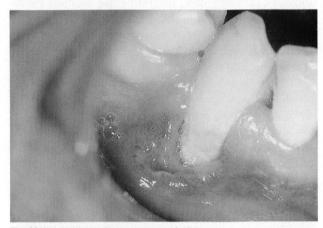

Fig. 93.4. Cytomegalovirus gingival ulceration.

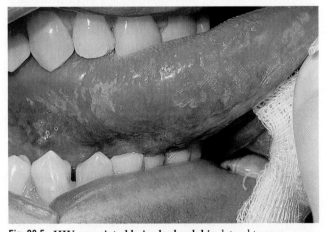

Fig. 93.5. HIV-associated hairy leukoplakia: lateral tongue.

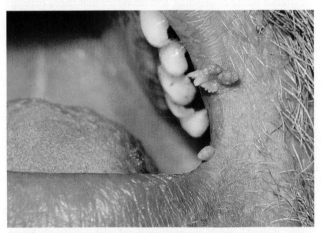

Fig. 93.6. HIV-associated condyloma acuminata.

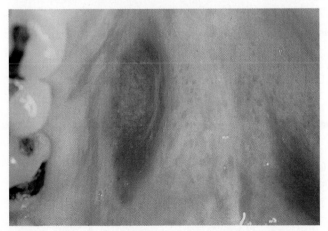

Fig. 93.7. HIV-associated Kaposi sarcoma: purple macules.

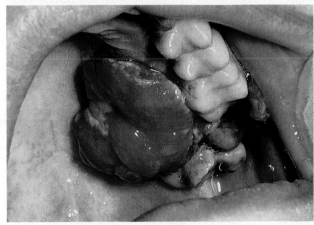

Fig. 93.8. HIV-associated non-Hodgkin lymphoma.

11

Meth Mouth (Figs. 94.1 and 94.2) Methamphetamine is a highly addictive substance that affects the central nervous system, causing euphoria and stimulation. It is a Schedule II narcotic that has a high potential for abuse. Common street forms of the drug are powder and crystal. The crystal form (also known as "ice," "crystal," and "glass") has higher purity and more potential for abuse. Crystal is typically smoked, producing an immediate and intense sensation. The drug is also taken orally, by snorting, or injected. The effects are rapid and generally last 4 to 12 hours. About 3% of young adults report use of crystal methamphetamine. Methamphetamine use is associated with risky and antisocial behaviors, including other illicit drug use, criminal behavior, and several adverse health consequences, such as mood disturbances, insomnia, cardiovascular problems (hypertension), convulsions, weight loss, psychotic symptoms that can be long term, and risk for Parkinson disease.

Chronic "meth" use can have devastating effects on the mouth. It is associated with rampant caries (**meth mouth**), which results from the drug's ability to decrease salivary flow and/or create the perception of a dry mouth and cause cravings for carbonated soft drinks. Chronic exposure of the teeth to carbonated drinks produces class V caries, especially on multiple anterior teeth. Key signs include malnourished individuals (teenagers and young adults) who have accelerated class V decay that is often stained a characteristic brownish color. Clinicians should inform patients to obtain substance abuse counseling and be aware that these patients (typical of drug abusers) may have a higher tolerance for local and general anesthetics.

Graft Versus Host Disease (GVHD; Figs. 94.3 and 94.4) is a frequent and potentially serious complication of allogeneic bone marrow transplant. Allogeneic transplant involves transfer of tissue (in this case hematopoietic stem cells) from different individuals of the same species. Donors are human leukocyte antigen (HLA) matched, as close as possible with the patient. The disease develops within the first 2 years of transplant as a result of cytotoxic T cells that target the graft as well as the skin, liver, lacrimal and salivary glands, and oral mucosa.

Oral GVHD is common and, in some cases, may be the only affected site. Presentations vary and are divided into acute (develops within the first 100 days) and chronic (after 100 days). **Acute oral GVHD** appears as mucosal erythema, atrophy, erosions, or severe sloughing of the tongue, buccal mucosa, or lips. **Chronic oral GVHD** often results in a lacy network of white lines or plaques that resemble lichen planus. A burning sensation may accompany the condition. Affected salivary glands exhibit reduced function resulting in dry mouth and can result in small superficial mucoceles inside the lip or on the palate. Attempts are made to prevent the disease with proper HLA matching and the use of immunosuppressive drugs. Treatment is directed at reducing pain and inflammation as well as improving moisture and salivary flow.

Medication-Related Osteonecrosis of the Jaw (Figs. 94.5–94.7), or **MRONJ**, is defined as the presence of exposed bone in the maxillofacial region that does not heal within eight weeks after diagnosis and there is no history of radiation therapy, or obvious metastasis, to the jaw. Drugs that inhibit bone formation and/or angiogenesis (denosumab, bevacizumab) are causative. The classic drugs first involved in this condition were the bisphosphonates. These drugs inhibit osteoclast function; thus, they inhibit bone resorption. They are used in the management of osteoporosis, osteogenesis imperfecta, Paget disease, and cancers involving bone. Bisphosphonates are administered orally (alendronate, ibandronate, risedronate) for osteoporosis or intravenously (pamidronate, zoledronate) to help slow the destruction from bony metastases arising from breast and prostate cancer or multiple myeloma. Bisphosphonate drugs, especially the IV forms, are more potent and associated with higher risk for MRONJ than the orally administered types, which are used to treat osteoporosis.

Although the exact cause of bisphosphonate osteonecrosis is not well defined, the most common trigger is oral trauma (dental extraction, implant placement, osseous surgery). Increased duration of drug use, smoking, alcohol use, corticosteroid therapy, diabetes, periodontal disease, and poor oral hygiene increase the risk of developing the disease. The most common site is the posterior mandible; however, tori and the maxilla can be involved.

MRONJ lesions begin as delayed healing after an extraction or trauma or in an area of periodontal disease. Early features can be recognized radiographically as widened periodontal ligament and sclerotic lamina dura surrounding an affected tooth. As the condition progresses, an ulcer that contains an area of exposed, underlying dead bone is seen. Early-stage disease causes little or no discomfort; however, progression leads to pain in most cases and can lead to fistula or perforation. Lesions are characterized by their persistent nature and poor response to treatments. Management involves implementation of preventive measures (perform extractions and invasive procedures) before initiating drug therapy and good oral hygiene measures and the performance of endodontic procedures in lieu of extractions during the course of therapy. Once MRONJ is established, oral antimicrobial rinses, pain medications, and surgical debridement are used to control infection and bone necrosis.

Drug-Induced Hyperpigmentation (Fig. 94.8) Many drugs and conditions can cause hyperpigmentation of the mucosa (see **Pigmented Lesions**, Figs. 77.1–78.8, for additional information). In this example, oral pigmentation is associated with administration of doxorubicin (Adriamycin). This chemotherapy drug is used in the treatment of many types of cancers. Other drugs that can cause oral pigmentation include bleomycin, minocycline, tetracycline, estrogen, imatinib (Gleevec), antimalarial drugs, as well as drugs associated with management of HIV infection such as clofazimine, ketoconazole, pyrimethamine, and zidovudine (AZT).

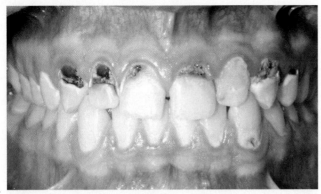

Fig. 94.1. **Meth mouth:** rampant decay incisors.

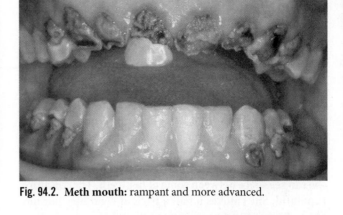

Fig. 94.2. **Meth mouth:** rampant and more advanced.

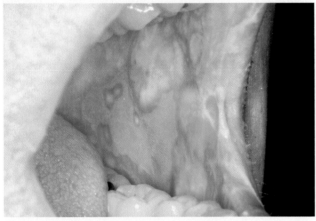

Fig. 94.3. **Graft versus host disease:** lichenoid mucosa.

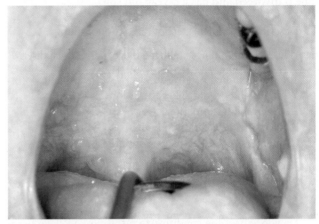

Fig. 94.4. **Graft versus host disease:** mucoceles on palate.

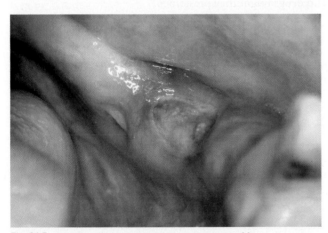

Fig. 94.5. **Bisphosphonate osteonecrosis:** exposed bone.

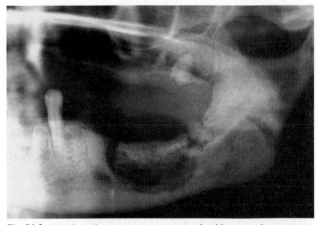

Fig. 94.6. **Bisphosphonate osteonecrosis:** dead bone molar region.

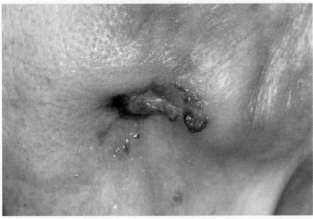

Fig. 94.7. **Bisphosphonate osteonecrosis:** draining onto the face.

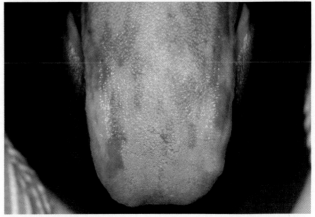

Fig. 94.8. **Drug-induced hyperpigmentation:** Adriamycin.

CASE 51. (FIG. 94.9)

This 27-year-old woman presents to your office as a new patient. Her intake forms do not list an employer. Her health history form indicates illicit drug use in the past, but no illicit drug use for the past 3 years. She has anterior crowns and with no visible decay. She claims her gums recently began hurting around several front teeth and now she can see space between some of her teeth. The condition is painful. She smokes a half a pack of cigarettes per day. She is divorced and has a 3-year-old son.

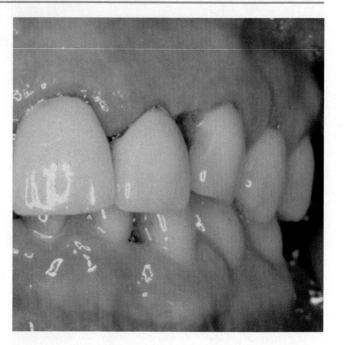

1. Describe the clinical state of the periodontium.

2. What clinical findings are suggestive of periodontal disease?

3. You detect bone loss around several of these teeth. Which term best describes the lesion?
   A. Necrotizing stomatitis
   B. Necrotizing ulcerative gingivitis
   C. Necrotizing ulcerative periodontitis
   D. Desquamative gingivitis

4. What factors (or condition) are associated with the oral findings?

5. Do you expect the condition to resolve if you clean her teeth?

6. If you refer this patient to a physician, what laboratory tests and drugs might they prescribe?

7. Would you expect her periodontal condition to resolve with periodontal instrumentation (scaling and root planing) and through daily self-care by the patient?

8. Do you believe that the patient should be referred to her primary care physician in regard to this periodontal condition? If so, how would you communicate this suggestion to the patient?

CASE 52. (FIG. 94.10)

This 21-year-old college student presents for his 6-month cleaning. He is a senior at the local university and finishing his degree in business. He has a girlfriend who attends the same university. He has no significant medical findings and reports only a slightly sore throat.

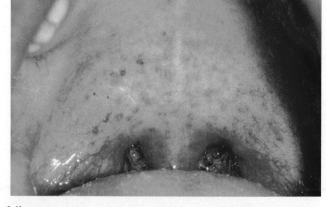

1. Describe the oral findings.

2. How is the patient's medical history potentially relevant to the clinical condition?

3. What questions could you ask regarding the information provided that might provide a diagnostic clue of what this condition is?

4. The presence of this oral findings is suggestive of all of the following *except*:
   A. Coughing
   B. Fellatio
   C. Bleeding disorder
   D. Viral infection
   E. Sturge-Weber syndrome

5. What is the most likely diagnosis of this condition?

6. What is the cause of this condition?

7. Why is knowledge of this sign important?

8. What complications can occur with this condition?

9. Should this patient be referred to his primary care physician for evaluation? If so, why?

10. What information should be provided to the patient when making this referral?

Additional cases to enhance your learning and understanding of this section are available Online through the book's Navigate 2 Advantage Access site.

11

Clinical Applications and Resources

Abbreviation	English	Latin Derivative
ad lib	at pleasure	ad libitum
a.c.	before meals	ante cibum
p.c.	after meals	post cibum
aq.	water	aqua
d.	a day, daily	dies
b.i.d.	twice a day	bis in die
t.i.d.	three times a day	ter in die
q.i.d.	four times a day	quater in die
h.	hour	hora
h.s.	at bedtime	hora somni
q.h.	every hour	quaque hora
q.3h.	every three hours	quaque tertia hora
q.4h.	every four hours	quaque quarta hora
q.6h.	every six hours	quaque sexta hora
n.r.	do not repeat	non repetatur
p.r.n.	as needed	pro re nata
stat.	immediately	statim
Sig.	label	signetur
c.	with	cum
gtt.	drops	guttae
tab	tablet	tabella
caps.	capsule	capsula
q.d.	every day	quaque die
p.o.	orally	per os

PRESCRIPTIONS AND THERAPEUTIC PROTOCOLS

Analgesics

Generic Name and Concentration	Trade Name	Disp:	Sig:
For Relief of Mild to Moderate Acute Pain			
Acetaminophen (Tylenol) 325 mg [OTC]	Tylenol	25	Take 2 tablets q.4h. p.r.n. for pain, not to exceed 12 tablets in 24 hours.
Aspirin 325 mg [OTC]		25	Take 2 tablets q.4h. p.r.n for pain.
Ibuprofen (Motrin) 400 mg	Advil, Motrin	25	Take 2 tablets q.4h. p.r.n for pain.
Propoxyphene napsylate 50 mg and acetaminophen 325 mg	Darvocet-N 50	25	Take 2 tablets q.4h. p.r.n. for pain.
Naproxen sodium 220 mg [OTC] Naprosyn 375 mg	Aleve	50	Take 2 tablets b.i.d p.r.n. for pain.
Celecoxib 200 mg	Celebrex	18	Take 1 tablet q.d. for pain. Note: Do not prescribe if allergic to sulfa medications.
Diflunisal 500 mg	Dolobid	18	Take 1 tablet b.i.d. for pain.
For Relief of Moderate Acute Pain			
Acetaminophen 300 mg, with codeine 30 mg	Tylenol with Codeine No. 3	20	Take 1 to 2 tablets q.4h. p.r.n. for pain.
Aspirin 325 mg, with codeine 30 mg	Empirin with Codeine No. 3	20	Take 1 to 2 tablets q.4h. p.r.n. for pain.
Aspirin 325 mg, butalbital 50 mg, caffeine 40 mg	Fiorinal	20	Take 1 to 2 tablets q.4h. p.r.n. for pain.
Aspirin 325 mg, butalbital 50 mg, caffeine 40 mg, codeine 30 mg	Fiorinal with Codeine 30 mg	20	Take 1 to 2 tablets q.4h. p.r.n. for pain.
Acetaminophen 325 mg, butalbital 50 mg, caffeine 40 mg	Margesic	20	Take 1 to 2 tablets q.4h. p.r.n. for pain.
Hydrocodone bitartrate 5 mg, with acetaminophen 500 mg	Lortab 5, Anexsia 5/500, Vicodin, Zydone	20	Take 1 tablet q.4–6h. p.r.n. for pain.
Dihydrocodeine bitartrate 16 mg, aspirin 356.4 mg, caffeine 30 mg	Synalgos-DC capsules	20	Take 1 to 2 tablets q.4h. p.r.n. for pain.
Hydrocodone 5 mg, ibuprofen 200 mg	Ibudone, Xylon 5	20	Take 1 to 2 tablets q.4–6h. p.r.n. for pain.
Hydrocodone 7.5 mg, ibuprofen 200 mg	Vicoprofen	20	Take 1 to 2 tablets q.4–6h. p.r.n. for pain.
Acetaminophen 325 mg, tramadol 37.5 mg	Ultracet	20	Take 2 tablets q.4–6 h. p.r.n. pain (not to exceed 8 tablets in 24 h)
For Relief of Moderate to Severe Acute Pain			
Hydrocodone bitartrate 7.5 mg, with acetaminophen 500 mg	Lortab 7.5/500	30	Take 1 tablet q.6h. p.r.n. for pain.
Hydrocodone bitartrate 7.5 mg, with acetaminophen 650 mg	Lorcet Plus	30	Take 1 tablet q.6h. p.r.n. for pain.
Hydrocodone bitartrate 10 mg, with acetaminophen 325 mg	Norco 10 mg–325 mg	30	Take 1 tablet q.6h. p.r.n. for pain.
Hydrocodone bitartrate 10 mg, with acetaminophen 650 mg	Lorcet 10/650	30	Take 1 tablet q.6h. p.r.n. for pain.
Oxycodone HCl 5 mg, with acetaminophen 325 mg	Percocet, Roxicet	24	Take 1 tablet q.6h. p.r.n. for pain.
Oxycodone HCl 5 mg, with acetaminophen 500 mg	Tylox	24	Take 1 tablet q.6h. p.r.n. for pain.
Oxycodone HCl 4.5 mg, oxycodone terephthalate 0.38 mg, aspirin 325 mg	Percodan	24	Take 1 tablet q.6h. p.r.n. for pain.
Meperidine HCl 50 mg, with promethazine HCl 25 mg	Mepergan Fortis Capsules	24	Take 1 tablet q.4–6h. p.r.n. for pain.

12

ANTIBIOTIC PROPHYLAXIS

To Prevent Infective Endocarditis—American Heart Association Guidelines Regimens for Dental Procedures (Single Dose 30 to 60 Minutes Before Procedure)			
Situation	*Agent*	*Adults*	*Children*
Oral dosage	Amoxicillin	2 g	50 mg/kg
Unable to take oral medication	Ampicillin or	2 g IM or IV	50 mg/kg IM or IV
	Cefazolin or ceftriaxone	1 g IM or IV	50 mg/kg IM or IV
Allergic to penicillins or ampicillin—oral	Cephalexin*† or Clindamycin or Azithromycin or clarithromycin	2 g 600 mg 500 mg	50 mg/kg 20 mg/kg 15 mg/kg
Allergic to penicillins or ampicillin and unable to take oral medication	Cefazolin or ceftriaxone† or Clindamycin	1 g IM or IV 600 mg IM or IV	50 mg/kg IM or IV 20 mg/kg IM or IV

*Or other first- or second-generation oral cephalosporin in equivalent adult or pediatric dosage.

†Cephalosporins should not be used in an individual with a history of immediate-type hypersensitivity to penicillin (i.e., anaphylaxis, angioedema of the airway).

Cardiac Conditions for which Prophylaxis Is Recommended during Dental Procedures

Prosthetic cardiac valve
Previous infective endocarditis
Congenital heart disease
- Unrepaired cyanotic congenital heart disease, including palliative shunts and conduits
- Completely repaired congenital heart disease defects with prosthetic material or device for the first 6 months after procedure
- Repaired congenital heart disease with residual defects at the site or adjacent site of prosthetic patch/device (which inhibits endothelialization)
- Cardiac transplantation recipients who develop cardiac valvulopathy

Dental Procedures for which Infective Endocarditis Prophylaxis Is Recommended

All dental procedures that involve "manipulation of gingival tissue or periapical region (root end) of teeth or perforation of the oral mucosa."

Dental Procedures for which Infective Endocarditis Prophylaxis Is NOT Recommended

Routine anesthetic injection through noninfected tissue
Placement of removable appliances
Placement of orthodontic brackets
Bleeding from trauma to lips/mucosa
Taking dental radiographs
Adjustment of orthodontic appliances
Shedding of deciduous teeth

To Eliminate Bacterial Organisms That Cause Oral Infection

Generic Name and Concentration	Trade Name	Disp:	Sig:
Phenoxymethylpenicillin 500 mg	Penicillin V	40	Take 2 tablets immediately and then 1 tablet q.6h. 1 hour a.c. Continue for 7 days.
Penicillin V potassium liquid 125 mg/5 mL	Penicillin VK*	200 mL	Children should take 1 teaspoonful q.6h.
Amoxicillin 500 mg	Amoxil*	30	Take 500-mg tablet t.i.d. Continue for 10 days.
Amoxicillin 500 mg, clavulanate potassium	Augmentin*	30	Take 1 tablet 3 times daily for 10 days.
Cephalexin 500 mg	Keflex*	40	Take 1 tablet q.6h. Continue for 10 days.
Dicloxacillin sodium 500 mg Note: For penicillinase-resistant infection.	Dynapen*	40	Take 1 tablet q.6 h. Continue for 10 days.
Erythromycin ethylsuccinate 400 mg	E.E.S.*	56	Take one 400-mg tablet q.6h. Continue for 7 days.
Trimethoprim 80 mg, with sulfamethoxazole 400 mg Note: For infections with Escherichia coli, Haemophilus influenzae, and Klebsiella and Enterobacter species.	Bactrim*	40	Take 1 tablet q.12h. Continue for 7 days.
Metronidazole 500 mg Note: For febrile patients with acute necrotizing ulcerative gingivitis involving anaerobic bacteria.	Flagyl*	40	Take 2 tablets immediately, then 1 tablet q.6h. until gone.
Clindamycin 300 mg Note: For bone infections involving anaerobic bacteria.	Cleocin	30	Take 1 capsule q.6–8 h. Continue for 7 days.
Tetracycline HCl V 250 mg Note: For infections of periodontal tissues.	Achromycin*	56	Take 1 tablet q.i.d. Continue for 7 days.

*Use with caution in patients with diminished or impaired liver function and in patients with diminished or impaired kidney function.

12

To Reduce Pathogenic Microbial Flora Often Associated with Periodontal Infections

Generic Name and Concentration	Trade Name	Disp:	Sig:
Chlorhexidine gluconate 0.12% oral rinse	Peridex, PerioGard	480 mL	Swish 1 teaspoonful for 1 minute; then expectorate. Perform b.i.d. daily (morning and evening) after brushing teeth. Avoid eating or drinking for 30 minutes.
Chlorhexidine gluconate 2.5 mg	PerioChip	Box of 10 chips	For office use only. Place in gingival sulcus in affected areas (≥5 mm). Administer once every 3 months if needed.
Doxycycline 20 mg *Note:* Not recommended for children.	Periostat	28	Take 1 or 2 tablets 1 hour before or 2 hours after a meal, q.d. for 14 days.
Doxycycline hyclate 10%	Atridox	450-mg syringe	Mix contents in syringes, then uncouple syringes, and express the product into the pocket until the formulation reaches the top of the gingival margin.
Metronidazole 500 mg	Flagyl	40	Take 2 tablets immediately, then 1 tablet q.6h. until gone.
Tetracycline HCl 125 mg/5 mL *Note:* May make skin sensitive to sunlight.	Sumycin	480 mL	Rinse with 2 teaspoonfuls for 3 minutes and swallow. Repeat q.i.d.

ANTIFUNGAL THERAPY

To Eliminate Pathogenic Fungal Organisms and Re-establish Normal Oral Flora

Generic Name and Concentration	Trade Name	Disp:	Sig:
Topical			
Nystatin topical powder 500,000 IU	Mycostatin	15-g squeeze bottle	Apply liberally to tissue side of clean denture p.c. Soak the clean denture in a suspension of 1 teaspoon of powder and 8 oz. of water overnight.
Nystatin oral tablets 500,000 IU	Nystatin, Nilstat	90	Dissolve 1 to 2 tablets as a lozenge in mouth 5 times d. for 14 consecutive days.
Clotrimazole 1% topical cream	Lotrimin	12 g	Apply liberally to affected area after meals.
Clotrimazole 10 mg	Mycelex Troches	60	Dissolve 1 tablet as a lozenge 5 times d. for 14 consecutive days.
Ketoconazole cream 2%	Nizoral	15-g tube	Apply liberally to affected area after meals.
Nystatin ointment 100,000 IU	Mycostatin	15- or 30-g tube	Apply liberally to affected area 4–6 times d.
Systemic			
Fluconazole* 100 mg	Diflucan	14	Take 2 tablets the first day, then 1 tablet q.d. for at least 2 weeks.
Itraconazole* 20 mg/mL	Sporanox Oral Solution	280 mL	Take 200 mg (20 mL)/day p.o. for 1 to 2 weeks. Vigorously swish solution in mouth for several seconds and swallow.
Ketoconazole† 200 mg	Nizoral	14	Take 1 tablet q.d. for 2 weeks.
Note: Should be used only if cannot use other antifungals. Can cause serious liver damage.			
Nystatin 500,000 U	Mycostatin	60	Take 1 tablet by mouth daily for 14 consecutive days.
Combination Topical Agents			
Betamethasone dipropionate 0.05% and clotrimazole 1%	Lotrisone	15- or 30-g tube	Apply liberally to affected area 4 or 5 times d.
Iodoquinol 10 mg and hydrocortisone 10 mg cream	Dermazene 1%	15- or 30-g tube	Apply liberally to affected area 4 or 5 times d.
Nystatin 100,000 U and triamcinolone acetonide 0.1%	Mycolog II	15-, 30-, or 60-g tube	Apply liberally to affected area t.i.d. to q.i.d.

These drugs are most effective when dentures are removed and treated, if applicable, and when intake of fermentable carbohydrates is reduced.

*Use with caution in patients with diminished or impaired liver function.

†Use with caution in patients with diminished or impaired liver function. Also, beware of multiple drug interactions.

12

To Prevent Oral Herpetic Infections (Daily Suppression)

Generic Name and Concentration	Trade Name	Disp:	Sig:
Sunscreen SPF 30 or higher		1 bottle	Applied daily to sun-exposed skin surface that are susceptible to recurrences.
Acyclovir 200 mg	Zovirax	100	Take 1 tablet 5 times d.
Acyclovir 800 mg	Zovirax	100	Take 1 tablet b.i.d.
Valacyclovir 500 mg	Valtrex	100	Take 1 tablet q.d. or b.i.d.

To Prevent Oral Herpetic Infections Associated with Dental Procedures

Valacyclovir 500 mg	Valtrex	30	Take 4 capsules b.i.d. on the day of dental treatment and 2 capsules b.i.d. the following 3 days.

To Treat Oral Herpetic Infections

Topical

Acyclovir cream 5%	Zovirax	15 g	Apply to oral lesions with a cotton-tipped applicator 6 times d.
Penciclovir 1% ointment	Denavir	15 g	Apply to lesions with a cotton-tipped applicator at least 5 times d.
Cidofovir 1% gel	Cidofovir	Compounded	Apply to lesions with a cotton-tipped applicator at least 5 times d.

Note: Used only if lesions are known to be acyclovir/valacyclovir resistant.

Foscarnet 3% cream	Foscavir	Compounded	Apply to lesions with a cotton-tipped applicator at least 5 times d.

Note: Used only if lesions are known to be acyclovir/valacyclovir resistant.

Docosanol 10% cream	Abreva	2 g	Apply to lesions with a cotton-tipped applicator at least 5 times d.
Benzalkonium chloride	Viroxyn	1 tube	Remove cap, squeeze tube, allow tip to saturate swab, then apply to developing lesion.

Systemic

Acyclovir 200 mg, 400 mg, 800 mg	Zovirax	50	Take 800 mg at onset of recurrence and 800 mg b.i.d. for at least 3 days.
Famciclovir 500 mg	Famvir	50	Take 1 capsule at onset of recurrence and t.i.d. for at least 3 days.
Valacyclovir 500 mg	Valtrex	50	Take 4 tablets at onset of recurrence and 2 to 4 tablets 12 hours later for at least 3 days.
L-Lysine 500 mg	Enisyl	100	Take 4 tablets q.4h. until symptoms subside.

Note: Treatment should begin during the early stage of the recurrence. Most effective if foods containing high content of arginine are avoided.

To Treat Oral Human Papillomavirus Infection

Generic Name and Concentration	Trade Name	Disp:	Sig:
Podofilox 0.5% gel	Condylox	3.5 g	Apply to lesions with a cotton-tipped applicator b.i.d. then withdraw for the next 4 days. Repeat cycle weekly up to 4 times, if needed.
Cidofovir 1% cream or 3% gel	Vistide	5 g	Apply and rub into lesions with a cotton-tipped applicator on q.o.d. for 1 week.
Imiquimod 5% cream	Aldara	5 g	Apply to lesions with a cotton-tipped applicator on a once-daily basis for 2 weeks.

Vaccines

To Prevent Recurrent Herpes Zoster (Shingles) Infections

Live, attenuated varicella-zoster virus (VZV; shingles) vaccine	Zostavax	Vial	Single-dose subcutaneous injection. For individuals 60 years of age and older.

To Prevent Oral Human Papillomavirus Infections and Related Disease

Quadrivalent HPV vaccine (low-risk HPV types 6 and 11 and high-risk HPV types 16 and 18)	Gardasil	Vial	3 injections given in 1 year at months 0, 1, and 6. For females and males 9–26 years.
Bivalent HPV vaccine (HPVs 16 and 18)	Cervarix	Vial	3 injections given in 1 year at months 0, 1, and 6. For females and males 9–26 years.

12

To Manage and Provide Short-Term Relief of Chronic Pain Associated with Mucosal Ulcerations			
Generic Name and Concentration	*Trade Name*	*Disp:*	*Sig:*
Diphenhydramine HCl 12.5 mg/5 mL elixir	Benadryl	4 fluid oz.	Rinse with 1 tablespoonful a.c. and p.r.n. for pain.
Benadryl elixir 12.5 mg/5 mL and Kaopectate (Upjohn) 50% mixture by volume		4 fluid oz of each; mix equal parts	Rinse with 1 tablespoonful for 2 minutes a.c. and p.r.n. for pain.
Lidocaine HCl 2% viscous solution HCl	Xylocaine	4 fluid oz.	Rinse with 1 tablespoonful a.c. and p.r.n. for pain.
Orabase with benzocaine (OTC)		5 or 15 g	Apply to affected area a.c. and p.r.n. for pain.
Dyclonine 0.5% or 1%		30 mL	Apply to affected area a.c. and p.r.n. for pain.
Lidocaine 4% gel	Topicaine-4	10 or 30 g	Apply to affected area a.c. and p.r.n. for pain.

ANTIANXIETY AGENTS

To Manage and Provide Short-Term Relief of the Symptoms of Anxiety Associated with Dental Procedures

Generic Name and Concentration	Trade Name	Disp:	Sig:
Alprazolam 0.25 mg	Xanax	20	Take 1 tablet in the evening before bed and 1 tablet 1 hour before appointment.*
Chlordiazepoxide 10 mg	Librium	20	Take 1 tablet in the evening before bed and 1 tablet 1 hour before appointment.*
Triazolam 0.25 mg	Halcion	20	Take 1 tablet 1 hour before dental appointments.*
Diazepam 5 mg	Valium	20	Take 1 tablet in the evening before bed and 1 tablet 1 hour before appointment.*
Oxazepam 10 mg	Serax	20	Take 1 tablet in the evening before bed and 1 tablet 1 hour before appointment.*
Buspirone 5 mg	BuSpar	20	Take 1 tablet q.d. or b.i.d.
Lorazepam 0.5 mg	Ativan	20	Take 1 tablet q.d. or b.i.d.
Hydroxyzine 25 mg	Atarax, Vistaril	20	Take 2 capsules in the evening before bed and 2 capsules 1 hour before appointment.
Note: Dose of child (30–60 lb) is half the adult dose.*			
Hydroxyzine syrup 10 mg/5 mL	Atarax	50 or 100 mL	Take 2 teaspoonfuls 1 hour before dental appointment.
Diphenhydramine 25 mg	Benadryl	25	Take 1 tablet q.i.d.

Note: Use lower doses of these drugs in the elderly and in patients who have kidney or liver impairment.

*Caution: Patients should not drive themselves to or from the appointment.

To Prevent Dental Caries and Dentin Sensitivity in Susceptible Patients

Generic Name and Concentration	Trade Name	Disp:	Sig:
Stannous fluoride 0.4%	Gel-Kam	4.3 fluid oz.	Apply 5–10 drops in a carrier and place carrier on teeth daily for 5 minutes.
Sodium fluoride 0.11%	Luride	60-mL bottle with dropper	6 months to 3 years of age: apply one-half dropperful (0.5 mL) daily to mouth of child.

3 to 6 years: apply one dropperful daily in mouth of child
Consider using when drinking water fluoride content is less than 0.3 ppm fluoride.

Generic Name and Concentration	Trade Name	Disp:	Sig:
1.1% neutral sodium fluoride (5,000 ppm)	PrevDent, ControlRx, Neutracare	2 oz.	Apply 5 drops in a custom-made tray and place tray over teeth daily for 5 minutes.
1.1% neutral sodium fluoride	NUPRO	12 oz.	Apply to susceptible tooth surfaces using cotton tip in dental office every 6 months.
5% sodium fluoride varnish (22,600 ppm)	CavityShield, Duraflor, DuraShield, PreviDent Varnish, Vella	1-oz tube	Apply to susceptible tooth surfaces using cotton tip in dental office every 6 months.
5% sodium fluoride varnish (22,600 ppm) with amorphous calcium phosphate	Enamel Pro Varnish with ACP, MI Varnish with RECALDENT	0.4 mL	Apply to susceptible tooth surfaces using cotton tip in dental office every 6 months.
5% sodium fluoride varnish (22,600 ppm) with tricalcium phosphate	Vanish White Varnish	0.5 mL	Apply to susceptible tooth surfaces using cotton tip in dental office every 6 months.

HEMOSTATIC AGENTS

To Help Stop Bleeding in the Oral Cavity

Generic Name and Concentration	Trade Name	Disp:	Sig:
Absorbable gelatin sponge	Gelfoam Gelfoam-plus	2 × 2 cm Box of 12	Place in extraction socket. Can place topical thrombin on sponge.
Absorbable collagen	Instat, Helistat	1 × 2 inch Box of 24	Place in extraction socket.
Absorbable dressings from bovine collage	CollaCote, CollaTape, CollaPlug	10 packs	Place in extraction site, biopsy site, or under stents or dentures when bleeding is present.
Chitosan-based hemostatic dressing	Hemcon Dental Dressing	10 × 12 mm	Place in contact with bleeding site for oral mucosal tissue wounds.
(N-butyl-2) cyanoacrylate	Histoacryl	0.5-mL ampules/10 box	Topical application (flow) into extraction or wound site
Microfibrillar collagen	Avitene	0.5 or 1 g	Place in extraction socket.
Oxidized regenerated cellulose	Oxycel, Surgicel	0.5 × 2 inch	Place in extraction socket.

Steroids

To Manage Mucosal Ulcers and Erosions Associated with Immunological and Skin Disorders

Generic Name and Concentration	Trade Name	Disp:	Sig:
Medium Potency Steroids			
Triamcinolone acetonide 0.1% ointment	Kenalog in Orabase	5-g tube	Apply to ulcerated area p.c. and h.s.
Betamethasone valerate 0.1% ointment	Valisone ointment	15-g or 30-g tube	Apply to ulcerated area p.c. and h.s.
Betamethasone syrup 0.1%	Celestone	50 mL	Rinse with 1 teaspoonful q.i.d., p.c. and h.s.
Triamcinolone 40 mg/mL solution	Kenalog-40	5-mL injectable vials	Mix 1 mL of steroid with 0.5 mL of anesthetic. Inject 0.25 mL at 4 locations around border of ulcer. Total 1 mL injected.
High-Potency Steroids			
Augmented betamethasone 0.05% ointment	Diprolene ointment	15- or 30-g tube	Apply to affected area p.c. and h.s.
Fluocinonide 0.05% ointment	Lidex ointment	15- or 30-g tube	Apply to mouth sore p.c. and h.s.
Dexamethasone elixir 0.5%	Decadron	100-mL bottle	Rinse with 1 teaspoonful q.i.d. for 2 minutes, then expectorate.
Very–High-Potency Steroids			
Budesonide 3-mg capsule	Budesonide*	40 capsules	Crush capsule; dissolve in 10 mL water. Rinse for 4 minutes t.i.d, and expectorate.
Dexamethasone elixir 0.75%	Decadron*	100-mL bottle	Rinse with 1 teaspoonful q.i.d. for 2 minutes, then swallow.
Clobetasol 0.05% ointment	Temovate ointment	15- or 30-g tube	Apply to affected area q.i.d.
Halobetasol propionate 0.05% ointment	Ultravate ointment	15- or 30-g tube	Apply to affected area q.i.d.
Methylprednisolone	Medrol* 4 mg Dosepak 21s	1 Dosepak (21 tabs)	Take graduated daily doses according to the manufacturer's directions listed on the Dosepak.
Prednisone* 10 mg		20	Take 4 tablets in the a.m. Continue daily for 4 d.
Prednisolone liquid 15 mg/5 mL	Prelone,* Orapred*	200-mL bottle	Rinse with 1 teaspoonful q.i.d. for 2 minutes, then expectorate.

More than 2 weeks of therapy of very–high-potency steroids may affect normal cortisol production and increase risk of candidiasis.

High-potency and very–high-potency steroids should be avoided in patients with gastrointestinal ulcers, diabetes, hematologic malignancy, and hepatitis and in women who are pregnant or nursing.

Immunomodulating Drugs

Generic Name and Concentration	Trade Name	Disp:	Sig:
Topical			
Cyclosporine 100 mg/mL Note: Black box warning	SandIMMUNE	200 mL	Rinse with 5 mL of 100 mg cyclosporine/mL t.i.d.
Pimecrolimus 1%	Elidel	30 g	Apply to affected area t.i.d.
Tacrolimus 0.1%	Protopic	30 g	Apply to affected area q.i.d.
Systemic			
Azathioprine 50 mg Note: Imuran can be prescribed to reduce the dose of prednisone.	Imuran	60	Take 1 tablet b.i.d.
Dapsone 25 mg Note: Dapsone requires checking complete blood count and liver function every month for 3 months.	Dapsone	60	Take 1 tablet t.i.d., 2 t.i.d., 3 t.i.d., 4 daily thereafter.
Mycophenolate mofetil Note: Black box warning.	Cellcept	500 mg	500–1,500 mg b.i.d.

Other Agents
Ulcer-Coating Agents

Diphenhydramine HCl with Kaopectate	Benadryl syrup (mix 50/50) with Kaopectate	8 oz	Rinse 1 tablespoonful in mouth for 1 minute then spit. Repeat as needed to relieve pain.

Cauterizer (for aphthous)

Active ingredient: sulfuric acid and phenolic solution	Debacterol	1 tube	Break tube to open; touch saturated cotton tip to ulcer for 20 seconds. Advise the patient it will hurt (burn).

12

To Replace Deficient Nutrients Necessary for Homeostasis

Generic Name and Concentration	Trade Name	Disp:	Sig:
Ferrous sulfate 250 mg	Iron	100	Take 1 tablet q.d. for 1 month, then reassess patient's hemoglobin level.
Folic acid 0.4 mg	Folate	30	Take 1 tablet q.d. for 1 month, then reassess patient's hemoglobin level.
Cyanocobalamin	Vitamin B12	10-mL vial	Inject 0.1 to 1 mL IM in deltoid; reassess patient's symptoms and blood profile monthly.
Water-soluble bioflavonoids 200 mg with ascorbic acid 200 mg	Peridin-C 500 mg	100	Take 1 tablet t.i.d.

SALIVA SUBSTITUTE

Generic Name and Concentration	Trade Name	Disp:	Sig:
Calcium phosphate (supersaturated) rinse	Caphosol, NeutraSal	30 mL	Use as a rinse p.r.n.
Carboxymethylcellulose 0.5% aqueous solution	Saliva substitute	120 mL	Use as a rinse p.r.n.
Carboxymethylcellulose	Moi-Stir,* Orex, Sage Moist Plus, Salivart,† Xero-Lube, Oasis Mouth Spray, MouthKote		Use as a rinse p.r.n.
Hydroxyethylcellulose, xylitol, citric acid	Optimoist	9 mL	Spray in mouth p.r.n. for dry mouth.
Glucose oxidase and lactoperoxidase	Biotene	120 mL	Rinse in mouth for 1 minute p.r.n. for oral dryness.
Oxidized glycerol triester	Aquoral	40-mL canister	2 sprays in mouth; swish with tongue q.4.h.
Pilocarpine 5 mg	Salagen	100	Take 1 tablet t.i.d. or q.i.d.
Caution: Contraindicated with glaucoma; precautions (eye, heart, obstructive lung diseases).			
Cevimeline HCl 30 mg	Evoxac	100	Take 1 tablet t.i.d. p.r.n. for oral dryness.
Caution: Contraindicated with glaucoma; precautions (eye, heart, obstructive lung diseases).			

Sugarless Chewing Gum and Mints

	MIGHTEAFLOW gum	1 pack	Chew gum q.i.d.
	Xerostom	1 pack	Chew gum q.i.d.
	Xylimelt mints with xylitol	1 pack	Take 1 mint q.i.d.

*120 mL with pump spray.
†75 mL with pump spray.

12

SEDATIVE/HYPNOTICS

To Produce a Sleeplike State for the Effective Dental Management of the Patient			
Generic Name and Concentration	*Trade Name*	*Disp:*	*Sig:*
Triazolam 0.25 mg	Halcion	30	Take 1 tablet 1 hour before appointment
Flurazepam 15 mg	Dalmane	30	Take 1 tablet 1 hour before appointment
Temazepam 15 mg	Restoril	30	Take 1 tablet 1 hour before appointment
Chloral hydrate 500 mg/5 mL	Noctec	1 pint	Take 1 teaspoonful 30 minutes before surgery.

Caution: Patients should not drive themselves to or from appointment.

To Aid the Patient in Quitting the Use of Tobacco

First: **A**sk about your patient's tobacco use
Advise them to quit
Assess their readiness to quit
Assist if ready to quit (medications, substitutes, and counseling)
Arrange for follow-up care

Generic Name and Concentration	Trade Name	Disp:	Sig:
Varenicline 1 mg	Chantix	60	Take 1/2 tablet per day for 3 days before quit date, then 1/2 tablet b.i.d. (>8 hours apart) for 4 days, then 1 tablet b.i.d. (>8 hours apart) for 12 weeks.
Wellbutrin SR 150 mg	Zyban	60	Take 1 tablet per day for 3 days before quit date, then 2 tablets per day (>8 hours apart) for 8 to 12 weeks.

12

Radiopacities (RO) (Section 6)

Entity	Age	Sex	Race/ Ethnicity	Cause	Radiographic Characteristics	Treatment
Tori	>30	F>M	Any	Hereditary overgrowth of the bone	Well-defined round/ oval RO	None required
Osteoma	>35	M–F	Any	Benign tumor of the bone	Well-defined RO, often in posterior mandible. Can be a component of Gardner syndrome	Excise, if needed
Retained root	>10	M–F	Any	Retention of a root	Trauma, failure of resorption, improper extraction	Removal
Socket sclerosis	>40	M–F	Any	Reaction of altered calcium metabolism associated with kidney disease	RO confined to and delineating an extraction socket	None
Osteosclerosis	>40	M–F	Any	Not determined	RO that obliterates marrow space; most in posterior mandible	None
Condensing osteitis	>20	M–F	Any	Pulpal inflammation	Focal RO that obliterates marrow space below apex of affected tooth; most in mandible	Endodontic therapy
Cementoblastoma	>20	M–F	Any	Cementoblastic benign tumor activity	Bulbous RO growth on the root of tooth; most mandibular molar	Surgical extraction
Osteoblastoma	15–35	M>F	Any	Osteoblast proliferation	RO, RL, or RL_RO circular mass	Excision
Cemento-osseous dysplasia	30–50	F	Blacks	Reactive process	3 stages: 1. RO, 2. mixed RL-RO, 3. RO with RL rim. Usually anterior mandible and multiple	None
Garre osteomyelitis	<20	M–F	Any	Chronic disease, periapical infection, bony fracture	RO layers laid down like "onion skin"	Remove source of infection; antibiotics

Radiolucencies (RL) (Section 6)

Entity	Age	Sex	Race/Ethnicity	Cause	Radiographic Characteristics	Treatment
Eruption cyst	<10	M–F	Any	Erupting tooth	Dome-shaped RL surrounding and overlying crown of unerupted tooth	Allow tooth to erupt; incise if needed
Dentigerous cyst	16–30	M–F	Any	Cystic degeneration of reduced enamel epithelium	Unilocular or sometimes multilocular RL, posterior mandible	Enucleation or excision
Inflammatory paradental cyst	16–30	M–F	Any	Cystic degeneration and proliferation of follicular epithelium	Unilocular RL with sclerotic rim, posterior mandible	Enucleation or excision
Keratocystic odontogenic tumor	10–40	M>F	Any	Cystic neoplasm with p53 and p63 mutations	Unilocular RL with smooth rim, posterior mandible; one third associated with impacted tooth. Associates with Gorlin-Goltz syndrome	En bloc excision

Periapical Unilocular Radiolucencies (Section 6)

Entity	Age	Sex	Race/Ethnicity	Cause	Radiographic Characteristics	Treatment
Periapical granuloma	>10	M–F	Any	Pulpal inflammation	Well-circumscribed unilocular RL at apex of nonvital tooth	Root canal therapy or extraction
Periapical cyst	>10	M–F	Any	Pulpal inflammation	Well-circumscribed unilocular RL at apex of nonvital tooth	Root canal therapy or extraction
Apical abscess	>10	M–F	Any	Pulpal inflammation	Unilocular RL at or near apex of nonvital tooth	Root canal therapy or extraction
Residual cyst	>10	M–F	Any	Cyst left behind after tooth extraction	Unilocular RL where root apex used to be	Excision
Apical scar	>20	M–F	Any	Nonhealing after extraction, surgery, or trauma	Unilocular RL at or near apex of nonvital tooth	None

12

233

Interradicular Unilocular Radiolucencies (Section 6)

Entity	Age	Sex	Race/ Ethnicity	Cause	Radiographic Characteristics	Treatment
Globulomaxillary cyst	>10	M–F	Any	Pulpal inflammation	Pear-shaped unilocular interradicular RL between maxillary lateral incisor and canine	Root canal therapy of affected tooth or excision
Lateral periodontal cyst	>40	M>F	Any	Proliferation of epithelial rests of dental lamina	Small corticated RL contacting and between premolar roots	Excision
Median mandibular cyst	>25	M–F	Any	Cystic degeneration of epithelium or from pulpal inflammation	Midline RL between central incisors, can extend posteriorly and cause root divergence	Excision
Incisive canal cyst (median palatal cyst)	>35	M>F	Any	Cystic degeneration of entrapped epithelium	Midline RL of anterior (or posterior) palate	Enucleation
Traumatic bone cyst	15–35	M>F	Any	Trauma	RL posterior mandible, scalloping superior radiopaque margin extending between roots	Curettage
Squamous odontogenic tumor	30–50	M–F	Any	Proliferation of epithelial rests of Malassez	Well-defined unilocular and triangular or semicircular RL between tooth roots	Enucleation or excision

Unilocular Radiolucencies: Root Bearing Regions (Section 6)

Entity	Age	Sex	Race/ Ethnicity	Cause	Radiographic Characteristics	Treatment
Periapical cemento-osseous dysplasia	30–50	F	Blacks	Reactive process	3 stages: 1, RL; 2, mixed RL-RO; 3, RO with RL rim. Usually anterior mandible and multiple	None
Submandibular salivary gland depression	>45	M>F	Any	Major salivary gland exerting pressure	Well-defined round RL below mandibular canal	None
Hematopoietic bone marrow defect	>40	F	Any	Accumulation of bone marrow	RL enlarged trabeculae with thin sclerotic border; mandibular molar region	None
Surgical ciliated cyst of maxilla	30–60	M–F after sinus surgery	Any	Implantation of respiratory epithelium	≤1-cm round RL above roots of maxillary teeth and in close proximity with maxillary sinus	Enucleation
Cemento-ossifying fibroma	30–50	F>M	Any	Reactive growth	Well-demarcated RL, near roots, two thirds in body of mandible	Enucleation

Entity	Age	Sex	Race/ Ethnicity	Cause	Radiographic Characteristics	Treatment
Neural sheath tumor	5–70	M–F	Any	Tumor of neural origin	RL posterior mandible	Excision
Ameloblastoma	18–50	M>F	Any	Aggressive tumor of ameloblasts	Uni- or multilocular RL posterior mandible; less common in anterior	Resection or enucleation
Ameloblastic fibroma	10–20	M–F	Any	Proliferation of ameloblasts	Small uni- or multilocular RL posterior mandible; no bone expansion	Enucleation

Multilocular Radiolucencies (Section 6)

Entity	Age	Sex	Race/ Ethnicity	Cause	Radiographic Characteristics	Treatment
Botryoid lateral periodontal cyst	20–80	M–F	Any	Proliferation of entrapped odontogenic epithelium	Multilocular RL in mandibular canine-premolar region	Enucleation
Central giant cell granuloma	Most <30	M–F	Any	Proliferation of mesenchymal cells and osteoclast-like giant cells	Well-defined unilocular RL below roots of teeth in the anterior jaw	Excision by curettage
Ameloblastoma	18–50	M>F	Any	Aggressive tumor of ameloblasts	Uni- or multilocular RL posterior mandible; less common in anterior	Resection or enucleation
Odontogenic myxoma	<35	M–F	Any	Benign tumor of odontogenic epithelial and mesenchymal cells	Multilocular RL, which has soap bubble appearance and internal septa	Excision
Central hemangioma	Most <20	M–F	Any	Proliferation of endothelial cells	Ill-defined or multilocular RL, more common in mandible, with tooth displacement	Surgical removal, sclerosis
Glandular (sialo) odontogenic cyst	>40	M>F	Any	Proliferation of odontogenic epithelium with mucus-laden cells	Demarcated RL of mandible. Thin sclerotic rim along portions of the border, remainder has dense border, and buccal-lingual expansion	Excision
Cherubism	1–8 also seen in adolescents	M–F	Any	Genetic mutation on chromosome 4 that leads to replacement of osseous tissue by fibrous connective tissue	Multilocular RL divided by bony septae with bilateral jaw enlargement	Cosmetic recontouring or none

12

Mixed Radiolucent-Radiopaque Lesions (Section 6)

Entity	Age	Sex	Race/ Ethnicity	Cause	Radiographic Characteristics	Treatment
Odontoma	6–30	M–F	Any	Hamartomas of incomplete tooth development	One or more RO with RL rim in posterior mandible/anterior maxilla	Excision
Ameloblastic fibro- odontoma	<20	M>F	Any	Proliferation	Unilocular mixed density RO-RL lesion in posterior jaw, with delayed tooth eruption or displacement	Excision
Adenomatoid odontogenic tumor	12–16	F	>Asians	Tumor of odontogenic epithelium	RL lesion in anterior jaw with RO flecks, 2/3 in maxilla, 75% with unerupted canine	Excision
Cemento- ossifying fibro- ma	30–50	F>M	Any	Reactive growth	Well-demarcated RL, near roots, 2/3 in body of mandible. Mature lesions are unilocular RL with RO foci.	Enucleation
Calcifying odontogenic (Gorlin) cyst	20–50	M–F	Any	Cystic proliferation of odontogenic epithelium	Demarcated unilocular RL with internal RO structures. Some are multilocular, about 1/3 associated with an impacted tooth or odontoma	Excision
Calcifying epithelial odontogenic (Pindborg) tumor	8–92; most 40	M–F	Whites > Blacks	Tumor of odontogenic epithelium	RL with calcific foci, most in mandibular molar region, with unerupted tooth and tumor-induced migration of an unerupted molar	Excision

Generalized Rarefactions (Section 6)

Entity	Age	Sex	Race/ Ethnicity	Cause	Radiographic Characteristics	Treatment
Osteoporosis	>60	F>M	>Whites	Aging-associated deficiency of organic bone matrix	Thin mandibular cortex and lamina dura, resorption of edentulous areas, enlarged radiolucent medullary spaces	Calcium, vitamin D, bisphosphonates
Rickets	<12			Deficiency or impaired metabolism of vitamin D, phosphorous, or calcium	Cortical bone thinned or absent, enamel hypoplasia, dentin fissures	Vitamin D or calcium therapy

Entity	Age	Sex	Race/Ethnicity	Cause	Radiographic Characteristics	Treatment
Hyperparathyroidism				Overproduction of parathormone	Thinned, granular trabecular pattern	Excise parathyroid tumor
Osteomyelitis	>30	M–F	Any	Bone infection	Irregular RL, moth-eaten pattern with or without FT	Antibiotics
Sickle cell anemia	<20	M–F	Blacks	Amino acid change in beta chain of hemoglobin	Stepladder configuration of the jaw trabeculae, hair-on-end skull cortex	Hydroxyurea, antibiotics
Thalassemia	<20	M–F	Mediterranean, SE Asia	Deletion or mutation in globin gene	Increased spacing in jaw trabeculae	Blood transfusion, marrow stem cell transplant
Leukemia	<25 or >55	M–F	Any	Proliferation of neoplastic WBCs	Destruction of tooth crypts, tooth displacement, irregular radiolucent areas of alveolar bone resembling periodontal disease	Chemotherapy, bone marrow/stem cell transplant
Osteoradionecrosis	>50	M–F	Any	Trauma and ischemia that leads to bone necrosis	Irregular RL with indistinct border	Antibiotics, curretage, surgery, hyperbaric oxygen

Floating Teeth (FT) (Section 6)

Entity	Age	Sex	Race/Ethnicity	Cause	Radiographic Characteristics	Treatment
Chronic periodontitis	>35	M–F	Any	Subgingival bacteria	Loss of alveolar bone with FT	Curettage, antibiotics
Langerhans cell disease	<20	M–F	Any	Proliferation of Langerhans cells	Loss of alveolar bone with FT	Chemotherapy, steroids
Osteomyelitis	>30	M–F	Any	Bone infection	Irregular RL, moth-eaten pattern with or without FT	Antibiotics
Malignancy	>50	M–F	Any	Neoplasia	Localized or infiltrative RL that lacks margin of sclerotic bone with or without FT	Chemotherapy and radiation
Multiple myeloma	>50	M–F	Any	Plasma cell tumors	Multiple, painful punched-out RL with or without FT	Chemotherapy and immunomodulators

12

Disease	Age	Sex	Race/ Ethnicity	Cause	Clinical Characteristics	Treatment
Fordyce granules	Any	M–F	Any	Ectopic sebaceous glands	Whitish yellow granules clustered in plaques located on buccal mucosa (bilaterally), labial mucosa, retromolar pad, lip, attached gingiva, tongue, and frenum. Lesions are nontender and rough to palpation and do not rub off. Onset after puberty; persists for life.	None required.
Linea alba buccalis	Any	M–F	Any	A type of frictional keratosis caused by persistent rubbing of buccal mucosa with interdigitating maxillary and mandibular teeth	White wavy line of varying length located on buccal mucosa, bilaterally. Lesions are nontender and smooth to palpation and do not rub off. Variable onset; persists with oral habits.	Eliminate bruxism and clenching.
Leukoedema	Any	M–F	Melo-derms	Unknown	Grayish white patch of variable size located on buccal mucosa (bilaterally), labial mucosa, and soft palate. Lesions are nontender and smooth to palpation and disappear when the mucosa is stretched. Leukoedema becomes more evident with increasing age.	None required.
Morsicatio buccarum	Any	M–F	Any	Chronic irritation caused by cheek biting	Asymmetric white plaque located on buccal mucosa and labial mucosa, often bilaterally. Lesions are nontender and rough to palpation and peel slightly when rubbed. Variable onset; persists with cheek-biting or lip-biting habit.	Eliminate cheek-biting or lip-chewing habit.
White sponge nevus	Any	M–F	Any	Autosomal dominant condition (mutation in keratin 4 or 13 genes) that results in defect in epithelial maturation and exfoliation	Solitary or confluent raised white plaques that may appear on buccal mucosa, labial mucosa, alveolar ridge, floor of the mouth, or soft palate. Lesions are nontender and rough to palpation and do not rub off. Onset at birth; persists for life.	None required.

Disease	Age	Sex	Race/ Ethnicity	Cause	Clinical Characteristics	Treatment
Traumatic white lesions	Any	M–F	Any	Acute chemical or physical trauma resulting in epithelial sloughing	White surface slough (eschar) usually located on the less-keratinized alveolar mucosa. Palate common for food burns. Lesions are tender to palpation and rub off, leaving a raw or bleeding surface. Onset within hours of trauma; regression in 1–2 weeks.	Eliminate irritant; use topical anesthetics and analgesics.
Leukoplakia	45–65	2:1 (M:F)	Any	Frequently related to tobacco or alcohol use	White patch that varies in size, homogeneity, and texture. High-risk locations include floor of the mouth, ventral tongue, lateral tongue, and uvulopalatal complex. Lesions do not rub off and usually are nontender. Onset occurs after prolonged contact with an inducing agent; persists as long as the inducing agent is present.	Biopsy and histologic examination. Close follow-up mandatory.
Cigarette keratosis	Elderly	M	Any	Heat and smoke from frequent smoking of non-filtered cigarettes	White pebbly circular patches located on upper and lower lips (kissing lesions). Keratoses are firm and nontender and do not rub off. Onset in conjunction with a prolonged cigarette smoking habit; persists with habit.	Use filtered cigarettes or stop smoking. Biopsy if lesion changes in color or becomes ulcerated or indurated.
Nicotine stomatitis	40–70	M	Any	Epithelial reaction to tobacco smoke or heat	White cobblestoned papules located on hard palate, excluding the anterior third. Papules have red centers, are nontender, and do not rub off. Onset varies according to degree of smoking; lesions are long-standing.	Stop pipe or cigar smoking, or reverse smoking habit.
Snuff dipper's patch	Teenagers and adult	M	Any	Chronic irritation of smokeless tobacco products	Corrugated whitish yellow patch located on mucobuccal fold, most prominent unilaterally. Patch is rough and nontender and does not rub off. Long-standing habit precedes lesion; patch persists with continuation of habit.	Discontinue tobacco use. Biopsy if color changes or if lesion becomes ulcerated or indurated.

(Continued)

12

Disease	Age	Sex	Race/ Ethnicity	Cause	Clinical Characteristics	Treatment
Verrucous carcinoma	>60	M	Any	Neoplastic changes induced by long-term use of tobacco, smokeless tobacco, and human papillomavirus infection	Papulonodular whitish red mass located on buccal mucosa, alveolar ridge, gingiva. Lesion is firm, nontender, and rough to palpation and does not rub off. Long-standing tobacco habit precedes onset; human papillomavirus present in 30%; lesion enlarges unless treated.	Biopsy to confirm diagnosis, then surgical excision. AVOID RADIATION THERAPY.
Squamous cell carcinoma (see "Red and Red-White Lesions")						

Disease	Age	Sex	Race/Ethnicity	Cause	Clinical Characteristics	Treatment
Purpura	Any	M–F	Any	Rupture of blood vessel caused by trauma or vascular abnormality	Red spot or patch consisting of extravasated blood that develops soon after trauma. Lesions do not blanch on diascopy and size varies (petechiae < ecchymosis < hematoma). Petechiae are common on soft palate; other purpura typically occurs on buccal or labial mucosa, depending on site at which blood pools. Lesions fade away.	Eliminate underlying cause.
Varicosity	>55	F	Any	Dilated veins caused by loss of elasticity	Reddish purple papule or nodule located on ventral tongue, lip, or labial mucosa. Lesions are asymptomatic and blanch on diascopy. Varicosities increase in size and number with increasing age and are persistent.	None necessary. Surgery for aesthetics.
Thrombus	>30	M–F	Any	Blood clot caused by stagnating blood or clotting abnormality	Red to blue-purple nodule located on labial mucosa, lip, or tongue. Lesions are firm and may be tender to palpation. Onset after traumatic bleeding; lesion is negative on diascopy and persists until treatment. Thrombi sometime spontaneously regress.	Surgical removal and histologic examination, if persistent or symptomatic.
Hemangioma	Child-adolescent	F	Any	Congenital abnormality resulting in a network of blood vessels in bone or soft tissue	Two types described: capillary and cavernous. Red to purple, soft, smooth-surfaced, or multinodular exophytic mass located on dorsal tongue, buccal mucosa, or gingiva. Lesions are positive on diascopy. Develops early in life, persists until treated. Hemangiomas sometimes spontaneously regress.	No treatment is necessary if present since youth, no functional disability, and no changes in size, shape, or color. Otherwise, surgery or histologic examination.

(Continued)

Disease	Age	Sex	Race/ Ethnicity	Cause	Clinical Characteristics	Treatment
Hereditary hemorrhagic telangiectasia	Postpuberty	M–F	Any	Autosomal dominant condition associated with multiple dilated end capillaries that results from a defect in a transmembrane protein (endoglin)—a component of the receptor complex for transforming growth factor beta (TGF-β)	Multifocal red macules located on palms, fingers, nail beds, face, neck, conjunctiva, nasal septum, lips, tongue, hard palate, and gingiva. Lesions are present at birth, become more visible at puberty, and increase in number with age. Telangiectasias lack central pulsation and blanch on diascopy; if they rupture, severe bleeding may result.	Avoid trauma and intubation. Monitor for hemorrhage or anemia.
Sturge-Weber syndrome	Birth	M–F	Any	Nonhereditary congenital disorder that results in multiple venous angiomas at various anatomic sites	Syndrome associated with seizures, mental deficits, gyriform brain calcifications, and a red to purple flat or slightly raised facial hemangioma. Vascular lesion often affects lips, labial or buccal mucosa, and gingiva along branches of trigeminal nerve, stops at midline. Abnormal oral enlargements may be concurrent.	None required. Elective surgery for aesthetics
Kaposi sarcoma	20–45* and >60	M	Jewish, Mediterranean, or *HIV infected	Associated with human herpesvirus type 8, a virus capable of promoting angiogenesis	Asymptomatic red macule of mucocutaneous structures that enlarges and becomes raised, then darkens in color. Advanced lesions are red-blue-violet nodules that ulcerate and cause pain. The hard palate, gingiva, and buccal mucosa are the most common oral locations.	Palliative, consisting of radiation therapy, laser surgery, chemotherapy, sclerosing agents, or a combination thereof.
Erythroplakia	>50	M>F	Any	Increased vascularity associated with carcinogen-induced epithelial changes and inflammation	Red patch of variable size located on any oral mucosal site. High-risk areas include floor of the mouth, soft palate-retromolar trigone, and lateral border of the tongue. Erythroplakias do not rub off and are usually asymptomatic. Lesions develop after prolonged contact with carcinogens or human papillomavirus; duration varies. Regression is rare.	Biopsy and histologic examination. Close follow-up.

Disease	Age	Sex	Race/Ethnicity	Cause	Clinical Characteristics	Treatment
Erythroleukoplakia and speckled erythroplakia	>50	M>F	Any	Increased vascularity associated with carcinogen-induced and *Candida*-induced epithelial changes and inflammation	Red patch with multiple foci of white. Nontender, do not rub off, often superficially infected with *Candida* organisms. Common locations include lateral tongue, buccal mucosa, soft palate, and floor of the mouth. Onset after prolonged exposure to carcinogens or human papillomavirus. Regression unlikely even if inducing agent is removed.	Biopsy and histologic examination. Examine for candidiasis. Close follow-up.
Squamous cell carcinoma	>50	2:1 M:F	Any	Prolonged exposure to carcinogens (tobacco, alcohol, or human papillomavirus high risk genotypes) and decreased immune surveillance	Red or red and white lesion or ulcer commonly located on the lateral tongue, ventral tongue, oropharynx, floor of the mouth, gingiva, buccal mucosa, or lip. Carcinoma often asymptomatic until it becomes large, indurated, or ulcerated. Onset after prolonged exposure to carcinogens. Persistence results in metastasis, usually apparent as painless, firm, matted, fixed lymph nodes.	Biopsy and histologic examination. Complete surgical removal, radiation therapy, or chemotherapy. Close follow-up.
Lichen planus	>40	F	Any	T-cell infiltration and cytokine-induced changes in epithelium; exact inducer unknown	Purple, polygonal, pruritic papules on flexor surfaces of the skin; fingernails sometimes affected. Intraoral lesions are often symptomatic and consist of white linear papules, reddish patches, and ulcerated regions of mucosa. Affected surfaces are often bilateral. Most common locations: buccal mucosa, tongue, lips, palate, gingiva, and the floor of the mouth. Lesions develop with stress and liver disease; they persist for many years with periods of remission and exacerbation.	Rest, anxiolytic agents, topical corticosteroids. Evaluate for liver disease; close follow-up for occasional malignant transformation in the erosive type.

(Continued)

12

243

Disease	Age	Sex	Race/Ethnicity	Cause	Clinical Characteristics	Treatment
Electrogalvanic white lesion	>30	F	Any	Metal antigen of a dental restoration that induces a hyperimmune T-cell response	Reddish white patches that resemble lichen planus located on buccal mucosa adjacent to metallic restorations. Lesions do not rub off and are usually tender or cause a burning sensation. Onset after weeks to years of exposure to metallic restoration; duration varies depending on the persistence of the allergen.	Replace metallic restoration or clasp that is causing the hypersensitive response.
Lupus erythematosus	>35	F	Any	Autoantibodies (antinuclear) that attack normal cells leading to perivascular inflammation	Reddish butterfly rash on bridge of nose. Maculopapular eruption with hyperkeratotic periphery and atrophic center. Affected areas may involve the lower lip, buccal mucosa, tongue, and palate. Intraoral lesions invariably have red and white radiating lines emanating from the lesion. Lesions do not rub off but are tender to palpation. Lesions often develop after short-term sun exposure. Lesions persist and require drug treatment.	Topical and systemic steroids; antimalarial agents in conjunction with adequate medical treatment.
Lichenoid and lupuslike drug eruption	Adult	M–F		Drug molecules act as allergens or haptens that stimulate immune reaction	Red-white patches that resemble lichen planus and lupus. The lesions are often atrophic or ulcerated centrally. Buccal mucosa, bilaterally, is the most common site. Onset varies and may be weeks or years after an allergenic medication is begun. Regression occurs when offending drug is eliminated.	Withdraw offending drug and substitute medication.

Disease	Age	Sex	Race/ Ethnicity	Cause	Clinical Characteristics	Treatment
Candidiasis	Newborns, adults	M–F	Any	Opportunistic infection with *Candida* species (most commonly C. *albicans*)	Variable appearance; white curds, red patches, white patches with red margins. Any oral soft tissue site is susceptible, but the attached gingiva is rarely affected. Onset often coincides with neutropenia, immune suppression, and frequent use of steroids or antibiotics. Lesions persist until adequate antifungal therapy is provided.	Antifungal therapy. Eliminate sucrose from diet. Medical control of diabetes, endocrinopathy, and immunosuppression.

12

Disease	Age	Sex	Race/ Ethnicity	Cause	Clinical Characteristics	Treatment
Melanoplakia	Any	M–F	Melanoderms	Melanin deposition in the basal layer of the mucosa and lamina propria	Generalized constant dark patch located on attached gingiva and buccal mucosa. Pigmentation varies from light brown to dark brown and is often diffuse, curvilinear, and asymptomatic and does not rub off. Melanoplakia is present at birth and persists for life.	None required.
Tattoo	Teenagers, adults	M–F	Any	Implantation of dye or metal in mucosa	Amalgam tattoo is the most common type of intraoral tattoo. Appears as a blue-black macule on gingiva, edentulous ridge, vestibule, palate, or buccal mucosa. Radiographs may demonstrate radiopaque foci. Lesions are asymptomatic, do not blanch, and persist for life.	None required.
Ephelis	Any	M–F	Light-skinned persons	Deposition of melanin triggered by exposure to sunlight	Light to dark brown macule that appears on facial skin, extremities, or lip after sun exposure. Ephelides are initially small but may enlarge and coalesce. Lesions are nontender and do not blanch or rub off.	None required.
Smoker melanosis	Older adult	M–F	Any	Accumulation of melanocytes and deposition of melanin in epithelium associated with tobacco smoking	Diffuse brown patch with diameter of several centimeters, usually on posterior buccal mucosa and soft palate. History of heavy tobacco smoking precedes development of the lesion. Features may decrease with discontinuation of the habit. Melanosis is asymptomatic and non-palpable.	Diminish or stop smoking.

Disease	Age	Sex	Race/ Ethnicity	Cause	Clinical Characteristics	Treatment
Oral melanotic macule	24–45	Slight male predilection	Any	Focal deposition of melanin along the basal layer, usually after trauma	Asymptomatic brown to black macule usually located on lower lip near midline; also occurs on palate, buccal mucosa, and gingiva. Onset is postinflammatory, and the lesion persists until treatment.	Biopsy and histologic examination to rule out other similar-appearing pigmented lesions.
Nevus	Any	F	Any	Accumulation of nevus cells in a distinct location, probably controlled by genetic factors	Nevi vary greatly in appearance. They may be pink, blue, brown, or black but do not blanch on diascopy. Usually appear as a bluish or brownish smooth-surfaced papule located on the palate. Other common sites include the buccal mucosa, face, neck, and trunk. Many lesions are present at birth. They increase in size and number with increased age.	Excisional biopsy and histologic examination.
Melanoma	25–60	M	White persons, especially light-skinned persons	Malignant neoplasm of melanocytes associated with chronic ultraviolet light exposure; unknown for oral melanomas	Painless, slightly raised plaque or patch that has many colors, especially foci of brown, black, gray, or red. Ill-defined margins, satellite lesions, and inflammatory borders are characteristic. Usually located on the maxillary alveolar ridge, palate, anterior gingiva, and labial mucosa. Thirty percent arise from pre-existing pigmentations. A recent change in size, shape, or color is particularly ominous.	Excisional biopsy, surgical removal, and referral for complete medical workup to rule out metastasis.

(*Continued*)

12

Disease	Age	Sex	Race/ Ethnicity	Cause	Clinical Characteristics	Treatment
Peutz-Jeghers syndrome	Child, young adult	M–F	Any	Autosomal dominant condition probably caused by a germline mutation in the *LKB1* gene (19p13.3)	Multiple, asymptomatic melanotic oval macules, prominently located on the skin of the palmar or plantar surfaces of the hands and feet, around the eyes, nose, mouth, lips, and perineum. In the mouth, brown discolorations occur on the buccal mucosa, labial mucosa, and gingiva. Lesions do not increase in size, but cutaneous lesions often fade with age; mucosal pigmentation persists for life. Colicky intestinal symptoms are probable.	Oral: none required. Gastrointestinal evaluation and genetic counseling.
Addison disease	Adult	M–F	Any	Adrenal hypofunction	Diffuse intraoral hypermelanotic patches occurring in conjunction with bronzing of the skin, especially of the knuckles, elbows, and palmar creases. Patches are nontender and nonraised and vary in shape. The buccal mucosa and gingiva are most commonly affected. Onset of the disorder is insidious and associated with adrenal gland hypofunction. Patient may report gastrointestinal symptoms and fatigue.	Systemic corticosteroids and mineralocorticoids.
Heavy metal pigmentation	Adult	M–F	Any	Prolonged exposure (vapors or ingestion) to metals (arsenic, bismuth, mercury, silver, or lead)	Blue-black linear pigmentation of marginal gingiva, prominently viewed along anterior gingiva. Spotty gray macules may be apparent on buccal mucosa. Neuralgic symptoms, headache, and hypersalivation are common. Argyria: blue-gray skin pigmentation, especially in sun-exposed areas.	Terminate exposure to heavy metal; provide medical referral. Oral lesions require no treatment but may be permanent.

Disease	Age	Sex	Race/Ethnicity	Cause	Clinical Characteristics	Treatment
Retrocuspid papilla	Child, young adult	M–F	Any	Developmental anomaly of connective tissue	Smooth-surfaced pink papule, 1–4 mm in diameter, located on the lingual attached gingiva apical to the marginal gingiva of the mandibular cuspids. These papules appear early in life, are often found bilaterally, and regress as the patient ages. The retrocuspid papilla is firm to palpation, asymptomatic, and nonhemorrhagic.	None required.
Lymphoepithelial cyst	Child, young adult	M–F	Any	Epithelium entrapped in lymphoid tissue that undergoes cystic transformation	Well-circumscribed, soft, fluctuant yellowish swelling that ranges in size from a few millimeters to 1 cm. Common locations for this nontender cyst include the lateral neck just anterior to the sternocleidomastoid muscle, floor of the mouth, lingual frenum, and ventral tongue. Lesion develops during childhood or adolescence and persists until treatment.	Excisional biopsy and histologic examination.
Torus, exostosis, and osteoma	Adult	F	Any	Unknown hereditary factors	Torus: bony hard nodule or multinodular mass located on the palate at the midline or mandibular lingual alveolar ridge. Exostosis: bony hard nodule, often multiple, located on buccal or labial alveolar ridge. Osteoma: bony hard nodule located adjacent to the jaws, often embedded in soft tissue. All three types are firm, painless (unless traumatized), slow growing, and long standing. Osteomas have the greatest growth potential.	Torus and exostosis: none required unless functional problems arise. Osteomas plus impacted and supernumerary teeth: gastrointestinal evaluation to rule out Gardner syndrome (gene defect on chromosome 5). If test results are positive, then gastrointestinal surgery and genetic counseling.

(Continued)

12

Disease	Age	Sex	Race/ Ethnicity	Cause	Clinical Characteristics	Treatment
Fibroma	Adult	M–F	Any	Usually a chronic irritant that produces a reactive hyperplasia of connective tissue	Irritation fibroma is a smooth-surfaced, pink, firm, symmetric papule or nodule that arises at a site of chronic irritation, such as the buccal mucosa, labial mucosa, and tongue. The gingiva is the common location for the peripheral odontogenic fibroma. Both lesions have sessile bases and are nontender and nonhemorrhagic.	Excisional biopsy and histologic examination.
Lipoma	>30	M–F	Any	Unknown genetic mutation possibly involving dysfunction proteins that regulate chromatin structure and function	Well-circumscribed, smooth-surfaced, dome-shaped, yellowish to pink nodule commonly located on buccal mucosa, lip, tongue, floor of the mouth, soft palate, or mucobuccal fold. Lesion is slightly doughy on palpation and grows slowly.	Excisional biopsy and histologic examination.
Lipofibroma	>30	M–F	Any	Unknown genetic mutation	Well-circumscribed, smooth-surfaced, dome-shaped, pinkish nodule commonly located on buccal or labial mucosa. Lesion is painless, movable, and rather firm. Slow growth and persistence are characteristic.	Excisional biopsy and histologic examination.
Traumatic neuroma	>25	M–F	Any	Trauma to large nerve that results in abnormal healing and aberrant neural conduction	Small, slightly raised, firm, pressure-sensitive papule that is commonly located in the mandibular mucobuccal fold near the mental foramen, facial to mandibular incisors, lingual retromolar regions, and ventral tongue. Visualization of the lesion may be difficult if the neuroma is subjacent to normal-appearing mucosa. Palpation elicits an electric shock sensation. Onset occurs after trauma; lesions persist until treated.	Excisional biopsy and histologic examination; if lesion recurs, corticosteroid injections may be effective.

Disease	Age	Sex	Race/ Ethnicity	Cause	Clinical Characteristics	Treatment
Neurofibroma	Childhood	M–F	Any	Gene dysregulation resulting in uncontrolled growth of peripheral nerves and neural sheaths	Firm pink nodules that are often deep seated. These tumors are located in skin, bones, buccal mucosa, tongue, or lips. Lesions are nontender but movable. Continued enlargement can lead to deformity. Multiple lesions and skin pigmentations are associated with von Recklinghausen disease (neurofibromatosis).	Excisional biopsy and histologic examination; in cases of neurofibromatosis: excisional biopsy, histologic examination, and follow-up for malignant transformation.
Papilloma	20–40	M	Any	Epithelial growth induced by chronic human papillomavirus infection (primarily types 6 and 11)	Small, pink, pebbly, slow-growing papule located on uvula, soft palate, tongue, frenum, lips, buccal mucosa, or gingiva. The base is pedunculated and well circumscribed, whereas the surface is most often rough to palpation.	Excisional biopsy and histologic examination.
Verruca vulgaris	Child, young adult	M–F	Any	Epithelial growth induced by chronic human papillomavirus infection (primarily types 2 and 4)	Rough, whitish pink papule located on the skin of the hands and perilabially on the lips, labial and buccal mucosa, and attached gingiva. Lesions are slow growing and have a sessile base. Verrucae may regress spontaneously or spread to adjacent mucocutaneous surfaces.	Excisional biopsy and histologic examination.
Condyloma acuminatum	20–45	M	Any	Epithelial growth induced by chronic human papillomavirus infection (primarily types 6 and 11)	Small, pink-to-dirty gray papule with rough, papillary surface that resembles a cauliflower. Base of condyloma is sessile, and the borders are raised and rounded. Lesions occur in multiples, and onset rapidly occurs after inoculation from affected sexual partner. Most common location is genitalia, labial mucosa, labial commissure, attached gingiva, and soft palate. Lesions can spread and coalesce into extensive clusters.	Surgical excision; depending on size and location, surgery may require general anesthesia.

(Continued)

12

Disease	Age	Sex	Race/Ethnicity	Cause	Clinical Characteristics	Treatment
Lymphangioma	Child, adolescent	M–F	Any	Congenital hamartoma of lymphatic channels	Soft, compressible, pinkish white swelling that may be superficial or deep seated. Superficial lesions resemble papillomas; deep-seated lesions cause diffuse enlargement. Lymphangiomas may occur in neck (cystic hygroma), dorsal or lateral tongue, lip, or labial mucosa. Long-standing lesions can cause functional problems or regress spontaneously.	Surgical excision; depending on size and location, surgery may require general anesthesia.

Disease	Age	Sex	Race/ Ethnicity	Cause	Clinical Characteristics	Treatment
Primary herpetic gingivostomatitis	Infant, child, young adult	M–F	Any	Primary herpes simplex virus (type 1) infection of oral epithelium; infection with type 2 is less likely.	Multiple vesicles that rupture, coalesce, and form ulcers of the lip, buccal and labial mucosa, gingiva, palate, and tongue. Ulcers are painful and initially are small and yellow and have red inflammatory borders. Onset is rapid, several days after contact with person harboring the virus. Lesions persist for 12–20 days.	Fluids, antivirals, antipyretics; antibiotics to prevent secondary infection, oral anesthetic rinses, analgesics.
Recurrent herpes simplex	Teenagers and adults	M–F	Any	Recrudescence of herpes simplex virus from sensory neuron, resulting in infection of orofacial epithelium, trauma, and stress associated	Multiple small vesicles that rupture and ulcerate. Lesions occur repeatedly at same site: usually the lip, hard palate, and attached gingiva. Onset is rapid and is preceded by prodromal burning or tingling. Lesions last 5–12 days and heal spontaneously.	Antivirals (acyclovir, famciclovir, valacyclovir), bioflavonoids, sunscreens (lip), lysine.
Herpangina	Child, young adult	M–F	Any	Coxsackievirus (types A1–6, A8, A10, A22, B3) and echovirus infection of oropharynx	Light gray vesicles that rupture and form many discrete shallow ulcers. Lesions have erythematous border and are limited to the anterior pillars, soft palate, uvula, and tonsils. Pharyngitis, headache, fever, and lymphadenitis are often concurrent. Lesions heal spontaneously in 1–2 weeks.	Palliative; vesicles heal spontaneously.

12

(Continued)

Disease	Age	Sex	Race/Ethnicity	Cause	Clinical Characteristics	Treatment
Chickenpox	Child	M–F	Any	Primary varicella-zoster virus infection	Vesicles on the skin and face that, after rupturing, resemble a dewdrop. Ulcers may be seen on soft palate, buccal mucosa, and mucobuccal fold. Skin lesions crust over and heal without scar formation. Condition often accompanied by chills, fever, nasopharyngitis, and malaise. Spontaneous healing occurs in 7–10 days.	Vaccination; palliative; vesicles heal spontaneously. Avoid scratching to limit scar formation.
Herpes zoster	>55, >35 in HIV positive	M–F	Any	Recrudescence of varicella-zoster virus from sensory neuron, resulting in infection of epithelium	Unilateral vesicular and pustular eruptions that develop over 1–3 days. Lesions occur along dermatomes and especially along the trigeminal nerve tract. Lesions are vesicular, ulcerative, and intensely painful and commonly affect the lip, tongue, and buccal mucosa extending up to the midline. Neuralgia may persist after healing.	Vaccination; palliative; lesions heal spontaneously. Antivirals (e.g., valacyclovir, famciclovir) in severe cases or immunosuppressed patients.

Disease	Age	Sex	Race/Ethnicity	Cause	Clinical Characteristics	Treatment
Hand-foot-and-mouth disease	Child, young adult	M–F	Any	Coxsackievirus (types A5, A9, A10, B2, B5) infection	Crops of multiple small yellowish ulcers that occur on palms and soles of hands and feet. The tongue, hard palate, and buccal and labial mucosa are affected. Total number of lesions may approach 100. Healing occurs spontaneously in about 10 days.	Palliative; ulcers heal spontaneously.
Allergic reactions immediate	Any	M–F	Any	Immediate immunologic reaction involving an allergen, IgE and the release of histamine from mast cells	Red swellings or wheals that occur periorally or on lips, buccal mucosa, gingiva, lips, and tongue. Contact with allergen usually precedes episode by a few minutes to hours. Warmth, tenseness, and itchiness are concurrent. Lesions regress if the allergen is withdrawn.	Remove allergen; antihistamines.
Allergic reactions delayed	Any	M–F	Any	Immunologic reaction after 24 to 48 hours involving an allergen, T cells, and a cytotoxic reaction	Itchy erythematous papules or vesicles that may eventually ulcerate. May occur on any cutaneous or mucocutaneous surface. The lips, gingiva, alveolar mucosa, tongue, and palate are affected. Erythema develops slowly over 24–48 hours. Fissuring and ulceration may result.	Remove allergen; corticosteroids.

12

(*Continued*)

Disease	Age	Sex	Race/Ethnicity	Cause	Clinical Characteristics	Treatment
Erythema multiforme	Young adult	M	Any	Complement-mediated and white blood cell–mediated cytopathic effects provoked by pathogens and drug allergens	Skin: target lesions. Oral: hemorrhagic crust of the lips, painful ulcerations of the tongue, buccal mucosa, and palate. Attached gingiva rarely affected. Headache, low-grade fever, and previous respiratory infection often precede lesions.	Topical analgesics, antivirals, antipyretic agents, fluids, corticosteroids, antibiotics to prevent secondary infection, if needed.
Stevens-Johnson syndrome	Child, young adult	Slight preference for males	Any	Complement-mediated and white blood cell–mediated cytopathic effects provoked by pathogens and drug allergens occurring at more than one location	Skin: target lesions. Eye: conjunctivitis. Genital: balanitis. Oral: hemorrhagic crust of the lips, painful ulcerations, and weeping bullae of the tongue and buccal mucosa. Attached gingiva rarely affected. Stevens-Johnson syndrome is the fulminant form of erythema multiforme. Eating and swallowing are often impaired.	Topical analgesics, antipyretic agents, fluids, corticosteroids, antibiotics to prevent secondary infection; hospitalization.
Toxic epidermal necrolysis	Older adults	F	Any	Severe complement-mediated and white blood cell–mediated cytopathic effects provoked by drugs	Severe large coalescing bullae	IV fluids, corticosteroids, hospitalization.

Disease	Age	Sex	Race/ Ethnicity	Cause	Clinical Characteristics	Treatment
Pemphigus vulgaris	46–60	2:1 (F:M)	Light-skinned persons, Jewish and Mediterranean persons	Autoimmune antibodies directed against desmoglein 3 and 1 (a component of the desmosome)	Multiple skin and mucosal bullae that rupture, hemorrhage, and crust. Lesions tend to recur in the same area, have circular or serpiginous borders, and tend to spread to adjacent areas. The Nikolsky sign is positive. Collapsed bullae are white and necrotic and produce fetid oris. Dehydration can occur if lesions are extensive.	Medical (and ophthalmologic) referral, systemic steroids, oral topical steroids, steroid-sparing and immunosuppressive agents.
Benign mucous membrane pemphigoid	>50	2:1 (F:M)	Any	Autoimmune antibodies directed against hemidesmosomal basement membrane antigens (BP 180 and 230)	Bullous type produces blisters and ulcers on skin folds and inguinal and abdominal areas. Cicatricial type produces bullae and ulcers affecting the mucosa of the eyes, mouth, and genitals, which can lead to scarring. Bullae are often hemorrhagic and persist for days, then desquamate. Oral lesions that occur on the gingiva, palate, and buccal mucosa are painful and limit oral hygiene. Nikolsky sign is positive.	Topical steroids, occlusive topical steroids, dapsone, or tetracycline and niacinamide. Medical referral and systemic steroids if severe; rule out corneal involvement and internal malignancy.

12

Disease	Age	Sex	Race/Ethnicity	Cause	Clinical Characteristics	Treatment
Traumatic ulcer	Any	M–F	Any	Traumatic insult to epithelium and underlying layers	Symptomatic, yellow-gray ulcer of variable size and shape, depending on inducing agent. Ulcers are often depressed and usually oval in shape, with erythematous border. Commonly located on labial and buccal mucosa, tongue at the borders, and hard palate. Ulcer lasts 1–2 weeks.	Palliative; remove traumatic influence.
Recurrent aphthous stomatitis	Young adult	F	Any	Instigating factor often unknown; related to defect in T-cell response; stress, trauma, and epithelial thinning	Small yellowish oval ulcer(s) with red border, located on movable nonkeratinized mucosa. Common sites include labial mucosa, buccal mucosa, floor of the mouth, tongue, and occasionally soft palate. Ulcers are tender and may be associated with a tender lymph node. Lesions develop rapidly and disappear in 10–14 days without scar formation.	Spontaneous healing in 10–14 days. If acute symptoms or recurrent and symptomatic, topical anesthetics, coagulating agents, or topical steroids may be used.
Pseudoaphthous	25–50	F	Any	Unknown immune defect associated with folic acid, iron, or vitamin B_{12} deficiencies, inflammatory bowel disease, Crohn disease, gluten intolerance	Depressed yellowish round or oval ulcer located on movable nonkeratinized mucosa. Common sites include labial mucosa, buccal mucosa, floor of the mouth, tongue, and occasionally soft palate. Tongue may demonstrate atrophied papillae. Ulcers are tender, develop during deficiency state, and disappear with replacement therapy within 20 days.	Evaluate for deficiency state. If patient is deficient, then nutritional supplements (e.g., iron, vitamin B_{12}, folate) are recommended. Gluten abstinence may be required.

Disease	Age	Sex	Race/Ethnicity	Cause	Clinical Characteristics	Treatment
Major aphthous stomatitis	Young adult	F	Any	Instigating factor often unknown; related to defect in T-cell response	Asymmetric unilateral large ulcer with necrotic and depressed center. Ulcers have a red inflammatory border and are extremely painful. Located on soft palate, tonsillar fauces, labial mucosa, buccal mucosa, and tongue; may extend onto attached gingiva. Rapid onset. Underlying tissue is often destroyed. Lesions heal in 15–30 days with scar formation. Recurrences are common.	Spontaneous healing, sometimes with scar formation. Topical anesthetics, topical steroids, stress management; identify allergens.
Herpetiform ulceration	Late 20s	M	Any	Variant form of recurrent aphthous stomatitis; cause unknown	Multiple pinhead-sized yellowish ulcers located on movable nonkeratinized mucosa. Common sites include anterior tip of tongue, labial mucosa, and floor of the mouth. No vesicle formation. Ulcers are painful and may be associated with several tender lymph nodes. Lesions develop rapidly and disappear in 10–14 days without scar formation.	Tetracycline rinses.

(*Continued*)

12

Disease	Age	Sex	Race/ Ethnicity	Cause	Clinical Characteristics	Treatment
Behcet syndrome	20–30	3:1 (M:F)	Asian, Mediterranean, Anglo	Delayed hypersensitivity reaction and vasculitis triggered by the presentation of human leukocyte antigens (HLA-B51) or environmental antigens, such as viruses, bacteria, chemicals, and heavy metals	Eye: conjunctivitis, iritis; genital: ulcers; oral: painful aphthouslike ulcers on labial and buccal mucosa; skin: maculopapular rash and nodular eruptions. Oral ulcers are often an initial sign of the disease onset. Arthritis and gastrointestinal symptoms may be concurrent. Recurrences, exacerbations, and remissions are likely.	Topical and systemic steroids.
Granulomatous ulcer (tuberculosis, histoplasmosis)	Older adult	M–F	Any	Infection by *Mycobacterium tuberculosis* or *Histoplasmosis capsulatum*	Asymptomatic, cobblestoned ulcer that usually occurs on dorsum of tongue or labial commissure. Cervical lymphadenopathy and primary respiratory symptoms often are concurrent. Onset of oral disease follows lung infection lasting several weeks to months. Oral ulcer may persist for months to years if underlying disease not treated.	Biopsy, histologic examination. Tuberculosis: drug combination of isoniazid, rifampin, rifapentine, ethambutol, streptomycin, and pyrazinamide. Histoplasmosis: amphotericin B.

Disease	Age	Sex	Race/Ethnicity	Cause	Clinical Characteristics	Treatment
Squamous cell carcinoma	>50	2:1 (M:F)	Any	Mutagenesis of genes that regulate cell growth and apoptosis caused by carcinogens (tobacco, alcohol, and human papillomavirus type 16 or 18)	Nonpainful yellowish ulcer with raised red indurated borders commonly located on posterior third of the lateral border of the tongue, ventral tongue, lips, and floor of the mouth. Associated features may include numbness, leukoplakia, erythroplakia, induration, fixation, fungation, and lymphadenopathy. Carcinoma has a slow onset and is often noticed after a recent increase in size.	Surgery, radiation therapy, or chemotherapy. Smoking and alcohol cessation.
Chemotherapeutic ulcer	15–30 and older adult	M–F	Any	Inhibition of rapidly reproducing cells by chemotherapeutic drugs	Irregular ulcerations of the lips, labial and buccal mucosa, tongue, and palate. Red inflammatory border is often lacking. Hemorrhage is likely when ulcers are deeply situated. Lesions are extremely painful and usually limit mastication and swallowing. Develops during second week of chemotherapy. Secondary infection with oral microorganisms is likely.	Antimicrobial rinses to prevent secondary infection. Topical anesthetics, palliative elixirs, and intravenous fluids.

Glossary

Abdomen: The part of the body lying between the thorax (chest) and pelvis.

Abfraction: Means "to break away," a term used in dentistry to define the loss of tooth structure at—or under—the cementoenamel junction caused by abnormal tooth flexure. The condition is controversial, and current evidence suggests that it exists only as a hypothetical component of cervical wear.

Abrasion: Wearing down or rubbing away by friction.

Abscess: A collection of pus that results from an infection and the body's defense reaction.

Acantholysis: Loss of coherence between epidermal or epithelial cells.

Acquired hypodontia: The absence of one or several teeth as a result of trauma, caries, periodontal disease, extraction, or other factors that occur after birth.

Acquired pellicle: A thin coating, derived mainly from salivary glycoproteins, which forms over the surface of a tooth crown when it is exposed to saliva.

Acromegaly: An abnormal endocrine condition where the pituitary gland produces too much growth hormone after the growth plates have closed resulting in enlarged and deformed bones, abnormal facial appearance, and enlarged tongue.

Acute: Having severe symptoms and a short course.

Adrenal gland: A small endocrine gland located above the kidney that secretes (a) endogenous glucocorticosteroids, which control digestive metabolism; (b) mineralocorticoids, which control sodium and potassium balance; (c) sex hormones; and (d) catecholamines (epinephrine and norepinephrine), which alter blood pressure and heart function.

Adrenalectomy: Surgical removal of the adrenal gland.

Aerobic: Requiring oxygen.

Aesthetic: Pertaining to the appearance of oral or dental structures or the pleasing effect of dental restorations or procedures.

Afunctional: Not functioning or working.

Agenesis: Complete absence of a structure or part of a structure caused by failure of tissue development.

AIDS: Acronym for *acquired immune deficiency syndrome*, reserved for patients infected with human immunodeficiency virus (HIV). It also refers to the terminal stage of the disease.

Allergen: A substance that induces hypersensitivity or an allergic reaction.

Amalgam: An alloy used to restore teeth, composed mainly of silver and mercury.

Ameloblastoma: A rare, locally aggressive tumor of odontogenic epithelium that occurs in the jaws and has a propensity to recur.

Amelogenesis: The formation of the enamel portion of the tooth.

Amelogenesis imperfecta: An autosomal dominant or X-linked disorder that leads to improper development of the dental enamel. The enamel can be lacking, hypoplastic, or hypocalcified. In this condition, the enamel is very thin and friable and frequently stained in various shades of brown.

Amputation: Strictly, this term refers to the removal of a limb, such as an arm, or of an appendage, such as a finger. With reference to a neuroma, however, amputation means a tumor of nerve tissue that results from severing of a nerve.

Amputation caries: Severe caries that results in complete loss of the tooth crown, often at the level of the gingiva.

Anaerobic: Lacking oxygen.

Analgesic: A drug or substance used to relieve pain.

Analogous: Having similar properties.

Anaplastic: Pertaining to adult cells that have changed irreversibly toward more primitive cell types. Such changes are often malignant.

Anergy: State of immune unresponsiveness. In allergy testing, this state occurs when the skin does not respond to an allergen.

Angioedema: Swelling of the soft tissues under the skin/mucosa caused by release of bradykinins and histamine. It can be a result of a hypersensitivity reaction or due to a medication or underlying medical condition, such as a congenital deficiency in an enzyme involved in the complement system.

Angiogenesis: The process of developing new blood vessels.

Angioma: A tumor made up of blood or lymph vessels.

Ankylosis: A condition marked by fusion of bones, often as a result of injury or inflammation, that results in loss of function. In dentistry, the term is used to mean when a tooth root is fused to the alveolar bone.

Anodontia: Congenital condition in which all the teeth fail to develop.

Anomaly: Deviation from normal.

Anorexia: A lack or loss of appetite for food.

Anterior: Located toward the front (opposite of *posterior*).

Antibiotic: A chemical compound that inhibits the growth or replication of certain forms of life, especially pathogenic organisms, such as bacteria or fungi. Antibiotics are classified as either biostatic or biocidal.

Antibiotic sensitivity: Testing a suspected organism to see whether it is sensitive to destruction by one or more specific antibiotics.

Antibody: A protein produced in the body in response to stimulation by an antigen. Antibodies react specifically to antigens in an attempt to neutralize these foreign substances.

Antigen: A substance, usually a protein, that is recognized as foreign by the body's immune system and stimulates formation of a specific antibody to the antigen.

Antipyretic: A drug or substance used to relieve fever.

Antiretroviral: An agent or drug that targets and works against retroviruses (e.g., HIV).

Aphthous: An ulcer that appears on the mucous membranes of the mouth, is painful, and typically heals spontaneously in 7 to 10 days.

Aplasia: Absence of an organ or organ part resulting from failure of development of the embryonic tissue of origin.

Apposition: Cell growth in which layers of material are deposited on already existing ones.

Arthralgia: Pain in one or more joints.

Aspiration: The withdrawal of fluid, usually into a syringe.

Asymptomatic: A lack of symptoms in the patient.

Atherosclerosis: A condition of degeneration and hardening of the walls of arteries caused by fat deposition.

Atopy: Hypersensitivity or allergy caused by hereditary influences.

Atrophic: A normally developed tissue that has decreased in size.

Attrition: The loss of tooth structure (wear) by mechanical forces from frequent occlusal loading from opposing teeth.

Atypical: Pertaining to a deviation from the normal or typical state.

Autoimmune disorder: A condition that occurs when the immune system mistakenly attacks and destroys healthy body tissue. To date, there are more than 80 types of autoimmune disorders.

Autoinoculation: To inoculate with a pathogen, such as a virus from one's own body. An example would be to spread herpesvirus from one's own mouth or lips to one's finger.

Autosomal dominant: One of several ways that a trait (features of a disorder) can be passed down through families. It occurs when an abnormal *gene* (from one of the 22 pair of nonsexual chromosomes) from one parent is passed down to a son or daughter such that the child inherits the disease and the gene is passed down to their children.

Axial inclination: The tilt the long axis of the tooth root has in the jaw in the anteroposterior plane.

Bacterial plaque: A collection of bacteria, growing in a deposit of material on the surface of a tooth, that can cause disease.

Bacteriostatic: The property of inhibiting the growth of bacteria.

Basal cell layer: The bottommost layer of the epidermis composed of *dividing cells* that are anchoring the epithelium to the deeper *dermis*.

Benign: A tumor that does not metastasize; generally not dangerous to health, and treatment cures the condition.

Bifid uvula: A cleft or split (small or large) in the uvula (fleshy mass that hangs from the soft palate).

Bilateral: On both sides of the body or mouth.

Biofilm: A well-organized community of bacteria that adheres to surfaces and is embedded in an extracellular slime layer.

Biopsy: Excision of living tissue for the purpose of examination by a pathologist.

Bosselated: Covered with bumps.

Bruxism: A habit related to stress or a sleep disorder characterized by grinding one's teeth.

Bulbous root: Enlarged rounded root.

Bulimia: An eating disorder characterized by frequent periods of excessive food consumption followed by the purging of the ingested food by vomiting or the use of laxatives.

Bulla: A circumscribed, fluid-containing, elevated lesion of the skin that is greater than 1 cm in diameter.

Cadherin: A family of adhesion proteins that makes up the desmosome and other structures.

Caliculus angularis: A slightly enlarged soft tissue fold on the buccal mucosa near the corner of the mouth.

Cancerization: The transformation of susceptible tissue into cancer; the spread of cancer.

Candida albicans: A diploid fungus (form of yeast) that causes opportunistic oral and genital infections.

Candidiasis: An infection, typically of the mucosa or skin, caused by *Candida albicans*.

Carcinogen: An agent that induces cancer.

Carcinoma: A malignant growth made up of epithelial cells that are capable of infiltration and metastasis. Carcinoma is a specific form of cancer.

Cellulitis: A spreading, diffuse, edematous, and sometimes suppurative (pus-producing) inflammation in cellular tissues.

Cervical enamel extensions: Spicules of enamel that project beyond the cementoenamel junction.

Cervical lymphadenopathy: Abnormally large lymph nodes in the neck, often caused by lymphocyte replication in response to an allergen or infectious organism.

Chancre: Painless ulceration formed during the primary stage of *syphilis*.

Cheilitis: Inflammation of the lips.

Chemotaxis: Taxis or movement of cells in response to chemical stimulation.

Chemotherapy: Treatment by chemical substances that have a specific effect on the microorganisms causing the disease. This term is usually reserved for the treatment of cancer with the use of drugs that inhibit rapidly reproducing cells. Side effects are possible.

Choristoma: A lesion that contains histologically normal tissues in an ectopic (abnormal) location.

Chromogenic bacteria: Bacteria that produce various colors during growth.

Chronic: Persisting for a long time; when applied to a disease, *chronic* means that there has been little change or extremely slow progression for a long period.

Cicatricial: Pertaining to a scar.

Cicatrix: A scar; the fibrous tissue that is formed after a wound heals.

Circumscribed: Encircled; curved boundaries of a lesion.

Cirrhosis: A chronic disease of the liver characterized by degenerative changes in the liver cells, the deposition of connective tissue, and other changes. The result is that the liver cells stop functioning and the flow of blood through the liver decreases. There are many causes of cirrhosis, including infection, toxic substances, and long-term alcohol abuse.

Class I caries: Decay affecting the fissural surface of the occlusal portion of a posterior tooth.

Class II caries: Decay affecting the interproximal surface of a posterior tooth below the contact point between teeth.

Class III caries: Decay affecting the interproximal surface of an anterior tooth below the contact point between teeth.

Class IV caries: Decay affecting the interproximal surface of an anterior tooth, including the incisal line angle.

Class V caries: Decay affecting the facial or lingual surface of a tooth, often at the gingival margin where plaque accumulates.

Clavicle: The collar bone, connecting the shoulder bone (scapula) to the chest bone (sternum).

Cleft lip: A developmental abnormality resulting in a split in the lip that is evident at the time of birth. Drug intake and smoking tobacco during pregnancy, as well as genetic factors, are contributory.

Cleft palate: A developmental abnormality resulting in a split in the palate that is evident at the time of birth. Delayed eruption and missing teeth often accompany this condition.

Cleidocranial dysplasia: A disorder involving the abnormal development of bones in the clavicle (cleido = collar bone) and skull (cranial = head).

Coagulation: The process of clotting, usually of blood. Clotting is the natural means by which bleeding ceases when a vessel has been severed.

Collagen: A protein present in the connective tissue of the body.

Coloboma: A developmental defect that may affect various parts of the eye, characterized by a missing part of the structure affected. For example, a coloboma of the lower eyelid means a missing part of the lower eyelid.

Commissural lip pits: Small, dimplelike depressions or pits found at the corner of the lips. Although rare, it is one of the more commonly occurring congenital malformations of the lower lip. The condition may be inherited.

Commissure: The junction of the upper and lower lips at the corner of the mouth.

Complement: A series of enzymatic proteins in normal serum that, in the presence of a specific sensitizer, can destroy bacteria and other cells. C1 through C9 are the nine components of complement that combine with the antigen-antibody complex to produce lysis.

Complete cleft lip: A congenital condition involving a large split in the lip that involves the structures of the nose and often cleft palate.

Complete cleft palate: A congenital condition involving a large split in the palate that permits communication between the oral and nasal cavities, typically involving the incisive foramen.

Concrescence: A condition in which the *cementum* of two adjacent tooth roots are fused together.

Concretion: A hardened mass, such as calculus.

Concurrent: One or more conditions, events, or findings occurring at the same time.

Congenital: Present at, or existing from, the time of birth.

Congenital epulis: A proliferation of cells resulting in a soft tissue mass of the alveolar ridge, palate, or tongue.

Congenital lymphangioma: A benign enlargement consisting of a mass of lymphatic vessels that are present at the time of birth.

Congenital syphilis: An infectious disease caused by a spirochete (*Treponema pallidum*) that is transmitted from mother to fetus during pregnancy. If untreated, the child is born with the infection that can damage many organs and tissues.

Connective tissue: The tissue that comprises the dermis and layers under the epithelium, characterized by collagenous, elastic, and reticular fibers; adipose tissue; blood vessels; cartilage; and bone. It forms the supporting and connecting structures of the body.

Constitutional symptoms: Symptoms affecting the whole body, such as fever, malaise, anorexia, nausea, and lethargy.

Cornified: A process whereby a tissue, usually epithelium, becomes rough and thickened in its outer coating.

Culture: The propagation of an organism in a medium conducive to growth.

Cunnilingus: Oral sex of the female genitalia.

Cusp of Carabelli: A small additional cusp on the mesiolingual surface of the maxillary *molars*.

Cyst: A pathologic epithelium-lined cavity, usually containing fluid or semisolid material.

Cytokines: A group of signaling proteins involved in inflammation and cell-to-cell communication.

Cytologic: Pertaining to the scientific study of cells.

Cytopathic: Pertaining to or characterized by pathologic changes in cells.

Cytotoxic: Damaging and toxic to living cells.

Debilitation: The process of becoming weakened.

Deciduous tooth: A primary or baby tooth. The normal number of deciduous teeth is 20.

Deglutition: The process of taking a substance through the mouth and throat into the esophagus. Deglutition is a stage of swallowing.

Dehiscence: An opening within an organ. In dentistry, the term is used to mean the loss of alveolar bone over the buccal or lingual aspect of the root, which leaves a characteristic oval root-exposed defect.

Dehydration: The removal of water from a substance. Prolonged fever and diarrhea cause dehydration.

Demineralization: A process whereby mineral substances (e.g., calcium, phosphate) are lost from a tissue such as enamel, dentin, or bone.

Dens evaginatus: A developmental anomaly that appears as a small, extra, dome-shaped, cusplike structure that emanates from the occlusal surface of a posterior tooth.

Dens in dente: A developmental anomaly that results from enamel and dentin folding inwardly toward the pulp. There are coronal and radicular forms.

Dental caries: A progressive destruction of the mineralized structures (enamel and dentin) of the teeth resulting from bacterial infection. The bacteria are found in plaque and use fermentable carbohydrates for food with the by-product being acid formation.

Dental lamina: The embryonic tissue of origin of the teeth.

Dental lamina cysts: Cysts that develop from the embryonic tissue that form teeth. Normally, the dental lamina disintegrates into small clusters of epithelium and is resorbed, but in this case, it becomes cystic.

Dentin dysplasia: A genetic (autosomal dominant) disorder involving abnormal dentin development of the primary and permanent teeth. Two types are described: type I is the radicular type and type II is the coronal type. In the radicular type, the roots of teeth are short, the *pulp* chambers are constricted, and spontaneous periapical radiolucencies may be evident. In the coronal type, the pulps have a "thistle tube" appearance.

Dentinoenamel junction (DEJ): The line or junction between the dentin and enamel.

Dermis: The connective tissue layer below the epidermis (skin) that contains nerve endings, sweat and sebaceous glands, blood vessels, and lymph vessels.

Desmosome: An intercellular bridge between epithelial cells. The bridge is made of proteins and tonofilaments.

Desquamation: Partial loss of the outer layer of skin or mucosa; peeling of the skin or mucosa.

Developmental: Pertaining to growth to full size or maturity.

Diascopy: The examination of tissue under pressure through a transparent medium. For example, suspected vascular lesions are examined by pressing a glass slide over an abnormality to see whether the reddish tissue turns white. Because blood flows through vascular lesions, pressure causes them to turn white and thus helps to confirm the diagnosis.

Diastema: A gap or spacing between two teeth.

Dilaceration: A bent root, usually affecting the apical half or third of the root.

Distal: Farthest from a point of reference. In dentistry, *distal* describes the surface farthest from the midline of the patient.

Distal drift: A tooth that moves distally often because of available space that results from a missing adjacent tooth.

Dorsal: Directed toward or situated on the back surface (opposite of *ventral*).

Ducts of Rivini: Ducts that lie beneath the tongue and permit saliva to enter the mouth from the sublingual glands.

Dysphagia: Difficulty swallowing.

Dysphonia: Difficulty speaking.

Dysplasia: An abnormality of development and maturation characterized by the loss of normal cellular architecture.

Dysplastic: Pertaining to an abnormality of development. This term is often used to describe the appearance of abnormal, premalignant cells under the microscope. The cells begin to lose their normal maturation pattern and have abnormally shaped, hyperchromatic nuclei.

Dyspnea: Labored or difficult breathing.

Ecchymosis: A large reddish-blue bruise (i.e., greater than 1 cm) caused by the escape of blood into the surrounding tissues. Ecchymoses do not blanch on diascopy.

Ecosystem: The interaction of living organisms and nonliving elements in a defined area.

Ectodermal: Pertaining to the outermost of the three primitive germ layers of an embryo. The middle layer is the mesoderm, and the innermost layer is the endoderm. Ectodermal structures include the skin, hair, nails, oral mucous membrane, and the enamel of the teeth.

Ectodermal dysplasia: A hereditary condition characterized by abnormal development of the skin, hair, nails, teeth, and sweat glands.

Ectopic: Located in an abnormal place. The ectopic tissue or structure may or may not be normal.

Ectopic eruption: Abnormal eruption location of a tooth.

Edema: Abnormal amounts of fluid in the intercellular spaces, resulting in visible swelling.

Edematous: An excessive accumulation of serous fluid in tissue spaces or a body cavity that produces swollen soft tissues.

Edentulism: A condition without teeth. The complete loss of all natural teeth.

Emanate: To give off or flow away from.

Embryologic: Pertaining to the development and maturation of an embryo during pregnancy.

Embryonic: Pertaining to the earliest stage of development of an organism.

Enamel hypoplasia: A disturbance in the development of enamel marked by deficient or defective enamel matrix formation, resulting in thin and hypocalcified enamel.

Enamel pearls: A concretion of enamel that is often dome shaped in an abnormal location. Pearls can appear at the cementoenamel junction or root surface and contribute to periodontal disease; rarely, they appear within dentin.

Encephalitis: Inflammation of the brain.

Endocrinopathy: A disease or abnormal state of an endocrine gland.

Endodermal: Pertaining to the innermost of the three primitive germ layers of an embryo. Endodermal structures include the epithelium of the pharynx, respiratory tract (except the nose), and the digestive tract.

Enostosis: Bone deposition within the marrow spaces of the jaws.

Epidermis: The outermost layer of the skin made of stratified squamous epithelium that protects the body surface.

Epistaxis: Bleeding from the nose.

Epithelium: The cellular makeup of skin and mucous membranes.

Epitope: The antigenic target of antibodies (IgG, IgM, IgA).

Epulis: A generic term used to describe any nodular or tumorous enlargement of the gingiva or alveolar mucosa.

Erosion: The wearing away of teeth through the action of chemical substances or a denudation of epithelium above the basal cell layer.

Eruption: An emergence from beneath a surface. For teeth, *eruption* means growth into the oral cavity; it may also refer to the development of skin lesions.

Eruption cyst: A fluctuant, fluid cyst that can appear 2 to 3 weeks before the eruption of a tooth. They are most often bluish, soft, associated with primary tooth eruption, and disappear upon tooth eruption.

Erythema: Redness in a tissue area.

Erythematous: Characterized by a redness of the tissue because of engorgement of the capillaries in the region. Erythematous lesions blanch on diascopy.

Erythroplastic: Characterized by a reddish appearance. This term implies abnormal tissue proliferation in the reddish area.

Eschar: A slough of epithelium often caused by disease, trauma, or chemical burn.

Esophagus: The flexible muscular tube that connects the mouth with the stomach.

Esthetic: Pertaining to the appearance of oral or dental structures or the pleasing effect of dental restorations or procedures.

Everted: Folded or turned outward.

Exacerbation: An increase in severity.

Exanthema: Skin eruption or rash.

Excisional biopsy: To completely remove a mass of tissue for the purpose of scientific (histologic) analysis.

Exophytic: An outwardly growing lesion.

Exostosis: A benign bony outgrowth on the surface of bone.

Extensor surface: Because the arms and legs can be extended or tensed by the appropriate extensor or tensor muscles, the anterior surface is referred to as the extensor surface, and the posterior surface is referred to as the tensor surface.

Extirpate: To completely remove or eradicate.

Extremity: A limb of the body, such as an arm or leg.

Extrinsic stains: Stains that come from external sources.

Exudate: Material that has escaped from blood vessels into tissue or onto the surface of a tissue, usually because of inflammation.

Factitial: Self-induced, as in factitial injury.

Fascial plane: Spaces between adjacent bundles of fascia that cover muscles. Infection often spreads along these planes.

Fellatio: Oral stimulation of the penis.

Fenestration: A perforation or opening in a tissue.

Fetor oris: An unpleasant or abnormal odor emanating from the oral cavity.

Fibroma: A benign tumor of fibrous (collagen) tissue.

Field cancerization: Malignant growths occurring in multiple sites of the oral cavity. The oral tissues have often been exposed to a carcinogen for a long time.

Fissural caries: Dental decay of the occlusal surface of a posterior tooth along enamel fissures and groves.

Fissure: A narrow slit or cleft.

Fluctuant: Strictly, this term describes a palpated, wavelike motion that is felt in a fluid-containing lesion. In this text, the term is frequently used to describe a soft, readily yielding mass on palpation.

Fluorosis: An abnormal condition caused by excess intake of fluorine or fluoride that is characterized by mottling and discoloration of the teeth.

Focal: A specific location or focus.

Fontanelle: One of several soft spots on the skull of infants and children in which the bones of the skull have not yet completely united. In these areas, the brain is covered only by a membrane beneath the skin.

Foramen: An opening that allows passage of tissues such as nerves or blood vessels between one area and another.

Fovea palatinae: Minor salivary gland openings close to the junction of the soft and hard palate.

Frenum: A fold of mucous membrane that limits the movement of an organ or organ part. For example, the lingual frenum limits tongue movement, and the labial frenula limit lip movements.

Frontal bone: The skull bone that forms the forehead. The frontal bone contains an airspace called the frontal sinus.

Furcal: Pertaining to or associated with the part of a multi-rooted tooth where the roots join the crown.

Fusion: An abnormality caused by the joining of two teeth during embryologic development resulting in one large tooth.

Ganglion: A collection of cell bodies of neurons outside of the central nervous system. A ganglion is essentially a terminal through which many peripheral circuits connect with the central nervous system.

Gardner syndrome: An inherited autosomal dominant disease that has the features of osteomas and intestinal polyps. The polyps have a propensity to become malignant during early adulthood.

Gastroenterologist: A medical specialist whose field is disorders of the stomach and intestines.

Gastrointestinal: Pertaining to the stomach and intestine.

Gemination: To arrange or occur in pairs. A tooth that splits during embryologic development into two teeth that remain connected.

Genetic counseling: A form of patient counseling in which the transmission of inherited traits is discussed.

Genial tubercles: Bony spines located on the lingual aspect of the mandible at the midline below the incisor roots that serve as the attachment of the geniohyoid and genioglossus muscles.

Genodermatosis: A hereditary skin disease.

Gingival crevicular fluid: Serum fluid emitted from the periodontal pocket. It contains inflammatory proteins (cytokines). The amount of fluid increases during periodontal disease.

Gingival recession: The result of migration of the free gingival margin to a position apical to the cementoenamel junction.

Gingivectomy: Surgical removal of gingival tissue.

Gingivitis: Inflammation of the gums, typically because of the accumulation of dental plaque.

Glaucoma: A disease of the eye characterized by increased intraocular pressure. This condition is often asymptomatic and, if not recognized or treated, leads to blindness.

Glossal: Pertaining to or associated with the tongue.

Glossodynia: Burning sensation of the tongue.

Glucan: A sticky substance (polysaccharide) secreted by bacteria in dental plaque that is composed of chains of D-glucose monomers linked by glycosidic bonds.

Glucose: A form of sugar that is the most important carbohydrate in the body's metabolism.

Glucosuria: The presence of an abnormal quantity of glucose in the urine. A sign of diabetes mellitus.

Granuloma: A collection of epithelioid macrophages surrounded by a ring of lymphocytes. They can form small nodules and are an outcome of a necrotic pulp.

Granulomatous: Pertaining to a well-defined area that has developed as a reaction to the presence of living organisms or a foreign body. The tissue consists primarily of histiocytes.

Gravid: Pregnant.

Gutta-percha points: An inelastic natural latex produced from the sap of trees that is shaped into cylindric points that are used in endodontics to fill a cleaned and shaped root canal.

Halitosis: An unpleasant odor of the breath or expired air.

Hamartoma: A tumorlike nodule consisting of a mixture of normal tissue usually present in an organ but existing in an unusual arrangement or an unusual site.

Hapten: An incomplete allergen. When combined with another substance to form a molecule, a hapten may stimulate a hypersensitivity or allergic reaction.

Hemangioma: A benign, reddish collection of blood vessels that can enlarge and bleed, regress, or be associated with the development of calcifications within the lesion known as phleboliths.

Hematoma: A large ecchymosis or bruise caused by the escape of blood into the tissues. Hematomas are blue on the skin and red on the mucous membranes. As hematomas resolve, they may turn brown, green, or yellow.

Hematopoietic: Pertaining to the production of blood or of its constituent elements. Hematopoiesis is the main function of the bone marrow.

Hematuria: The presence of blood in the urine.

Hemidesmosome: An intercellular bridge between epithelial cells and the basement membrane.

Hemihypertrophy: The presence of hypertrophy on one side only of a tissue or organ. In facial hemihypertrophy, for example, one half of the face is visibly larger than the other.

Hemoglobin: The iron-containing pigment of the erythrocytes. Its function is to carry oxygen to the tissues. One of the causes of anemia is a deficiency of iron, causing patients to look pale and feel tired.

Hemolysis: Generally speaking, this term refers to the disintegration of elements in the blood. A common form of hemolysis occurs during anemia and involves lysis or the dissolution of erythrocytes.

Hemorrhage: Bleeding; the escape of blood from a severed blood vessel.

Hemostasis: The stoppage of blood flow. This can occur naturally by clotting or artificially by the application of pressure or the placement of sutures.

Hepatosplenomegaly: The simultaneous enlargement of the liver and spleen.

Hereditary: Transmitted or transmissible from parent to offspring; determined genetically.

Herpes simplex virus (HSV): A transmissible DNA virus belonging to the human herpesvirus family that causes gingivostomatitis, mucosal ulcers, and perioral disease. This virus establishes latency in neurons and reactivates to cause recurrent ulcers (fever blisters).

Hertwig (epithelial) root sheath: A collection of epithelial cells located at the cervical loop of the enamel organ (i.e., DEJ) in a developing tooth. This sheath migrates downward to form the root of the tooth.

Hiatal hernia: Protrusion of any structure through the hiatus of the diaphragm. Affected patients are prone to indigestion.

Histiocyte: A large phagocytic cell from the reticuloendothelial system. The reticuloendothelial system is a network made up of all of the phagocytic cells in the body, which include macrophages, Kupffer cells in the liver, and the microglia of the brain.

Histology: The microscopic study of the structure and form of the various tissues making up a living organism.

Histoplasmosis: A disease caused by the fungus *Histoplasma capsulatum* that primarily affects the lungs but also affects the eyes and infrequently the tongue.

Human papillomavirus (HPV): A small transmissible DNA virus that causes human disease. More than 100 different HPVs have been identified. The "low-risk" types cause benign growths, such as warts and papillomas; the "high-risk" types can cause cancer.

Hutchinson triad: A pattern of presentation for congenital syphilis that consists of abnormal teeth (Hutchinson incisors and mulberry molars), interstitial keratosis, and deafness as a result of damage to the eighth cranial nerve.

Hypercementosis: A condition characterized by increased cementum deposition on the roots of teeth. Any part of the root may be affected; however, the apical two thirds is most common. Local or systemic factors may cause this condition.

Hyperdontia: A condition or circumstance characterized by one or more extra (or supernumerary) teeth.

Hyperemia: The presence of excess blood in a tissue area.

Hyperglycemia: The presence of excessive sugar or glucose in the bloodstream.

Hypermenorrhea: Excessive uterine bleeding of unusually long duration at regular intervals.

Hyperorthokeratosis: Keratin is the outermost layer of the epithelium as seen under the microscope and is seen in two forms: orthokeratin and parakeratin. Orthokeratin has no visible nuclei within the outer layer, whereas nuclei are present in parakeratin. Hyperorthokeratosis is the presence of excess orthokeratin.

Hyperplasia: An increase in the size of a tissue or organ caused by an increase in the number of constituent cells.

Hyperplastic: Pertaining to hyperplasia; tissue that displays hyperplasia features.

Hypersensitivity: Generally, this term means an abnormal sensitivity to a stimulus of any kind; however, it is often used with specific reference to some form of allergic response.

Hypertension: High blood pressure.

Hypertrophy: An increase in the size of a tissue or organ caused by an increase in the size of constituent cells.

Hypocalcification: Less than normal amount of calcification.

Hypodontia: The congenital absence of one or several teeth as a result of agenesis.

Hypoplasia: Incomplete development of a tissue or organ; a tissue reduced in size because of a decreased number of constituent cells.

Hypopyon: Pus in the anterior chamber of the eye.

Hyposalivation: Low salivary flow that can result in the perception of a dry mouth (xerostomia).

Hypotension: Low blood pressure.

Hypotrichosis: A condition of lack of hair growth.

Iatrogenic: A condition or disorder resulting from a complication of medical treatment.

Idiopathic: Arising from an obscure or unknown cause.

Ileum: The distal or terminal portion of the small intestine, ending at the cecum, which is a blind pouch forming the proximal or first part of the large intestine.

Ilium: The lateral or flaring part of the pelvic bone, otherwise known as the hip.

Immunofluorescence: A laboratory assay used by pathologists and researchers that applies known antibodies to tissue to identify the presence and location of specific antigens or proteins.

Immunosuppressant: An agent or drug that suppresses or prevents the immune response.

Implant: A titanium structure inserted into alveolar bone that serves as a root for the prosthetic reconstruction of a missing tooth.

Incipient lesion: A beginning lesion; in an initial stage.

Incisional biopsy: The removal of a portion of suspected abnormal tissue for microscopic study.

Incisive canal: The bony canal located within the palatal bone that supports the nasopalatine nerve and blood vessels and exits at the incisive foramen behind the maxillary central incisors.

Incisive papilla: A slightly elevated papule of normal tissue on the palate in the midline immediately posterior to the central incisors. Immediately beneath this structure lies the incisive canal.

Induration: Characterized by being hard; an abnormally hard portion of a tissue with respect to the surrounding similar tissue, often used to describe the feel of locally invasive malignant tissue on palpation.

Infant: A human baby from birth to 2 years of age.

Infarct: A localized area of ischemic necrosis resulting from a blockage of the arterial supply or the venous drainage of tissue. Ischemic necrosis is dead tissue resulting from an inadequate blood supply. An example is a heart attack, which is an infarct of heart muscle.

Inflammation: A bodily process involving white blood cells and chemicals that results from infection, irritation, or injury and produces tissue redness, warmth, swelling, and pain.

Insulin: A protein hormone secreted by the islets of Langerhans of the pancreas that helps move glucose from the blood to tissues. Insulin deficiency produces hyperglycemia, otherwise known as diabetes mellitus.

Integrins: A large group of heterodimeric transmembrane proteins that serve as receptors for extracellular matrix and cell surface proteins.

Intrinsic staining: A term used in dentistry to indicate discoloration from staining that occurs from within the tooth.

Invaginate: To fold and grow within, in the manner of a pouch.

Iris: The part of the eye that is blue, gray, green, or brown. It is a muscular tissue, and its function is to constrict and dilate the pupil. The pupil is the black-appearing portion in the middle of the iris that allows light into the eye.

Iritis: Inflammation of the iris that is often caused by viral infection or rheumatoid disease. The main symptom of iritis is photophobia (aversion to light).

Irreversible pulpitis: Inflammation of the pulp that cannot be reversed that eventually results in death of the pulp. Pain is a key feature of this condition.

Ischemia: A deficiency of blood to a body part, usually caused by constriction or blockage of a blood vessel.

Kaposi sarcoma: A malignant tumor of vascular tissue. Once rare in the Americas, it is now seen frequently in patients with AIDS. The lesions are red-purple in appearance and may be seen anywhere on the skin, especially on the face and in the oral cavity.

Keratin: A strong protein and major component of skin, hair, nails, and teeth.

Keratinization: The formation of microscopic fibrils of keratin in the keratinocytes (keratin-forming cells). In the oral cavity, the term is used to describe changes in the outer layer of the epithelium.

Keratotic: A condition of the skin characterized by the presence of horny growths. On the oral mucous membrane, keratotic tissue usually looks white; the term implies a thickening of the outer layer of the oral epithelium.

Kilodalton: A unit of mass being one thousand times that of a dalton. A dalton is one sixteenth the mass of an oxygen atom.

Lamina dura: The thin compact bone that surrounds the socket (alveolus) of a tooth.

Lamina propria: The layer of connective tissue immediately beneath the epithelium of the oral mucosa.

Laryngeal: Pertaining to the larynx, which is a part of the airway. It is located between the pharynx at the back of the oral cavity and the trachea at the beginning of the lungs. The larynx contains the vocal cords, which make audible sounds.

Lateral: Pertaining to or situated at the side.

Lateral vaults: The region of the palate adjacent to the posterior teeth.

Leptomeninges: The two more delicate components of the meninges: the pia mater and the arachnoid.

Lesion: A site of structural or functional change in body tissues that is produced by disease or injury.

Leukemia: A cancer of the blood-forming tissues.

Leukoplakia: A white patch that cannot be rubbed off and that does not clinically represent any other condition.

Lipid: Fat or fatty; a naturally occurring substance made up of fatty acids.

Lipoma: A benign soft tissue tumor composed of fat cells (adipocytes).

Lobulated: Made up of lobules, which are smaller divisions of lobes. Many structures are divided into lobes and lobules, such as the brain, lung, and salivary glands. Some pathologic lesions are described as lobulated when the lesion is divided into smaller parts.

Locular: Containing small, often rounded, compartments within an organ or tissue.

Lymphadenitis: Inflammation of lymph nodes generally resulting in enlargement and tenderness.

Lymphadenopathy: Enlarged lymph nodes that may or may not be tender. The enlargement results from increased number of lymphocytes presenting in the node.

Lymphatic: Pertaining to the lymph and vein-like vessels in which the lymph travels.

Lymphoblastic: Pertaining to a cell of the lymphocytic series; the term implies proliferation. Lymphoblastic is one of the forms of leukemic cancer of the leukocytes characterized by the presence of malignant lymphoblasts or immature lymphocytes.

Lymphocyte: A variety of leukocyte that is important to the immune response and that arises in the lymph nodes. Lymphocytes can be large or small; they are round and nongranular and are classified as either T or B lymphocytes.

Lymphoma: A neoplasm that develops from lymphoid cells (e.g., B cells, T cells, NK cells).

Macrocheilia: Abnormally large lips.

Macrodontia: Teeth that are considerably larger than normal.

Macroglossia: Abnormally large tongue.

Macule: A spot or stain on the skin or mucous membrane that is neither raised nor depressed. Some examples of macules include café au lait spots, hyperemia, erythema, petechiae, ecchymoses, purpura, oral melanotic macules, and many others illustrated in this atlas.

Malaise: A constitutional symptom that describes a feeling of uneasiness, discomfort, or indisposition.

Malignant: A neoplastic growth that is not usually encapsulated, grows rapidly, and can readily metastasize.

Marrow space: The space in the trabecular bone composed of red or yellow marrow. Red marrow is where hematopoiesis occurs. Yellow marrow is composed mostly of fat. The size of the marrow space can indicate pathologic processes (e.g., anemia, thalassemia, trauma, infection, or tumors).

Mastication: Chewing.

Medial: Situated toward the midline (opposite of lateral).

Median palatal raphe: A fibrous band of soft tissue that is found in the midline of the palate.

Melena: Darkened or black feces that are caused by the presence of blood pigments; a sign of intestinal bleeding.

Meningitis: Inflammation of the meninges, which are the three membranes covering the brain and spinal cord (the dura mater, arachnoid, and pia mater). Meningitis produces both motor and mental signs, such as difficulty in walking and confusion.

Mesenchymal: The meshwork of embryonic connective tissue in the mesoderm that gives rise to the connective tissue of the body (bone, cartilage, ligaments), blood vessels, and lymph vessels.

Mesial: Toward the front, anterior, or midline. The mesial surface of teeth is the side of the tooth closest to the midline. The five surfaces of teeth are mesial, distal, occlusal or incisal, labial or facial, and lingual or palatal.

Mesiodens: A midline supernumerary tooth commonly seen in the maxillary arch.

Metastasize: To spread or travel from one part of the body to another; a term usually reserved to describe the spread of malignant tumors.

Microdontia: Teeth that are considerably smaller than normal.

Micrognathia: Jaws that are small with respect to normal.

Migration: Movement from one location to another.

Mineralized: Characterized by the deposition of mineral, often calcium and other organic salts, in a tissue. The term *calcified* is used when the mineral content is known to be calcium, whereas the term *mineralized* is more general and does not specify the exact nature of the mineral.

Monocytic leukemia: Leukemia is cancer of the leukocytes; in this condition, the predominating leukocytes are monocytes.

Morphology: Descriptive of shape, form, or structure, or the science thereof.

Mucinous saliva: Saliva that contains mucin, a large glycosylated protein produced by salivary glands (primarily the submandibular gland).

Mucopurulent: Consisting of both mucus and pus.

Mucosa: The moist epithelial lining of endodermal structures, such as the mouth, eyes, gastrointestinal tract, lungs, and genitalia.

Mucositis: Inflammation of the mucosa.

Mutagenesis: The induction of genetic mutation.

Myelogenous leukemia: Leukemia is cancer of the leukocytes; in this instance, the predominating leukocytes are myeloid or granular (polymorphonuclear leukocytes).

Nasopharyngitis: Inflammation of the nasopharynx (the back of the nasal complex and upper throat). Sore throat, postnasal drip, and fever are common signs.

Natal teeth: Teeth that are present at birth.

Necrosis: The death of a cell as a result of injury or disease.

Neocapillary: New growth of capillaries, which are the smallest blood vessels and connect small arterioles to small venules.

Neoplasia: Characterized by the presence of new and uncontrolled cellular growth.

Neoplasm: A mass of newly formed tissue; a tumor.

Neoplastic: Tissue that has features of neoplasia.

Neural crest cells: Cells that originate from the neural crest (a transient ectodermal tissue found between the neural tube and the epidermis during embryologic development). Neural crest cells migrate from this region and differentiate into a wide variety of cell types throughout the body, giving rise to sensory and sympathetic neurons, glia cells, melanocytes, Schwann cells, adrenomedullary cells, and components of the enteric nervous system.

Neuralgia: Abnormal pain along the course of a nerve. The pain can be episodic or chronic.

Neurogenic: Originating in or from nerve tissue.

Neuroma: A tumor of nervous tissue that is usually benign and associated with numbness and pain.

Neuropathy: Any abnormality of nerve tissue.

Neutrophil: A medium-sized leukocyte with a nucleus consisting of three to five lobes and a cytoplasm containing small granules; one group of leukocytes is called *granulocytes*, and the others are *eosinophils* and *basophils*. Neutrophils make up about 65% of the leukocytes in normal blood. Also known as polymorphonuclear leukocyte, PMN, or "poly."

Neutrophil chemotaxis: Taxis or movement of neutrophils in response to chemical substances or agents.

Nevoid basal cell carcinoma syndrome (Gorlin-Goltz syndrome): An autosomal dominant syndrome caused by a mutation in a gene known as patched (PTCH), a tumor suppressor gene located on chromosome 9q. This syndrome is characterized by multiple jaw odontogenic cysts, basal cell nevi on the skin, skeletal anomalies (bifid and other rib anomalies), and soft tissue anomalies like prominent finger pads and palmar pitting of the hands.

Nevus: A small tumor of the skin containing aggregations or theques of nevus cells; a mole. It may be flat or elevated and pigmented or nonpigmented; it may or may not contain hair.

Nodule: A circumscribed, usually solid lesion having the dimension of depth. Nodules are less than 1 cm in diameter.

Noncaseating: A tissue-degenerative process that forms a dry, shapeless mass resembling cheese.

Noncornified: The lower layers of the epithelium (intermediate, parabasal, and basilar cells) that do not have a keratinized surface.

Nonvital tooth: A tooth with dead pulp tissue that is unable to transmit nerve signals effectively.

Nursing bottle caries: Dental decay that affects the primary teeth as a result of prolonged use of the nursing bottle that contains milk, juice, or soda pop. The maxillary anterior teeth are most commonly and can be severely affected.

Occipital bone: One of the bones that make up the skull; a thick bone at the back of the head.

Odontogenic: Pertaining to the development and formation of teeth.

Odontogenic epithelium: Epithelium that develops into teeth. After tooth development, this epithelium can remain within the jaws and become cystic.

Odontoma: A developmental anomaly (hamartoma) of enamel and dentin.

Oligodontia: Few teeth; the presence of fewer than the normal number of teeth.

Oncogenic: Capable of causing tumor formation.

Open contact: A term that describes the interproximal contact between teeth that normally touch each other. In this instance, the interproximal spaces between the teeth do not contact.

Operculum: The gingival flap of tissue surrounding the crown of a partially erupted tooth.

Opportunistic microorganism: Microorganisms that usually are not pathogenic but become so under certain circumstances, such as an environment altered by the action of antibiotics or long-term steroid therapy. Opportunistic microorganisms cause opportunistic infections.

Organism: Any viable life-form, such as animals, plants, and microorganisms, including bacteria, fungi, and viruses.

Orogenital: Refers to mouth contact with the genitalia.

Oropharynx: The area of the throat that is at the back of the mouth.

Otorhinolaryngologist: An ear, nose, and throat specialist.

Orthodontic tooth movement: The repositioning of teeth using removable or fixed appliances, such as braces, to straighten the alignment of teeth and improve the appearance and function of the teeth.

Osseointegration: The process of a foreign body such as an implant biologically connecting with the bone.

Osteogenesis imperfecta: A genetic disorder characterized by a defect in collagen that results in bones that break easily and defective dentin in teeth.

Osteoma: A benign tumor of bone most often found in the skull, sinuses, and facial bones.

Osteomyelitis: Inflammation accompanied by infection of the bone; often chronic.

Osteoporosis: A condition associated with aging caused by a deficiency of organic bone matrix. It causes bones to become weak and brittle.

Overhang: Defect in a restoration that extends beyond the interproximal surface of the tooth.

Palatogingival groove: A defect in cementum formation that results in a linear groove on the lingual surface of a tooth root, most commonly a maxillary incisor.

Palliative: Treatment to relieve symptoms; not the cause of a condition.

Pallor: Paleness of the skin or mucous membrane; an absence of a healthy color. This sign often accompanies constitutional symptoms and anemia.

Palpate: To feel with the fingers or hand.

Papilloma: A benign pebbly growth caused by infection with human papillomavirus.

Papillomatous: Pertaining to a benign pebbly growth.

Papule: A small mass, without the dimension of depth, that is less than 1 cm in diameter. When described as pedunculated, a papule is on a stalk; when described as sessile, a papule is attached at its base and does not have a stalk.

Papulonodular: A type of lesion elevated above the surface of the skin that has features both of a papule and nodule.

Parakeratin: A type of epithelium consisting of the outermost layer (stratum corneum) that demonstrates keratin and small residual nuclei.

Parakeratotic epithelium: Incomplete keratinization characterized by retention of nuclei of cells at the uppermost level of the epithelium (stratum corneum).

Paramedian lip pits: Small bilateral depressions in the mucosa of the lower lip adjacent to the midline. This condition is often inherited as an autosomal dominant trait associated with van der Woude syndrome.

Paramolar: A supernumerary or "fourth" molar positioned distal to the third molar.

Paresthesia: An abnormal tingling or pricking sensation caused by damage to peripheral nerves or restriction of nerve impulses.

Parietal bone: One of the bones that make up the skull; there is one parietal bone on each side of the skull, forming the skull's top and upper sides.

Partial eruption: A condition in which a tooth erupts through the gum tissue but not fully into occlusion.

Parturition: The delivery of the fetus from the mother; to give birth.

Parulis: A gumboil; a subperiosteal abscess arising from dental structures that emanates onto the gingival or alveolar mucosa.

Patch: Similar to a macule but larger; a large stain or spot, usually neither raised nor depressed, which may be textured.

Patent: The condition of being open; this term is often applied to ducts, vessels, and passages to indicate that they are not blocked.

Pathognomonic: Uniquely distinctive of a specific disease or condition; usually consists of signs or findings that, when present and recognized, enable the diagnosis to be made.

Pathologic: Pertaining to or caused by disease.

Pathosis: An abnormal state or condition.

Pedunculated: A tissue mass originating by a stalk from its base.

Periapical: Pertaining to or located at the apex (root end) of a tooth.

Periapical abscess: An abscess located at the apex (root end) of a tooth, generally as a result of infection.

Periapical inflammation (apical periodontitis): Inflammation located at the apex (root end) of a tooth.

Pericoronitis: Inflammation of the tissue overlying a partially erupted tooth.

Perifurcal: Pertaining to or located at the furca of a tooth, below the cementoenamel junction where the roots fuse together.

Perilabial: Pertaining to the region around or near the lips.

Perinatal: Pertaining to the time frame around childbirth.

Perineum: The lower surface of the trunk; when a patient is lying down with legs spread apart, the perineum is the area from the base of the spine to the anal region to the genital area and, finally, to the crest of the mons pubis.

Periodontal abscess: Abscess of the gingival or periodontal tissue secondary to periodontal infection.

Periodontitis: Inflammation resulting from microbial infection of the structures that support the teeth.

Perioral: In the proximity of or around the oral cavity.

Periorbital: In the proximity of or around the orbit, which is the bony socket of the eye.

Periosteum: The thin layer of dense, irregular, connective tissue membrane that covers the outer surface of bone, excluding the joints.

Peripheral: Pertaining to the outer part, such as the edge or margin.

Permanent dentition: Succedaneous (adult) teeth, which erupt after the primary teeth. As there are no replacements for the permanent teeth, they should be properly taken care of if they are to last a lifetime. There are 32 permanent teeth.

Petechiae: Little red spots, ranging in size from pinpoint to several millimeters in diameter. Petechiae consist of extravasated capillary blood.

Pharyngitis: Inflammation of the pharynx, which is often painful.

Physiologic: Refers to normal body function (opposite of *pathologic*).

Pilocarpine: A drug used to stimulate salivary flow or to produce constriction of the pupil of the eye.

Pink tooth of mummery: A pink, discolored nonvital tooth that obtains its color from absorption of blood products into the dentin.

Plaque: An area with a flat surface and raised edges.

Platelet: One of the elements found in circulating blood. A platelet has a circular or disklike shape and is small; hence the term *platelet*. Platelets aid in blood coagulation and clot retraction.

Plica fimbriata: Slight folds of mucous membrane tissue located bilaterally on the ventral surface of the tongue.

Polydipsia: Excessive thirst. A sign of disease.

Polypoid: A polyplike protruding growth with a base that is equal in diameter to the surface of the mucosal lesion.

Polyuria: Excessive amounts of urine. A sign of disease.

Posterior: Directed toward or situated at the back (opposite of *anterior*).

Primary tooth: Deciduous (baby) tooth; there are 20 primary teeth.

Prognathism: A developmental deformity of the mandible that causes it to protrude abnormally.

Protostylid: An extra cusp found on the buccal surface of a molar.

Pruritus: Itching.

Pseudo: Not real. Appears to be something it is not.

Pseudohyphae: Long, filamentous forms that can be seen under the microscope when *Candida albicans*, a fungal microorganism, assumes its pathogenic form.

Pulp polyp: An enlargement of pulp tissue beyond a broken down tooth crown in response to bacterial infection and inflammation. The condition is most common in primary or permanent molars in children.

Pulse: A patient's heartbeat, as felt through palpation of a blood vessel.

Punctate: Spotted; characterized by small points or punctures.

Purpuric: Pertaining to purpura, which are large bruises consisting of blood extravasated into the tissues. Bruises are bluish-purple in color.

Purulent: Containing pus.

Pustule: A well-circumscribed, pus-containing lesion, usually less than 1 cm in diameter.

Pyogenic granuloma: A mass of vascular granulation tissue produced in response to minor trauma or chronic irritation.

Qualitative: Of or pertaining to quality; descriptive information about what something looks and feels like.

Quantitative: Of or pertaining to quantity; descriptive information about how much of something there is or how big something is.

Radiation: In dentistry, electromagnetic energy or x-rays transmitted through space. Radiation also means divergence from a common center; one of the properties of x-rays is that like a beam of light, they diverge from their source.

Radiolucent: A term to describe anatomic structures that allow the passage of x-rays or other radiation to a film or sensor. Radiolucent structures appear dark on the film.

Radiopaque: A term to describe anatomic structures that do not allow the passage of x-rays or other radiation to a film or sensor. Radiopaque structures appear light on the film.

Radiotherapy: Radiation therapy; the use of radiation from various sources to treat or cure malignant disorders.

Rampant caries: A rapidly progressing form of decay affecting the teeth.

Recessive inheritance: A mode of passing a gene carried by both parents that does not cause any clinical manifestation until passed to their offspring.

Recrudescence: Recurrence of signs and symptoms of a disease after temporary abatement.

Recurrent caries: Decay affecting the teeth adjacent to surfaces where decay previously occurred and a restoration was placed. Caries adjacent to a restoration margin.

Reduced enamel epithelium: The epithelium (sulcular epithelium) that overlies a developing tooth and remains in the periodontal tissue around a tooth crown after enamel formation is complete. It is formed by two layers: an inner layer of ameloblastic cells that is adjacent to formed enamel and an outer layer of cuboidal cells (outer enamel epithelium). Cystic degeneration of this tissue results in a dentigerous cyst.

Refractory: Not readily responsive to treatment.

Regional odontodysplasia: A rare developmental abnormality of teeth resulting in defective (thinned) enamel and dentin. On radiographs, the teeth have reduced radiodensity, producing a ghostlike appearance.

Remission: Improvement or abatement of the symptoms of a disease; the period during which symptoms abate.

Renal failure: Inability of the kidneys to function properly. A patient whose kidneys completely fail will die without renal dialysis or a kidney transplantation. One of the causes of kidney failure is prolonged hypertension (high blood pressure).

Retinopathy: A disease or abnormality of the retina of the eye. The retina cannot be seen without special instruments and is the part of the eye that receives and transmits visual information coming in from the pupil and lens onto the brain via the optic nerve.

Retrognathia: A retruded mandible.

Rests of Malassez: The epithelial remains of Hertwig root sheath that reside in the periodontal ligament after a tooth develops and erupts.

Reversible pulpitis: Inflammation of the pulp that causes pain but is reversible if the cause of the inflammation is removed.

Root caries: Decay affecting the root surface of the tooth usually at the gingival margin. This condition only occurs when root surfaces are exposed, usually in association with gingival recession.

Rotated tooth: An erupted tooth that is positionally rotated from that of normal.

Sarcoma: A malignant growth of cells of embryonic connective tissue origin. This condition is highly capable of infiltration and metastasis.

Sarcomatous: Pertaining to sarcoma, which is a malignant tumor of mesenchymal tissue origin.

Scar: A mark or cicatrix remaining after the healing of a wound or other morbid process.

Sclera: The strong outer tunic of the eye, or whites of the eyes. When the sclera turns blue or yellow, it is a sign of systemic abnormality.

Sclerosis: Stiffening of tissue resulting from deposition of molecules that have hardening and fibrinous properties.

Sebaceous: Pertaining to glands that produce sebum that are often associated with hair follicles.

Sepsis: A morbid state resulting from the presence of pathogenic microorganisms, usually in the bloodstream.

Septicemia: The presence of pathogenic bacteria in the blood.

Sequestration: Abnormal separation of a part from the whole, such as when a piece of bone sequestrates from the mandible because of osteomyelitis; the act of isolating a patient.

Serosal: Pertaining to the lining of internal organs, such as the intestines.

Serpiginous: Characterized by a wavy or undulating margin.

Serum: The watery fluid remaining after coagulation of the blood. If clotted blood is left long enough, the clot shrinks and the fibrinogen is depleted; the remaining fluid is the serum.

Sessile: Attached to a surface on a broad base; does not have a stalk.

Shell teeth: Teeth lacking normal dentin, producing a shell appearance, which are often associated with dentinogenesis imperfecta.

Shovel-shaped incisors: A syndrome seen in Native Americans, Canadians, Eskimos, and Hispanics that is associated with prominent marginal ridges of the maxillary incisors.

Sign: An objective finding or observation made by the examiner that the patient may be unaware of or does not report.

Sinus: An airspace inside the skull, such as the maxillary sinus; an abnormal channel, fistula, or tract allowing the escape of pus.

Smooth surface caries: Decay affecting the smooth (interproximal, buccal, or lingual) surface of teeth.

Splenic: Of or pertaining to the spleen, which is a structure in the upper left abdomen just behind and under the stomach. The spleen contains the largest collection of reticuloendothelial cells in the whole body; its functions include blood formation, blood storage, and blood filtration.

Spontaneous: Occurring unaided or without apparent cause; voluntary.

Squamous epithelium: An uninterrupted layer of epithelium characterized by the top layer consisting of flat, scalelike cells. Squamous epithelium lines the oral mucosa and skin.

Stepladder trabecular pattern: A pattern of medullary bone that appears radiographically as successive linear increments or steps. This pattern is suggestive of extramedullary hematopoiesis that occurs with certain types of anemias.

Stomatitis: Inflammation of the mouth and lips that is often accompanied by redness and pain.

Subcutaneous: Below the cutaneous (epidermal) layer.

Submucosal palatal cleft: An incomplete cleft of the palate where the epithelium covers a defect in the subjacent connective tissue.

Sulcus terminalis: A shallow V-shaped groove in the dorsum of the tongue behind the circumvallate papillae.

Superficial: Located on or near the surface.

Supernumerary: In excess of the regular number.

Supernumerary roots: An excess number of roots.

Suppurative: The discharge of pus from infected tissue.

Supraeruption: A condition in which a tooth erupts beyond the normal plane of occlusion. This condition can result when the opposing tooth is missing.

Symptom: A manifestation of disease that the patient is usually aware of and frequently reports.

Syndrome: A combination of signs and symptoms occurring commonly enough to constitute a distinct clinical entity.

Talon cusp: An extra cusp on an anterior tooth that resembles eagle's talon.

Taurodont: A malformed, multirooted tooth characterized by an altered crown-to-root ratio, the crown being of normal length, the roots being abnormally short, and the pulp chamber being abnormally large.

Taurodontism: Pertaining to a condition in which there are taurodont teeth.

Telangiectasia: The formation of capillaries near the surface of a tissue. Telangiectasia may be a sign of hereditary disorder, alcohol abuse, or malignancy in the region.

Template bleeding time: The amount of time necessary for bleeding to stop after a skin incision of consistent length and depth.

Texture: Pertains to the characteristics of the surface of an area or lesion. Some descriptions of texture are as follows: smooth, rough, lumpy, and vegetative. The tiny bumps on the surface of a wart cause it to have a vegetative texture.

Therapeutic: Of or pertaining to therapy or treatment; beneficial. Therapy has as its goal the elimination or control of a disease or other abnormal state.

Thorax: That part of the body between the neck and abdomen, enclosed by the spine, ribs, and sternum. In the vernacular, the thorax is referred to as the chest. The main contents of the thorax are the heart and lungs.

Thrombocytopathia: A condition in which there is an abnormality in platelet function.

Thrombocytopenia: A condition in which there are less than the normal number of platelets.

Thrombophlebitis: The development of venous thrombi in the presence of inflammatory changes in the vessel wall.

Thrombosis: Formation of thrombi within the lumen of the heart or a blood vessel. A lumen is the space within a passage; a thrombus is a solid mass that can form within the heart or blood vessels from constituents in the circulating blood. Patients prone to the formation of thrombi should receive anticoagulant therapy.

Tonsillar pillars (fauces): The soft tissue folds derived from the second and third branchial arches that border and house the tonsils (lymphoid patches of tissue in the oropharynx).

Tooth bud: The embryonic tissue of origin of the teeth; tooth buds develop from the more primitive tissue of the dental lamina.

Torus: A bony nodule on the hard palate or on the lingual aspect of the premolars.

Tourniquet test: When pressure is applied to the blood vessels of the upper arm using a blood pressure cuff, a bleeding tendency is detected when petechiae develop in the region.

Trabeculae: Thin, anastomosing threads of bone or tissue.

Transient: Temporary; of short duration.

Translocation: Rearrangement of parts. In dentistry, the term is used when a tooth erupts into an abnormal location but remains within the dental arch.

Translucent: Somewhat penetrable by rays of light.

Transposition: Two teeth exchanging places.

Trauma: A wound or injury; damage produced by an external force.

Treacher Collins syndrome: An autosomal dominant disorder that results in characteristic head and face abnormalities, which include ear malformations, hearing loss, small jaws, malocclusion, and open bite.

Trismus: Tonic contraction of the muscles of mastication that limits jaw opening. It is also referred to as *lockjaw*. Trismus is caused by oral infections, salivary gland infections, tetanus, trauma, and encephalitis.

Trunk: The main part of the body, to which the limbs are attached. The trunk consists of the thorax and abdomen and contains all of the internal organs. This term is also used to describe the main part of a nerve or blood vessel.

Tumor: A solid, raised mass that is greater than 1 cm in diameter and has the dimension of depth. This term also describes a mass consisting of neoplastic cells.

Twinning: The complete division of a single tooth bud resulting in a divided tooth.

Ulcer: Loss of surface tissue caused by a sloughing of necrotic inflammatory tissue; the defect extends into the underlying lamina propria.

Umbilicated: Having a central mark or depression.

Unilateral: Affecting only one side of the body.

Uremia: A toxic condition caused by the accumulation of nitrogenous substances in the blood that are normally eliminated in the urine.

Urticaria: A vascular reaction of the skin characterized by the appearance of slightly elevated patches that are either more red or paler than the surrounding skin. Urticaria is also known as hives and may be caused by allergy, excitement, or exercise. These patches are sometimes intensely itchy.

van der Woude syndrome: An autosomal dominant syndrome characterized by a cleft lip or cleft palate and distinctive pits of the lower lips or both lips.

Vascular: Pertaining to vessels, particularly blood vessels.

Vasoconstriction: To decrease the diameter or caliber of a blood vessel.

Ventral: Directed toward or situated on the belly surface (opposite of *dorsal*).

Vermilion: That part of the lip that has a naturally pinkish red color and is exposed to the extraoral environment. The vermilion contains neither sweat glands nor accessory salivary glands.

Vermilion border: The mucocutaneous margin of the lip.

Vermilionectomy: Surgical removal of the vermilion border of the lip.

Vertigo: An unpleasant sensation characterized mainly by a feeling of dizziness or that one's surroundings are spinning or moving.

Vesicle: A well-defined lesion of the skin and mucous membranes that resembles a sac, contains fluid, and is less than 1 cm in diameter.

Visceral: Pertaining to body organs.

Viscous: Thick or sticky.

Wheal: A localized area of edema on the skin. The area is usually raised and smooth surfaced and is often very itchy.

Xerostomia: Perception of a dry mouth.

X-linked inheritance: A mode of transmitting a gene carried on the X chromosome from parents to their offspring.

Index